Eva Brehmer-Andersson

Dermatopathology

Eva Brehmer-Andersson

Dermatopathology

With 138 Figures in 445 Separate Illustrations and 5 Tables

Springer

Eva Brehmer-Andersson
Värtavägen 17
115 53 Stockholm
Sweden

ISBN-10 3-642-43996-9 Springer-Verlag Berlin Heidelberg NewYork
ISBN-13 978-3-642-43996-4 Springer-Verlag Berlin Heidelberg NewYork

Springer is a part of Springer Science+Business Media
springer.com

Softcover re-print of the Hardcover 1st edition 2006

Editor: Gabriele Schröder, Heidelberg
Desk Editor: Ellen Blasig, Heidelberg
Production and Typesetting: LE-TEX Jelonek, Schmidt & Vöckler GbR, Leipzig
Cover Design: Frido Steinen-Broo, EStudio Calamar, Spain

Printed on acid-free paper 24/3100/YL 5 4 3 2 1 0

Preface

The purpose of this book is to introduce future pathologists and dermatologists to the exciting field of dermatopathology. During the past 40 years dermatopathology has become a big and important topic. There are today many excellent and comprehensive textbooks on the subject, but the overwhelming amount of material and increasing number of this kind of textbook make it difficult to start to discover new fields. I have chosen to focus on relevant processes in basic pathology and discuss how they work or are supposed to work in both common and unusual skin diseases, which I have been confronted with during a life-long practice in pathology and dermatopathology. I also focus on some controversial concepts prevailing and on the diversity in nomenclature. My expectation is to promote the understanding of pathogenesis in diseases of the skin and arouse an appetite for further and more comprehensive studies, and hopefully even to inspire new fruitful investigations. In this respect, the book will even address those experienced in the specialty.

Eva Brehmer-Andersson
March 2006

Acknowledgement

This book is based on experiences acquired at the Departments of Pathology of the University Hospitals in Lund and Umeå, and at the Karolinska University Hospital and South Hospital in Stockholm, Sweden. In all these places I have had a close and inspiring collaboration with the respective Departments of Dermatology. I want to heartily thank all staff members who during the years, besides their own routine work, have willingly helped me with important things such as further sections and stainings, and searching for old slides, records and print-outs.

I am deeply indebted to Sven Lindskog, Professor at the Department of Oral Histology, Karolinska Institute, Stockholm, for generously having put his photo laboratory at my disposal, and to Karl Gabor, colleague and photographer, for valuable advice about adaptation of the photographic material.

Contents

6 Cell Death in the Living Body

7 Vasculitis

8 Skin Lesions due to Abnormalities in Blood Components

26 Recurrent Vesicular Eruptions

27 Profiles of the Epidermal/Dermal Area in some Vesicular/Bullous Dermatoses

28 Skin Lesions Due to Drugs

29 Artifacts

30 Glossary

Subject Index

Abbreviations

ACA	Acrodermatitis chronica atrophicans
AGEP	Acute generalized exanthematous pustulosis
AIDS	Acquired immunodeficiency syndrome
ALHE	Angiolymphoid hyperplasia with eosinophilia
B cells	B lymphocytes
BEA	Bacillary epithelioid angiomatosis
C	Complement
CAMs	Cell adhesion molecules
c-ANCA	Antineutrophilic cytoplasmic antibodies
CD	Common differentiation (antigen)
CD3	Molecular complex in T cells
CD4	Helper T cells
CD8	Suppressor T cells
CMV	Cytomegalovirus
CSHRH	Congenital self-healing reticulohistiocytosis
DIC	Disseminated intravascular coagulation
DNA	Deoxyribonucleic acid
EBV	Epstein-Barr virus
ECP	Eosinophilic cationic protein
EDN	Eosinophilic derived neurotoxin
EED	Erythema elevatum diutinum
ELAM	Endothelial leukocyte adhesion molecule
EM	Erythema multiforme
EORTC	European Organization for Research and Treatment of Cancer
ESR	Erythrocyte sedimentation rate
FBGC	Foreign body giant cell
GM-CSF	Granulocyte-macrophage colony-stimulating factor
H&E	Hematoxylin-eosin
HCMV	Human cytomegalovirus
HIV	Human immunodeficiency virus
HL	Hairy leukoplakia
HLA	Human leukocyte antigen
HPV	Human papilloma virus
HSV	Herpes simplex virus
ICAM	Intercellular adhesion molecule
IFN	Interferon
IgA	Immunoglobulin A
IgD	Immunoglobulin D
IgE	Immunoglobulin E
IgG	Immunoglobulin G
IgM	Immunoglobulin M
IL	Interleukin
kDa	kiloDalton
LCH	Langerhans cell histiocytosis
LFA	Leukocyte function antigen
LGC	Langhans giant cell
LPS	Lipopolysaccharide
MAC	Macrophage activation antigen
MBP	Major basic protein
MHC	Major histocompatibility complex
NK	Natural killer (cells)
PAS	Periodic-acid-Schiff
PLC	Pityriasis lichenoides chronica
PLEVA	Pityriasis lichenoides et varioliformis acuta
PSR	Polymerase chain reaction
RNA	Ribonucleic acid
S-100	Protein expressed on Langerhans cells
SJ	Stevens-Johnson (syndrome)
SLE	Systemic lupus erythematosus
T cells	T lymphocytes
TCR	T-cell receptor region
TEN	Toxic epidermal necrolysis
TGF	Transforming growth factor
TNF	Tumor necrosis factor
t-PA	Tissue plasminogen activator
t-PAI	Inhibitor of t-PA
TTP/HUS	Thrombotic-thrombocytopenic purpura /hemolytic-uremic syndrome
VCAM	Vascular cell adhesion molecule
VEGF	Vascular endothelial growth factor
vG	van Gieson
VLA	Very late activation (integrins)
vWF	von Willebrand factor
VZV	Varicella/herpes zoster virus

Magnification

Magnification [= the objective × the factor of the microscope × a factor of the magnification device (depending on the distance used)] is mentioned in legends only when considered of special interest (i.e., to make it possible to compare the size of different vessels as in Figs. 2.3 and 9.2 and to give an idea of the size of microorganisms and other small particles as in Figs. 19.1 and 29.7. Indications of size and staining only at the end of the legends include all micrographs in the figure.

Chapter 1

Requirements for a Good Diagnostic Result 1

The purpose of asking for a histopathologic investigation of a skin lesion is either to verify a diagnosis, already suspected clinically, or to get help and suggestions in difficult cases.

The clinical expression and the histopathologic pattern of a skin lesion are two aspects of the same pathologic process. To arrive at a correct or likely diagnosis, especially in unclear cases, a close collaboration between the dermatologist and the pathologist is essential. It is vital that the dermatologist has a basic knowledge of dermatopathology and that the pathologist knows enough dermatology to be able to propose a diagnosis, relevant in the context, but not suggested in the pathology consulting form. The investigation process starts in the consulting room with the taking of one or several biopsy specimens and is completed with an adequate consulting form. The samples are then processed and interpreted in the laboratory.

1.1 Sampling Technique

It is important to select a representative lesion without secondary alterations such as scratch marks or infection. Specimens from a vesicular eruption should, if possible, contain a whole vesicle. In bullous lesions, the margin of a fresh bulla is the best area to choose for a biopsy. If several biopsy specimens are taken from lesions of different kinds or ages they should be put in different and appropriately labeled jars.

The samples are best taken with a punch. Different sizes of punch are available. The selected area is infiltrated with a local anesthetic. This does not interfere with the microscopic investigation. It is important to handle biopsy specimens with care and not squeeze them. Tissue damage often renders interpretation difficult or impossible. To be complete, a biopsy specimen should include subcutaneous tissue. The reason is that changes often involve both the dermis and subcutis as in acrodermatitis chronica atrophicans, eosinophilic cellulitis and some kinds of vasculitis. Further examples are scleroderma and alopecia. To settle the diagnosis of scleroderma it is indispensable to be able to examine the dermal–subcutaneous interface, and in alopecia affected hair follicles are situated in the subcutaneous fat.

When the lesion is large and deep-seated, as in panniculitis, a knife biopsy is often recommended. This gives an oval piece of tissue. To get good sections, the ends of the specimen are usually trimmed after fixation, and only the central part is used. It is possible to get an equally good and deep sample with less tissue damage by freezing and using a large punch. After injection of local anesthetic an assistant freezes the area to be punched with ethyl chloride and the freezing is continued while the frozen and thus stable tissue pillar is taken out. The material received is then immediately put in 10% buffered formalin for fixation. If deep-frozen material is required for further special investigations, the pillar may be bisected; one half is fixed in formalin and the other half is put in a deep-freezer.

1.2 The Consulting Form

The consulting form should report on:

- Sex and age
- Profession and hobbies (if relevant)
- Previous illnesses (if relevant)
- Current diseases and treatments
- Pregnancy
- The start, progress and course of the eruption
- The appearance of the lesions with respect to localization, color, papules, vesicles, bullae, pustules, margins, hemorrhage, etc.
- The region from which the biopsy was taken
- The kind (age) of lesions if several specimens are taken
- Ongoing therapy for the skin disease
- One or several clinically conceivable diagnoses

1.3 Routine Processing

The fixed material is dehydrated and then put in molten paraffin and cooled. Specimens embedded in a solidified paraffin block are sectioned in a microtome at 5–7 μm. These are placed on glass slides, deparaffinized, rehydrated, and stained. The procedure takes about 24 h. Thus routinely processed specimens are ready to be examined and reported on at best on the day after they have been received in the laboratory. However, if special stainings, consultations and/or literature studies are required the report may be delayed for a week or more.

As a rule punch biopsy samples should be embedded whole and cut lengthwise. To get maximum information from the specimen the best way is to make serial sections. However, this is not possible in daily practice; step sections are generally used. A good routine is to take nine sections from each level and put them on three parallel glass slides for alternate staining with hematoxylin-eosin (H&E), van Gieson (vG), and periodic-acid-Schiff (PAS) stains.

The routine use of these three stains has benefits. It is possible to distinguish between different normal structures, and different pathologic changes. Fungal hyphae and spores are difficult or impossible to identify using H&E and vG stains, but are stained red with PAS (i.e., they are PAS-positive). Also small intracellular droplets of epithelial mucin (sialomucin) of metastatic adenocarcinomas, which are uncolored on H&E- and vG-stained sections, are PAS-positive. An area with fibrinoid necrosis is shiny red on H&E-stained sections, and yellow on vG-stained sections, and is PAS-positive. The finding of hyaline material in dermis–subcutis, adnexa and vessels, which is stained red like normal collagen (but less intensively) by H&E, yellow by vG, and red by PAS, should be suspected to be amyloid and checked for this material by means of a special stain. PAS is useful also in vascular lesions (Table 1.1).

Other special stains are used for identification of pigments (iron and melanin), dermal mucin, calcium, mast cells, elastic and reticular fibers, bacteria, etc. To reveal fat deposits in tissue, formalin-fixed frozen sections and special stains are used, whereas ordinary deparaffinized sections are useless. Polariscopic examination is utilized for recognition of doubly refractile material, such as foreign bodies or crystals.

Immunohistochemical investigations on paraffin-embedded or frozen material are often indispensable for identification of different kinds of tissue cells and blood cells, and are of paramount importance in tumor pathology. The use of this kind of investigation is increasing steadily and also includes identification of different kinds of molecular components such as adhesion molecules, cytokines and antigens (Sect. 4).

1.4 Interpretation of Histopathologic Changes

Recognition and evaluation of histopathologic changes always includes comparison with normal structures. The architecture of the skin differs with sex and age and from one area to another in the same individual with respect to, for example, the thickness and looseness of the dermis, the thickness of the epidermis, and the presence and size of rete ridges. It is therefore necessary that the dermatopathologist has good knowledge of the histology of the skin, as also implied in this book, which does not systematically deal with the architecture of the normal skin.

The capacity of tissues to respond to different kinds of pathogenic stimuli is restricted. This implies that several kinds of diseases can provoke similar histo-

Table 1.1 Staining characteristics of some tissues and structures for hematoxylin-eosin, van Gieson, and periodic-acid-Schiff stains

Tissue or structure	H&E	vG	PAS +/–
Collagen, normal	Red	Red	Blue –
Collagen, sclerotic	Red	Red	Blue –
Fibrin	Shiny red	Yellow	Red +
Fibrinoid necrosis	Shiny red	Yellow	Red +
Thrombi	Shiny red	Yellow	Red +
Muscles	Red	Yellow	Blue –
Nerves	Red	Yellow	Blue –
Amyloid	Red	Yellow	Red +
Epithelial mucin	Colorless	Colorless	Red +
Fungal structures	Transparent	Transparent	Red +

pathologic patterns. After all, many skin disorders have a histopathologic structure typical enough to allow the pathologist to suggest a diagnosis or a group affiliation. However, it is important to remember that although a skin disease is said to have a typical histopathologic pattern, this does not mean that this pattern is unique (pathognomonic) for this particular disease. In some cases it is possible to settle the correct diagnosis by demonstrating the presence in the tissue of causative agents such as fungi, bacteria, parasites and foreign bodies.

Very often the histopathologic changes are nonspecific, which means inconspicuous or basic and therefore common to many kinds of pathogenic stimuli. The reason could be that the expression of the disease is mild, or that the specimen is taken at the beginning or at the end of the life cycle of the lesion, or is not representative. The histopathologic pattern of a skin lesion, like those of all other pathologic processes, goes through a process of development, and therefore differs more or less from one time to another. What we see in a given biopsy specimen is analogous to a frozen picture in a film. The most typical histopathologic picture is most likely to be obtained from a specimen taken from a lesion in its prime. Discrepancy between the histopathologic findings and the clinical expression should be an incentive to perform new biopsies. If earlier biopsy material exists, this should always be reexamined and considered together with the new material. It is often necessary to make repeated biopsies during the course of a disease. The histopathologic findings have to be considered together with the clinical picture, laboratory findings, and the history and course of the disease.

The report should be as concise as possible, but circumstantial enough to evoke in the mind of the experienced reader a realistic image of the changes. It should contain a conclusion, and if possible a diagnosis or a suggestion of one or two conceivable diagnoses. For further education and development, feedback to the pathologist is very important.

2 The Dermal Blood Vasculature

2.1 General Architecture of Blood Vessels

To grasp the delicacy of the microvasculature of the skin it is necessary to review the organization of the body vasculature, and also the construction of arteries, capillaries, and veins.

2.1.1 Arteries

Arteries are classified with respect to their caliber and structure of their walls as:

- Large arteries of elastic type or conducting arteries (arteria pulmonalis, aorta and its large branches)
- Medium-sized arteries of muscular type or distributing arteries (for example the radial artery)
- Small arteries including small unnamed arteries and arterioles

Accordingly, arteries of elastic type give off branches that become medium-sized muscular arteries, and these in turn give off small arteries, which end up in arterioles of different sizes. Eventually arterioles merge into capillaries. In consequence, the caliber of an artery gradually decreases with increasing distance from the heart, while the sum of the diameters of the lumens of all of its branches greatly increases.

The wall of all arteries consists of three layers. These are from inside out: tunica intima, tunica media, and tunica adventitia. In all vessels the luminal surface is covered with a single layer of endothelial cells, which alone or together with a thin subendothelial sheet of fibrous and elastic tissue forms the intima. Usually the media is the thickest layer and its construction determines the type of artery. In arteries of elastic type both the subendothelial layer of the intima and the media are mainly built up of elastic membranes. In arteries of muscular type the media consists mainly of concentric layers of smooth muscle cells and the elastic tissue is confined to two distinct elastic membranes: one internal beneath the endothelium and one external between the media and adventitia. Depending on the size of the vessel, the media of small arteries and arterioles is composed of one or several layers of smooth muscle cells. Small arteries and arterioles have only one elastic membrane located directly below the endothelium. In all types of arteries the adventitia consists mainly of connective tissue, which merges with the connective tissue of the neighborhood. The modification of vessels from large arteries to arterioles is insidious and only gently progressive. It means that in each group of vessels the difference between the largest and the smallest is conspicuous.

2.1.2 Capillaries

Capillaries are tiny tubes composed of one layer of endothelial cells, which on the abluminal surface is covered with a basement membrane; between these two laminae there is a discontinuous layer of pericytes, cells which are provided with long branching processes and are able to contract. The caliber of the capillary is on average 9–10 μm, just large enough to permit the cellular components of the blood to pass. The capillaries have one arterial and one venous part, and in that way they connect the arterial and venous system.

Under normal conditions not all capillaries are open simultaneously. Arterioles act as functional sphincters and control the flow through the capillary bed with respect to the needs of the tissue of the area, caused by, for example, muscular movements, regulation of the body temperature and digestion. However, they also react to infections and other kinds of injury (Sect. 5.2.1).

2.1.3 Veins

The blood in the capillary bed drains into venules, the counterpart to arterioles, of the venous vascular system. Towards the heart the size of the veins gradually increases, while the wall becomes thicker. Like arteries they are categorized as large, medium-sized and small.

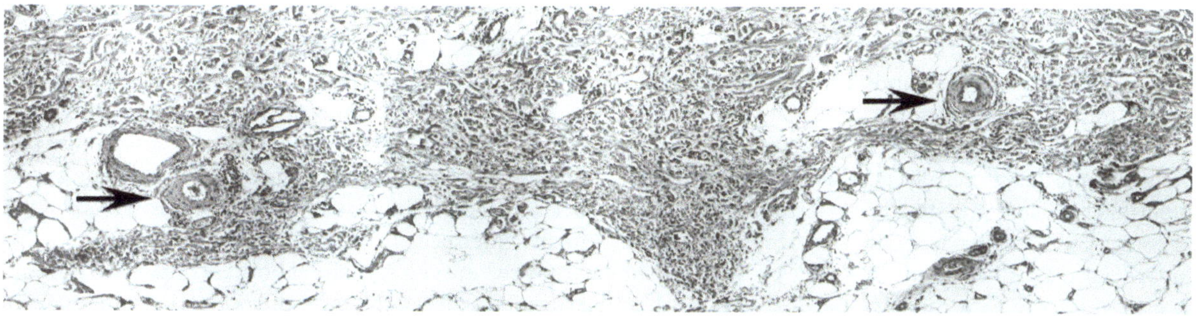

Fig. 2.1 Arterioles at the dermal–subcutaneous interface. There are only two ascending arterioles (*arrows*). Above and to the left of the left arteriole there is a dilated small vein and to the right there is a dilated lymphatic with valves. H&E, original magnification ×60

Usually veins accompany their corresponding arteries. The caliber and capacity of the vein are greater, but the wall of the vein is thinner and less elastic than that of the artery. Many medium-sized veins have valves, which prevent flow away from the heart.

2.1.4 The Endothelium

The endothelium is a huge organ of the body with many important properties. It has the capacity to control the passage of small and large molecules into the arterial wall and through the walls of capillaries and venules, to maintain the balance between coagulative and fibrinolytic activities, to regulate the vascular tone and blood flow, and to regulate immune and inflammatory reactions.

2.1.5 Arteriovenous Anastomoses

In addition to the connection between the arterial and venous blood system at the capillary level there are in many parts of the body arteriovenous anastomoses at the level of small arteries and veins. The connecting branches are profusely innervated, have a special architecture, and are provided with a contractile segment. When the segments are contracted the blood passes through the capillaries; when they are relaxed the blood is shunted directly into the venous system. The arteriovenous anastomoses play an important role in the regulation of body temperature.

Other temperature-regulating shunts are the abundantly innervated glomus structures (glomera) situated in the subcutaneous tissue and deep dermis. The glomus, which has a connective tissue capsule, is penetrated by an arteriole. Inside the capsule the vessel splits up into branches or becomes highly convoluted. Also epithelioid smooth muscle cells (glomus cells) replace the subendothelial elastic membrane. The arterial part of the glomus then connects with a short thin-walled venule, which leaves the glomus and drains to the subcutaneous or dermal venous plexus. Glomera are mainly found in the nail bed, and finger and toe pads, the central part of the face, and ears.

2.2 The Microvasculature of the Skin

Arteries in the skin belong to the group of small arteries, and are derived from vessels located below the muscles. They penetrate the muscles and continue through the subcutaneous connective tissue towards the dermal–subcutaneous interface, where they appear as ascending arterioles.

In the deep dermis ascending arterioles give off

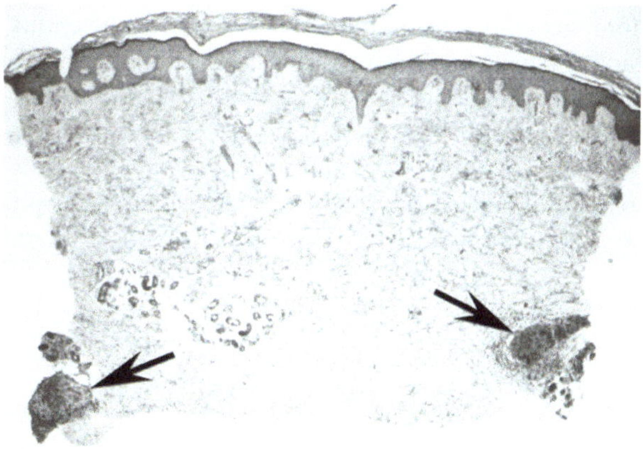

Fig. 2.2 Arterial vasculitis. A 4-mm punch biopsy specimen shows two affected ascending arterioles (*arrows*) at the dermal–subcutaneous border, one on each side of the specimen. The structures above the left arrow are sweat glands. H&E, ×25

branches, which create the deep vascular plexus. A dense capillary network, originating form the deep plexus, surrounds sweat glands and hair follicle bulbs. In the mid-dermis ascending arterioles anastomose with each other. On the way to the papillary dermis they become progressively smaller, give rise to the superficial plexus, and finally as terminal arterioles transform into capillaries. Like the deep plexus, the superficial plexus is arranged parallel to the skin surface. It gives rise to a capillary network around hair shafts and sends capillary loops into the dermal papillae. Approximately one loop supplies one papilla (Ryan 1983). The postcapillary venules drain into venules of the superficial plexus. Descending venules go from the superficial plexus to the deep plexus, which drains into veins in the subcutaneous tissue. Like arterioles, venules also anastomose. However, the venous part of the microvasculature is more profuse than that of the arterial part.

The dermal microvasculature has been studied by electron and light microscopy (Yen and Braverman 1976; Braverman and Yen 1977; Higgins and Eady 1981). The walls of ascending arterioles, arterioles in the superficial plexus, and descending venules contain smooth muscle cells arranged in one or several layers. Ascending arterioles, but not terminal arterioles, have an internal elastic membrane. In terminal arterioles, postcapillary venules and venules of the superficial plexus, muscle cells are replaced by a continuous sheath of pericytes. Capillaries have a discontinuous layer of pericytes. The capillary loop has three sections: one extrapapillary ascending, one intrapapillary, and one extrapapillary descending. The first two sections have arterial, and the third venous, characteristics. The main difference is that the arterial capillary has a homogeneous basement membrane, while the venous capillary has a multilayered one. This change appears abruptly at the border between the papillary and subpapillary areas. Also there is a close relationship between the capillary loops and the overlying epidermis. In areas of normal skin with high rete ridges the papillary loops are well developed and elongated, while in areas with low ridges the loops are short. Regardless of the length of the loop, the intrapapillary part is always arterial in character (Braverman and Yen 1977).

In histologic sections of normal skin, vessels are inconspicuous; also most observed vessels are venules. Figure 2.1 demonstrates the rather large space between ascending arterioles at the dermal–subcutaneous interface. In this punch biopsy specimen the distance between the lateral borders of the two present arterioles is about 2.8 mm. In another specimen taken with a knife, where three arterioles were identified, the distance between each vessel was at least 3 mm. Consequently, a biopsy taken with a 4-mm punch will include at the most two ascending arterioles (Fig. 2.2); using a 3-mm punch, affected vessels may be missed.

To identify elastic membranes in venules and small arterioles it is necessary to use a special staining such as vG-elastin, which stains the elastic membrane black. Small arterioles in the upper dermis may be visualized by immunohistochemical staining with antibodies against smooth muscle α-actin or smooth muscle myosin heavy chain (Fig. 2.3). In routinely stained specimens thickened veins may be difficult or impossible to differentiate from arterioles (Figs. 2.3e and 2.4c). Medium-sized veins in the upper subcutis may have valves (Fig. 2.4b).

References

1. Braverman IM, Yen A (1977) Ultrastructure of the human dermal microcirculation. II. The capillary loops of the dermal papillae. J Invest Dermatol 68:44–52
2. Higgins JC, Eady RAJ (1981) Human dermal microvasculature. I. Its segmental differentiation. Light and electron microscopic study. Br J Dermatol 104:117–129
3. Ryan TJ (1983) Cutaneous circulation. In: Goldsmith LA (ed) Biochemistry and physiology of the skin. Oxford University Press, Oxford, pp 817–877
4. Yen A, Braverman IM (1976) Ultrastructure of the human dermal microcirculation. The horizontal plexus of the papillary dermis. J Invest Dermatol 66:131–142

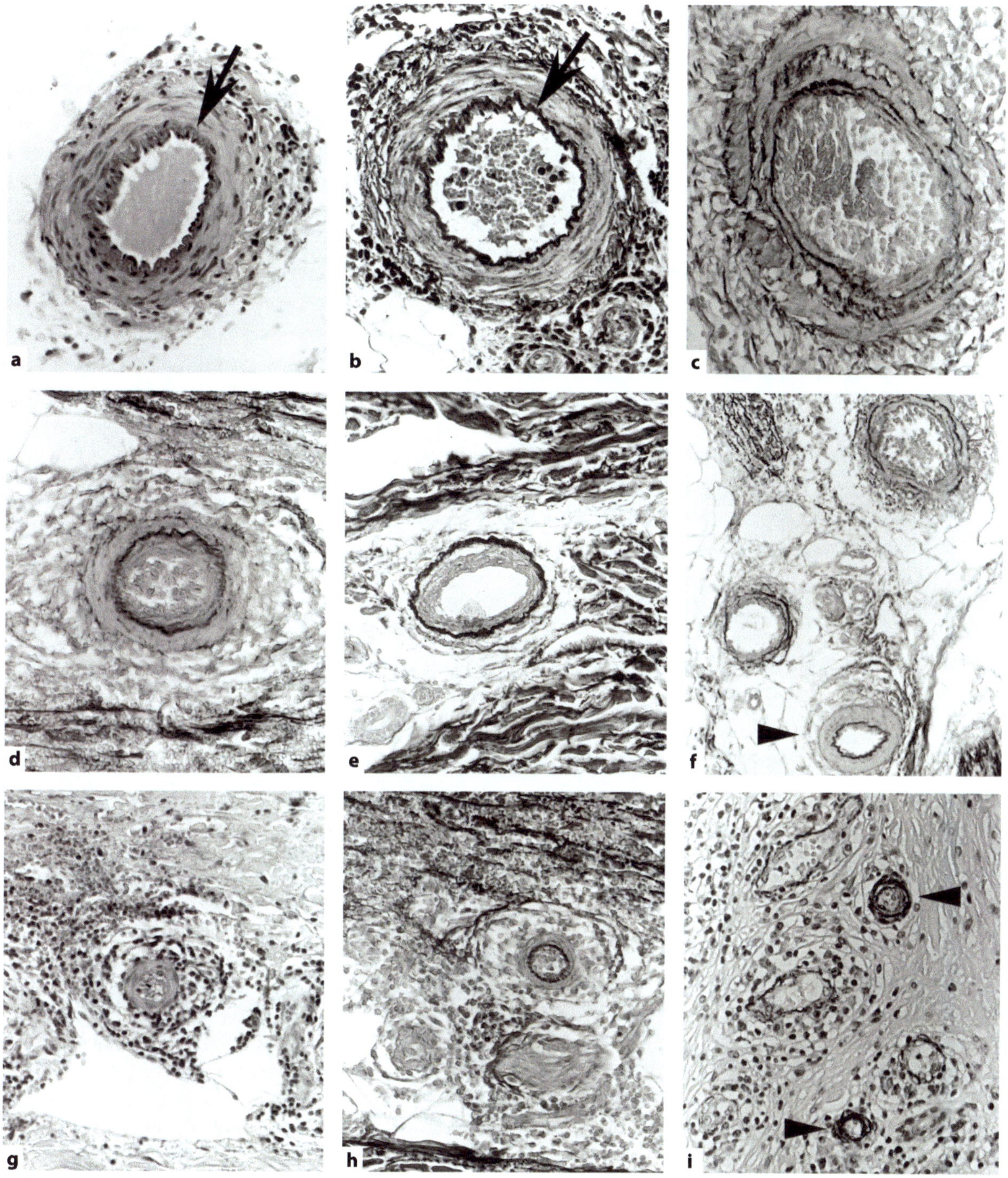

Fig. 2.3 Vessels in tissue with inflammatory changes. **a** A small artery in which the internal elastic membrane is seen as a pleated grayish band (*arrow*); H&E, ×200. **b** A small artery in which the internal elastic membrane is seen as a distinct black band (*arrow*); vG-elastin, ×200. **c** A small vein with several layers of disrupted elastic membranes; vG-elastin, ×200. **d** Arteriole; vG-elastin, ×200. **e** A sclerotic venule is encircled by a thick elastic membrane; vG-elastin, ×200. **f** Two venules and an arteriole (*arrowhead*); vG-elastin, ×100. **g** Small arteriole; H&E, ×200. **h** A small arteriole; vG-elastin, ×200. **i** Three small dilated venules and two small arterioles (*arrowheads*); smooth muscle α-actin, ×200

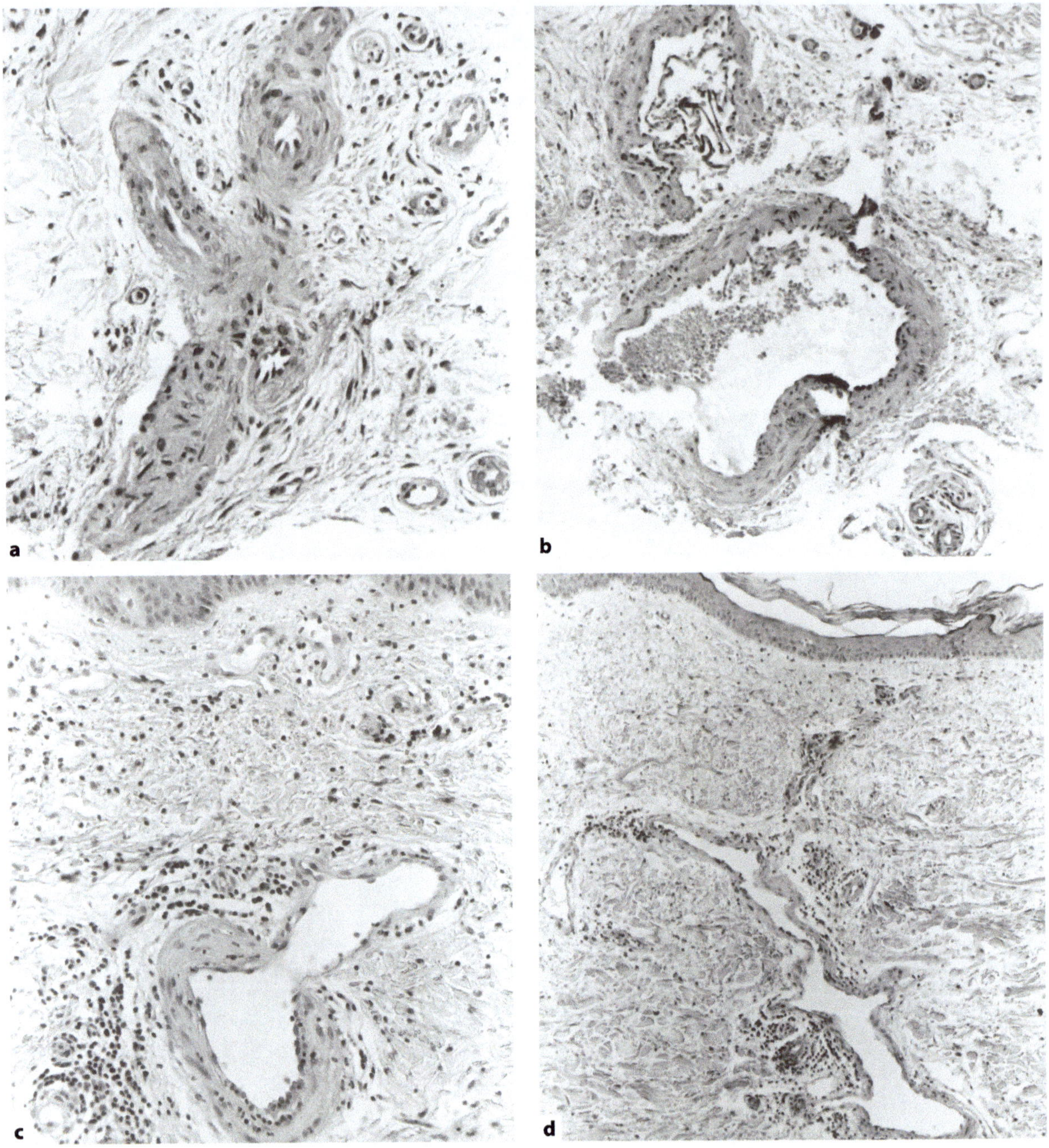

Fig. 2.4 Vessels in tissue with inflammatory changes. a A branching arteriole at the dermal–subcutaneous border (sole of the foot); ×200. b A vein in the superficial part of the subcutis, probably cut close to a junction with a smaller affluent branch. The smaller vein contains a pleated valve (border of the foot); ×125. c In the lower dermis a thin-walled dilated venule drains into a thick- walled one; ×200. d Dilated and winding venule in the lower part of the dermis; H&E, ×100

CHAPTER 3

The Dermal Lymphatic Vasculature 3

The main functions of the lymphatic system are to bring escaped proteins and fluid from the interstitial tissue back to the blood circulation and to carry macrophages to lymph nodes for presentation of antigens (Sect. 4.1.2). Lymphatic vessels form in the interstitial tissue as blind tubes, which link together and form capillaries. Towards the heart, postcapillary lymphatics of similar size unite and decrease in number while they increase in caliber. Finally, two main trunks are formed, which close to the heart merge with the venous system.

3.1 The Construction of Lymphatic Capillaries

Lymphatic capillaries have a discontinuous basal lamina. Smooth muscle cells and pericytes are lacking. Endothelial cells are connected with elastic and collagen fibers in the perivascular tissue. There are also actin-like microfilaments in the cytoplasm of the endothelial cells. These structures and the special construction of the vessel wall enable the vessel to change its form (collapse, dilate and fold) and the endothelial cells to interdigitate (see Glossary), slip over each other, or move from each other giving rise to gaps. There are several kinds of lymphatic valves:

- Joining valves and segment valves are large permanent intraluminal valves. They open and lock sections of the vessels and thus maintain the unidirectional (centripetal) lymph flow. Joining valves are situated where one vessel merges into another, and segment valves divide the wall lengthwise in sections. The part between two pairs of segment valves is called a lymphangion.
- Interendothelial (inlet) valves are temporarily formed when endothelial cells move from each other to give rise to the above-mentioned gaps, which directly connect the vessel lumen with the interstitial tissue.
- Unicellular valves and bunch valves are two smaller intraluminal structures, which are temporary and appear and disappear in harmony with the pressure gradients. They are supposed to support the lock-gate function of the segment valves (Daróczy 1988).

The large intraluminal valves have a core of connective tissue covered with endothelial cells like those of the vessel wall. However, the cells at the free end of the valves, the tip cells, are different. They have the capacity to seal the lymphangion by tightly connecting with each other and with the tip cells of the opposite valve (Fig. 3.1).

3.2 Lymphatic Capillaries in the Skin

In the skin, lymphatic capillaries arise as blind tubes in the papillary dermis, link together and form the superficial lymphatic plexus located in the subepidermal compartment. Vertical branches connect the superficial plexus with the deep lymphatic capillary plexus at the dermal–subcutaneous interface. Here the capillaries become postcapillaries, and merge into lymphatic collecting vessels. In both plexus the vessels are arranged parallel to the epidermis (Daróczy 1988).

Inactive lymphatic capillaries are collapsed and their endothelial cells cannot be differentiated microscopically from the surrounding connective tissue fibroblasts; thus they are invisible in sections from routinely processed and stained biopsy specimens. Open capillaries are thin-walled, have an irregular form, and contain intraluminal valves, not always visible in a given section. It may be difficult to differentiate lymphatics and thin-walled dilated blood vessels in routinely stained sections; however, valves in a thin-walled vessel in the upper half of the dermis always indicate a lymphatic (Ryan et al. 1986; Daróczy 1988). Because of the structure of the wall (lack of basal lamina and the presence of gaps) it is difficult or impossible to identify capillary lymphatics with enzyme- or immunohistochemical methods.

3.3 Prelymphatics and Initial Lymphatics (Lymphatic Sinusoids, Blind Tubes)

Investigations by Casley-Smith and Sims (1976) and others indicated that proteins and fluid are transported to initial lymphatics in preformed channels (prelymphatics; at that time not possible to visualize), and are walled off by ground substance. The radius of the channels was estimated to be about 60 nm. The statements have been verified. Modern techniques allow prelymphatics and initial lymphatics to be stained and investigated in animals (Zöltzer 2003; Ji and Kato 2003).

Zöltzer studied lymphatics in the endometrium of the uterus in rats and guinea pigs in different phases of estrogen stimulation. The author concluded that initial lymphatics do not exist in the luminal two-thirds of the endometrium. However, in estrus, post-estrus and pregnancy tissue, channels transporting fluid to the initial lymphatics at the basic endometrium, are frequently observed. The channels are less-often seen in the inter- and pre-estrus periods and thus seem to

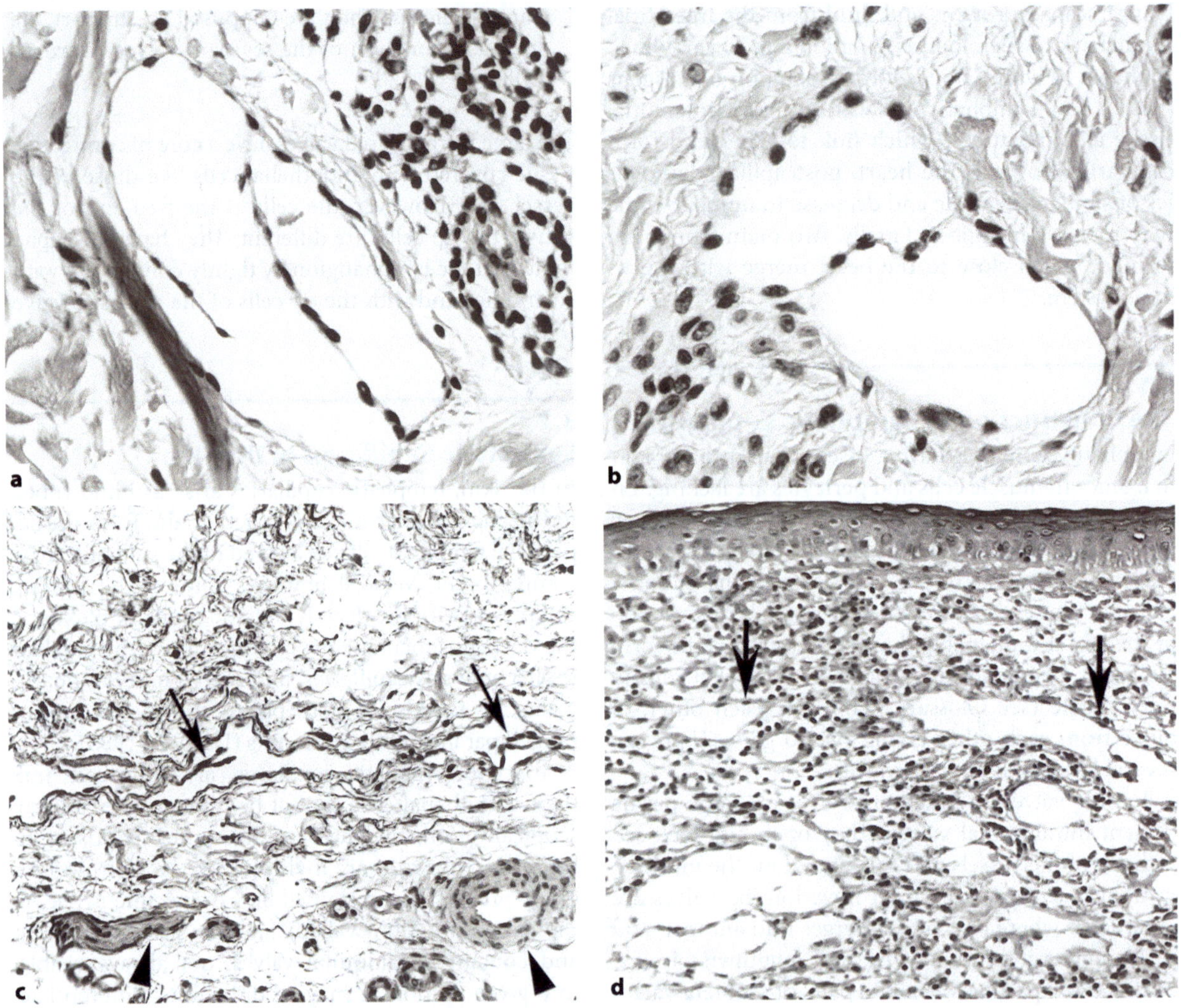

Fig. 3.1 Lymphatic vessels. **a** A lymphatic vessel with open valves is located close to the epidermis. **b** Another vessel in the same section has locked valves. Note the endothelial cells on the surface of the valves; H&E, ×400. **c** A postcapillary lymphatic vessel at the dermal–subcutaneous border. Two sets of segmental valves demarcate a lymphangion (*arrows*). *Left arrowhead* peripheral nerve, *right arrowhead* ascending arteriole. Between and below these structures there are blood capillaries; Bosma-Steiner silver stain, ×100. **d** A lesion of acrodermatitis chronica atrophicans. There is a longitudinally cut lymphatic vessel with a locked valve (*arrows*) and below it groups of "vacuoles"; H&E, ×200

be able to adapt to a more or less edematous endometrium.

By means of a silver staining it was possible to differentiate between initial lymphatics, precollectors, and collectors. The histologic pattern of initial lymphatics was distinctly different from those of precollectors and collectors. Initial lymphatics had markedly flattened oak-leaf-like endothelial cells, conspicuously attenuated basal membrane, and often so-called open interface formations, which directly connected them with draining channels. Zöltzer concluded that initial lymphatics might be extremely flexible structures that with higher lymphatic loads give rise to dilatation of both initial lymphatics and open junction formations.

Ji and Kato (2003) investigated the lymphatic network in the gastric wall of Japanese monkeys (*Macaca fuscata*) by histochemical stainings. They found fine lymphatics with many blind ends evenly distributed in the mucosa, which usually surrounded the basal portion of gastric glands. In the submucosa there were blind ends and capillaries with valves which drained directly or by a communicating branch into larger lymphatics—an arrangement very like that in the skin.

Probably the "vacuoles", resembling fat cells and occasionally observed in the upper dermis in acrodermatitis chronica atrophicans (Sect. 18.4.2.1; Figs. 18.4b–d), rarely in biopsies from other skin diseases, and in the mucous membrane of the colon, are dilated prelymphatics and/or dilated initial lymphatics and thus a kind of lymphedema (Åsbrink et al. 1986; Brehmer-Andersson et al. 1998; Lee et al.1995; Trotter and Crawford 1998; Snover et al. 1985).

References

1. Åsbrink E, Brehmer-Andersson E, Hovmark A (1986) Acrodermatitis chronica atrophicans. A spirochetosis. Clinical and histopathological picture based on 32 patients. Course and relationship to erythema chronicum migrans Afzelius. Am J Dermatopathol 8:209–219
2. Brehmer-Andersson E, Hovmark A, Åsbrink E (1998) Acrodermatitis chronica atrophicans. Histopathologic findings and clinical correlations in 111 cases. Acta Derm Venereol (Stockh) 78:207–213
3. Casley-Smith JR, Sims MA (1976) Protein concentrations in regions with fenestrated and continuous blood capillaries and in initial and collecting lymphatics. Microvasc Res 12:245–257
4. Daróczy J (1988) The dermal lymphatic capillaries. Springer-Verlag, Berlin
5. Ji R-C, Kato S (2003) Lymphatic network and lymphangiogenesis in the gastric wall. J Histochem Cytochem 51:331–338
6. Lee J, Bhawan J, Rothman K (1995) Massive papillary dermal fatty infiltration in a patient with psoriasis. J Cutan Pathol 22:182–184
7. Ryan TJ, Mortimer PS, Jones RL (1986) Lymphatics of the skin. Neglected but important. Int J Dermatol 25:411–419
8. Snover DC, Sandstad J, Hutton S (1985) Mucosal pseudolipomatosis of the colon. Am J Clin Pathol 84:575–580
9. Trotter MJ, Crawford RI (1998) Pseudolipomatosis cutis. Superficial dermal vacuoles resembling fatty infiltration of the skin. Am J Dermatopathol 20:443–447
10. Zöltzer H (2003) Initial lymphatics. Morphology and function of the endothelial cells. Lymphology 36:7–25

4 The Immune Response

The immune response includes two mechanisms: *adaptive* (specific or acquired) immunity and *innate* (natural or native) immunity.

4.1 Adaptive Immunity

Antigens are immunogenic substances, which, if foreign to the body and inserted into the tissue, are capable of provoking a specific immune response. Immunogenic substances are mainly proteins with a molecular weight of >10 kilo Daltons (kDa). However, even small molecules, so-called haptens, can be antigenic when conjugated with a larger antigenic molecule, usually a protein. The large molecule is called the carrier molecule.

The immune response is a kind of defense mechanism. Under normal conditions the body does not react to autologous (self) antigens. Occurrence of antibodies against components in the tissue of one's own body gives rise to autoimmune diseases. In this way, or by causing hypersensitivity reactions, the immune response is involved in the pathogenesis of a large number of skin diseases, some of which are discussed in Chapters 7, 22–25, and 28.

Foreign substances (antigens), which may be either microbes or some other kind of agent foreign to the body, initiate the adaptive immune defense mechanism. A specific immune response against the intruding antigen, such as a type of microbe, is provoked mainly by means of either the humoral antibody system or the cell mediated immune response. The majority of antigens cause both cell-mediated and humoral immune responses. The spleen, lymph nodes, tonsils, the lymphatic tissue of the gut, and also non-lymphoid tissue such as the skin and mucous membranes may be involved.

In the humoral antibody system the effector cells are plasma cells, which are developed from B-lymphocytes (B cells) and secrete antibodies. The specific antibodies bind to the antigen and form antigen–antibody complexes. Antibodies are immunoglobulins (glycoproteins) present in the plasma, which depending on their molecular weight and other characteristics are divided into five classes sharing a basic structure: IgG, IgM, IgA, IgD and IgE. The molecule looks like the letter Y and has a shaft, the Fc part, and two identical arms, the Fab parts. The Fab parts are the conventional antigen-binding sites. Every Ig class is composed of an indefinite number of subgroups of antigen molecules. This is the result of small variations occurring in the Fab portions during development with the aim of matching an indefinite number of possible antigens. However, some kinds of cells, for example monocytes, neutrophils, eosinophils, basophils, mast cells, and natural killer (NK) cells (see Sect. 4.2), have receptors for the Fc shaft.

In the cell-mediated immune response the effector cells are T-lymphocytes (T cells). In T cells, the various antigen-specific receptors are located in the T cell receptor region (TCR) (Sect. 4.1.2.2). B and T cells cooperate (Sect. 4.1.2.1).

4.1.1 B and T Cells

Immune response is triggered by binding of antigen molecules to specific receptors on the surface of B cells and T cells. B cells develop from stem cells in the bone marrow and T cells from stem cells in the thymus. From these organs lymphocytes migrate to lymphoid tissue in other parts of the body. During a step in development both kinds of lymphocytes become committed or specifically responsive (i.e., they become capable of responding only to a particular antigen, or closely related antigens). Committed B and T cells are also called naive, a term that is used here. It follows that the lymphoid tissue in various sites in the body consists of a high number of small groups of lymphocytes each of which responds only to one specific antigen. When naive B or T cells are stimulated by an appropriate antigen they undergo blast transformation, proliferate and give rise to a clone of genetically identical cells. B cells give rise to plasma cells, which are the effector cells of the humoral immune system and produce antibodies, and to memory B cells. T cells give rise to effector T cells and memory T cells.

The first time a specific antigen enters the lymphoid tissue, only a small number of naive lymphocytes are capable of binding the antigen. The reaction is weak and slow. However, the second, and every subsequent, time the same antigen is introduced to the body, due to the memory cells, which are said to be sensitized (immunocompetent, specifically primed), there will be a strong and quicker response. Also the activity lasts much longer than the first time.

4.1.2 The Lymph Node

On the way back from the interstitial tissue to the blood, the lymph is transported via the lymphatic vasculature to groups of lymph nodes strategically located in the subcutaneous tissue and inner organs. The lymph node is bean-shaped and has a convex surface and a hilus (Fig. 4.1). It is separated from the surrounding tissue by a connective tissue capsule from which radiating septa (trabeculae) run through the node towards the hilus and merge with the connective tissue of the hilus. The stroma between the trabeculae consists of a meshwork of delicate reticulin fibers.

At the convex surface of the node, several afferent lymphatics penetrate the capsule in the areas between

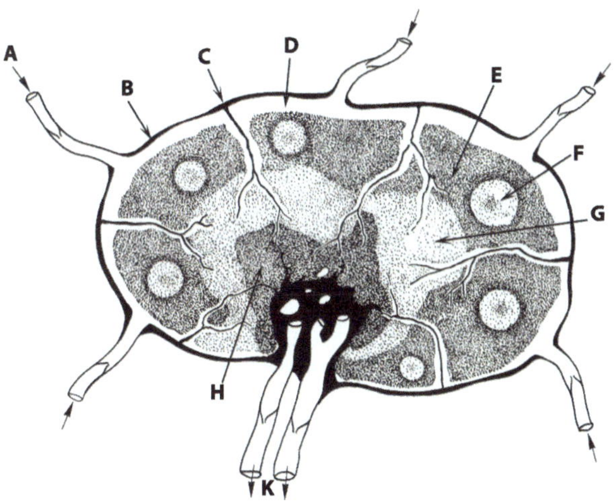

Fig. 4.1 The lymph node and its lymphatics. A Afferent lymphatic, B capsule, C radiating trabecula, D marginal sinus which gives rise to sinuses surrounding the radiating trabeculae, E cortex, F germinal center, G paracortex, H medulla, K efferent lymphatics (illustrator Edward Brehmer; reproduced from Brehmer-Andersson E (1988), with permission)

the trabeculae and drain into the subcapsular (marginal) sinus. From the marginal sinus the lymph flows through sinuses surrounding the trabeculae towards the hilus. Sinuses are wide and winding channels with net-like walls permitting free passage of fluid and cells from sinuses to parenchyma and vice versa. At the hilus the lymph leaves the node via two or three efferent lymphatics, somewhat larger than the afferent lymphatics. Because of the valves of the lymphatics, the flow of lymph is always directed from the convex surface of the node to the hilus. After passage through the lymph node the lymph continues towards the thoracic duct and enters the venous system at the junction of the left internal jugular and subclavian veins. Almost all blood vessels enter and leave the node at the hilus and the larger branches of both arteries and veins follow the connective tissue trabeculae. Postcapillary venules of the paracortical area have high cuboidal endothelial cells and therefore are called high endothelial venules (epithelioid venules). They are of importance for the recirculation of lymphocytes (Sect. 4.1.3).

The parenchyma of the lymph node mainly contains small mature lymphocytes, but there also are dendritic cells and macrophages. Dendritic cells are endowed with fine cytoplasmic processes and are non-phagocytic. There are two functionally different types of dendritic cells: follicular dendritic cells and interdigitating dendritic cells. Follicular dendritic cells are capable of binding, and for some time retain, antigen–antibody complexes on their surface and present the antigen to naive and sensitized B cells. Macrophages phagocytose, process and present antigen to sensitized T cells, which in contrast to B cells cannot be activated by soluble antigens. Interdigitating dendritic cells express high levels of class II MHC molecules (see Glossary) and therefore are well suited to present antigen to naive T cells. The lymph node may be divided into three more or less distinct areas: the cortex, the paracortex or deep cortex, and the medulla.

4.1.2.1 The Cortex—the Main Territory for B Cells

The B cells occupy the cortex, the area between the marginal sinus and the paracortex. The major part of the cortical parenchyma is made up of densely packed small B cells mixed up with follicular dendritic cells and macrophages; however, there are also a fair number of T cells.

In the cortex, germinal centers, which are well-demarcated areas surrounded by a rim of small dark lymphocytes, evolve as a response to antigen stimulation by, for example, intruding bacteria. Naive or sensitized B cells become activated, undergo blast transformation, proliferate and give rises to a clone of large immature centroblasts and centrocytes, which together with follicular dendritic cells and macrophages make up the germinal center. There are many mitotic figures. Macrophages found in all regions of the lymph node are especially conspicuous in the fully developed germinal center. They contain phagocytosed cells with pyknotic nuclei. Because of their abundant and light cytoplasm they are called starry sky cells (Fig. 18.2). Immature B cells differentiate into immature plasma cells and memory cells. Immature plasma cells migrate to the medulla where they mature and become competent to secrete antigen-specific antibodies (immunoglobulins) into the blood. They may also migrate to infected tissue. As mentioned above, the germinal centers contain some T cells. These belong to the subgroup T-helper cells and are necessary for the production of large amount of IgG antibodies in the secondary response.

4.1.2.2 Paracortex or Deep Cortex—the Main Territory for T Cells

The paracortex, the main territory for the T cells, occupies the area between the cortex and medulla. It contains mainly T cells and interdigitating dendritic cells. The lymphocytes are less densely packed than those in the cortex.

Induced by antigenic stimulation, naive or sensitized T cells give rise to large, clear T-lymphoblasts resulting in a diffuse hyperplasia of the paracortex without distinct germinal centers. The T-lymphoblasts differentiate into effector cells and memory cells. Each T cell is genetically programmed to recognize a specific cell-bound antigen by means of an antigen-specific T cell receptor (TCR) (see Glossary). TCR are linked to a cluster of protein molecules called the CD3 molecular complex. This complex is identical in all T cells. It is involved in the transduction of signals into the T cell after the cell has bound an antigen but does not itself bind to antigen.

There are subgroups of T cells, which express different kinds of function-associated molecules. The most important of these subgroups are those expressing CD4 ($CD4^+$) helper T cells and CD8 ($CD8^+$) suppressor/cytotoxic T cells. These membrane-associated molecules serve as coreceptors. During antigen presentation CD4 molecules bind to the class II MHC molecules on the antigen-presenting cells, while CD8 molecules bind to class I MHC molecules. It follows that $CD4^+$ cells can recognize antigen only in connection with class II MHC, and $CD8^+$ cells only in association with class I MHC. By secreting cytokines (Sect. 4.1.5) $CD4^+$ helper cells influence practically all cells of the immune system: other T cells, B cells, macrophages, and NK cells.

Recently two functionally different subgroups of $CD4^+$ cells have been detected. The T-helper-1 ($CD4^+$-1) cells produce and secrete the cytokines interleukin-2 (IL-2) and interferon gamma (IFN-γ), but not IL-4 or IL-5, while T-helper-2 cells manufacture IL-4 and IL-5, but not IL-2 or IFN-γ. T-helper-1 cells are involved in macrophage activation, synthesis of IgG antibodies, and delayed hypersensitivity reactions. The T-helper-2 ($CD4^+$-2) cells give rise to the production of IgE antibodies, and are involved in the defense against parasites (worms) and in the hypersensitivity reaction type 1. The $CD8^+$ cells act primarily as cytotoxic cells.

T cells go back to the circulation via efferent lymphatics and the main lymphatic ducts and eventually invade the infected tissue. $CD4^+$ cells are directed towards bacteria such as mycobacteria, which are able to survive in the cytoplasm of macrophages, and fungal infections. They may induce the formation of granulomas (Sect. 5.3). Cytotoxic T cells ($CD8^+$ cells) attack virus-infected cells, and potentially malignant tissue cells. The $CD8^+$ cell sensitized to a given virus recognizes an infected cell as non-self by identifying the virus antigen together with the autologous (self) class I MHC antigen on the cell surface. The lymphocyte gets in close contact with the infected cell, destroys it, and is thereafter free to attack another infected cell (Sect. 20.1.5). Malignant or potentially malignant cells are thought to be recognized by tumor antigens expressed on the cell surface together with the autologous class I MHC antigen and are destroyed by cytotoxic lymphocytes in the same way as virus-infected cells. This phenomenon is called immunologic surveillance.

4.1.2.3 Medulla—the Area Between the Paracortex and the Hilus

The medulla is composed of plasma cells in different stages of maturation and small lymphocytes.

4.1.3 The Recirculation of Lymphocytes

Large numbers of small lymphocytes recirculate continuously. About 80% of the recirculating cells are T cells. The majority of both T cells and B cells are memory cells with a long life span. Both types of recirculating lymphocytes enter the lymph node from the blood by moving through the wall of high endothelial venules of the paracortex, the mechanism of which is described in Sect. 5.2.1. The B cells migrate to the cortex, and the T cells to the paracortex. From these compartments the lymphocytes leave the nodule via the sinuses in the medulla and the efferent lymphatics, and eventually return to the blood via the thoracic duct. The recirculation of memory cells and the construction of lymph nodes, permitting a slow filtering of lymph in only one direction, facilitate the encounter between antigens and memory cells.

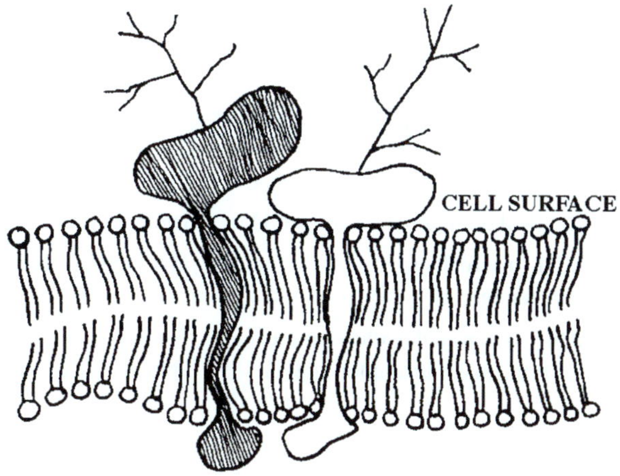

Fig. 4.2 Adhesion molecules. The cell membrane which is made up of two rows of lipid molecules contains two different transmembrane adhesion molecules. One is a protein, the other a glycoprotein (illustrator Edward Brehmer; reproduced from Brehmer-Andersson E (1988), with permission)

4.1.4 Immune Response in Non-Lymphoid Tissues

If antigen is inserted into non-lymphoid tissue it will be carried off to the local lymph nodes where it induces an immune response. However, if the antigen persists for a longer time at the site of insertion, B and T cells from the activated nodes migrate to the place of inoculation and induce a chronic inflammation. The main actors are B cells. Sometimes the appearance of the inflammatory tissue mimics that of the stimulated cortex in lymph nodes and displays germinal centers. This kind of reaction, called lymphocytoma, is rather common in inflammatory lesions of unknown origin in the oral and genital mucous membranes. The borrelial lymphocytoma in the skin is well known in regions where bites from spirochete-infested ticks are common (Fig. 18.2). Another example is cutaneous leishmaniasis infection (Fig. 19.1a).

A parallel phenomenon may appear with T cells as actors. In these cases a specific antigen present in the skin stimulates sensitized T cells to blast transformation and proliferation at the same place. The activated lymphocytes give rise to a clone of specific T cells (i.e., genetically identical T cells). These cells may be observed in herpes virus infection, vasculitis, and pityriasis lichenoides et varioliformis acuta (Figs. 7.14c, 20.5c and 26.3f).

4.1.5 Cytokines and Cell Adhesion Molecules

Cytokines are cell-secreted soluble proteins which act as messenger molecules of the immune system. On contact with antigen they are released from different kinds of cells, such as sensitized lymphocytes (lymphokines), monocytes (monokines) and keratinocytes (keratinocyte-derived cytokines). Interleukin is a general term for a group of multifunctional cytokines that are produced by a variety of lymphoid and non-lymphoid cells. At least 18 different interleukins have been identified (IL-1, IL-2, etc.). Other important cytokines are IFN-α, IFN-β and IFN-γ, tumor necrosis factor (TNF) alpha and beta, transforming growth factor (TGF) beta, and lipopolysaccharide (LPS).

Cell adhesion molecules (CAMs) are multifunctional integral membrane protein and glycoprotein molecules which when expressed on the cell surface allow cell to cell and cell to matrix interactions and signal transduction. The molecule consists of a major part that is extracellular, a transmembrane part, and a short intracellular part connected to the actin cytoskeleton (see Glossary) of the cell (Fig. 4.2). The extracellular part, the receptor, tightly and specifically binds to a counter-receptor (ligand), which is either another CAM or an extracellular matrix protein such as collagen, fibronectin or laminin. These bindings (receptor–ligand interactions) are transitory. The expression on the cell surface of CAMs taking part in the immune response is induced, modified (i.e., upregulated or downregulated) and inhibited by cytokines.

There are at least four families of CAMs: integrins, the immunoglobulin gene family, selectins, and cadherins. The most relevant are discussed in the sections below and summarized in Table 4.1 (Katz et al. 1991):

Integrins

Integrins include, among other subunits, beta 1 and 2. The beta 1 group includes the very late activation (VLA) integrins. These are distributed on several cell

Table 4.1 Cell adhesion molecules: abbreviation, expression, and binding

CAM	Expressed on	Binds to
VLA-4 (very late activation antigen 4)	Lymphocytes	VCAM-1
LFA-1 (leukocyte function antigen 1)	Lymphocytes	ICAM-1 and ICAM-2
MAC-1 (macrophage activation antigen 1)	Macrophages, monocytes, neutrophils	Endothelial cells
ICAM-1 (intercellular adhesion molecule 1; the major ligand for LFA-1)[a]	Always on endothelial cells, certain epithelial cells, antigen-presenting cells	LFA-1[b]
ICAM-2 (intercellular adhesion molecule 2)	Endothelial cells	LFA-1[b]
CD2 (common differentiation antigen 2)	T cells	LFA-3[b]
LFA-3 (leukocyte function antigen 3)	Endothelial, epithelial, and mesenchymal cells	CD2
VCAM-1 (vascular adhesion molecule 1)	Endothelial cells	VLA-4[c]
ELAM-1 (CLA, CD62 E) (endothelial leukocyte adhesion molecule 1)	Endothelial cells	Lymphocytes[d]

[a] Other cell types may be induced to express ICAM-1 by cytokines such as IL-1 and IFN-γ. For example, IFN-γ can induce expression of both class II HLA antigen and ICAM-1 molecules on the surface of keratinocytes. ICAM-1 molecules may then bind to LFA-1 molecules on $CD8^+$ T cells. In this way, $CD8^+$ cells are able to migrate into the epidermis (Nickoloff 1988).

[b] The main function of LFA-1/ICAM-1 and -2 and CD2/LFA-3 interactions is to closely appose antigen-presenting cells long enough to sensitize T cells and thereby activate them.

[c] The cytokines IL-1 and TNF-α can induce the expression of VCAM-1 on endothelial cells.

[d] ELAM-1, after activation by cytokines, is expressed on endothelial cells of venules in extracutaneous sites of inflammation and was thought primarily to mediate extravasation of neutrophils. However, at sites of chronic inflammation, ELAM-1 is also expressed on high endothelial cells of venules in the dermis. Investigations have shown that in this setting ELAM-1 exclusively binds to memory T cells. Also the binding is independent of acute activation events that regulate integrin-mediated adhesions. ELAM-1 is therefore thought to be the tissue-selective endothelial cell adhesion molecule for skin-homing memory T cells (Picker et al. 1991; Shimizu et al. 1991) (Sect. 4.4).

types including T cells and keratinocytes and bind to extracellular matrix. However, one of them (VLA-4) as well as binding to fibronectin, also binds to endothelial cells. The beta 2 integrins, also called the leukocyte integrins, are expressed only on cells of lymphoid and myeloid lineage, and those of interest here are leukocyte function antigen 1 (LFA-1) and macrophage activation antigen 1 (MAC-1).

Immunoglobulin Gene Family

The immunoglobulin gene family is a large group of molecules which structurally resemble immunoglobulins; only a few of them are CAMs. Those relevant here are intercellular adhesion molecule 1 (ICAM-1), intercellular adhesion molecule 2 (ICAM-2), common differentiation antigen 2 (CD2), leukocyte function antigen 3 (LFA-3) and vascular cell adhesion molecule 1 (VCAM-1).

Selectins

Selectins are calcium dependent. The group includes endothelial leukocyte adhesion molecule 1 (ELAM-1, CLA, CD62 E).

Cadherins

Cadherins are a group of CAMs which like selectins are calcium dependent. They are involved principally in the organization of cells in tissues and organs, and also form permanent connections between cells such as desmosomes.

4.2 Innate Immunity

The adaptive immunity described above is directed towards a specific antigen, which may be either a microbe or some other kind of agent, foreign to the body. It takes some time to develop. The time required depends on the presence or not of memory lymphocytes. In contrast to the adapted system, the innate system is directed only towards microbes and not to non-microbial antigen. Also it is capable of acting immediately. The main components of the innate system are neutrophils and macrophages, NK cells, and the complement system. Neutrophils contain a number of different inherited receptors which enable them to recognize and bind to the appropriate bacterial antigens. The antigens are common to several kinds of bacteria, but do not exist in human cells. The innate system may activate the adaptive system.

4.2.1 The Complement System

The components of the complement system act as chemical mediators. In inactive form it comprises nine different protein components, C1 through C9, present in the plasma. Activated by an antigen, for example a bacterium, these components attach successively to the target antigen and split up into several additional fragments, the complement cascade. The cascade triggers or enhances processes such as attraction of leukocytes, vascular leakage, phagocytosis, and cell destruction by lysis. The nine inactive components (molecules) may be divided into three groups C1→C423→C56789. With the exception of C4, they are numbered in the order in which they are activated and attached to the target. The activation of the complement cascade may be initiated by two different mechanisms: the classic pathway and the alternative pathway.

4.2.1.1 The Classic Pathway

In a setting where bacteria enter a body already exposed to this kind of bacteria, they evoke an inflammatory response and are rapidly covered by antibodies (IgM or IgG) which have leaked into the tissue from involved venules. Bacteria and antibodies form antigen–antibody complexes. The C1 molecules, also present in the leaked plasma, bind to antibodies on the surface of the bacteria and trigger the complement cascade. In the next step C4, C2 and C3 become activated and settle on the bacteria. Activated C3 and C4 split off small fragments C3a and C4a, which act as inflammatory mediators, called anaphylatoxins. The larger parts of these split molecules are called C3b and C4b. Together the assembly C2–C3b–C4b acts as an enzyme and splits the molecule C5 into a small and a large fragment. The small fragment C5a becomes the third and most powerful of the anaphylatoxins. The assembly C5b–C6–C7–C8–C9 forms the membrane attack complex, which acts as a kind of rod with the power to penetrate the surface of bacteria and other cells ending up in destruction of the target. The three anaphylatoxins degranulate mast cells and basophils; C5b is also a chemotactic factor for granulocytes and macrophages. C3b promotes phagocytosis.

4.2.1.2 The Alternative Pathway

If there are no antibodies against invading bacteria or the antibody is not IgM or IgG, C3b molecules (always present in a small amount in the plasma) settle on the bacteria. By interacting with a series of proteins also present in the plasma, C3b activates C3 and thereby starts the complement cascade.

In addition to its role as an assistant in the body defense, the complement takes part in adverse skin reactions.

4.3 Adverse Reactions of the Immune System

There are four main types of hypersensitivity reactions (i.e., adverse reactions) in which different components of the immune system take part.

4.3.1 Type I. Immediate Reactions

Antigens such as pollen or penicillin may in some individuals stimulate the production of antibodies of the IgE class which via their Fc part bind to mast cells in tissues and basophils in the blood without giving rise to symptoms. However, if a sensitized person is exposed anew to the antigen, it binds to the Fab parts of the IgE antibodies already attached to mast cells and basophils, which induces degranulation of these cells and release of histamine into the tissue. The release of histamine is followed by contraction of bronchial smooth muscles, increased vascular permeability and increased secretion by nasal, bronchial and gastric glands. The effect may occur rapidly in urticaria, allergic rhinitis, bronchial asthma, or anaphylactic shock.

4.3.2 Type II. Cytotoxic Antibody-Dependent Reactions

Antibodies bind to antigen present on the surface of cells or to extracellular matrix protein. Two types of mechanism are relevant in dermatopathology.

Cytotoxic Antibody-Dependent Complement-Mediated Reactions

These reactions occur via two different pathways. In the first pathway, antibodies (IgM or IgG) bind to antigen on the cell surface with their Fab parts and activate the complement system. Membrane attack complexes, mentioned above, are formed and attack the target. They puncture the cell membrane and thereby lyse the cell. In the second pathway, the split product C3b in the complement cascade or antibodies become attached to the target optimizing it for phagocytosis. Clinical examples are thrombocytopenia due to drugs, autoimmune bullous dermatoses, transfusion reactions, and rhesus incompatibility.

Cytotoxic Antibody-Dependent Cell-Mediated Reactions

The target cells get coated with low concentrations of antibodies, usually IgG. The Fc part of the immunoglobulin binds to receptors on monocytes, neutrophils, eosinophils, thrombocytes or NK cells and the target cells are killed without phagocytosis. This type of reaction may play a role in graft reactions.

4.3.3 Type III. Reactions due to Circulating Immune Complex Activated by Complement

IgG or IgM antibody–antigen complex circulating in the blood or deposited in tissue may be activated by complement and give rise to tissue destruction. The antigen may be foreign proteins or infectious agents. Clinical examples are leukocytoclastic vasculitis and serum sickness.

4.3.4 Type IV. Cell-Mediated Hypersensitivity Reactions

The delayed hypersensitivity reaction is initiated by $CD4^+$ cells. Clinical examples are immune granulomas (sarcoidosis, tuberculosis) and allergic contact dermatitis (see below).

The direct cytotoxicity reaction is mediated by $CD8^+$ cells, which cause lysis of virus-infected cells and probably also play a part in the pathogenesis of lichen planus (Sect. 24.1.3).

4.4 The Skin Immune System

As already mentioned above a fair number of lymphocytes are continuously recirculating. From the blood they migrate into tissues and then back to the circulation via lymphatics. Under normal conditions this is called trafficking or homing. Naive lymphocytes migrate into lymph nodes via the high endothelial venules in the paracortex, and memory cells preferentially to the type of tissue in which they were previously stimulated (sensitized). The migration into tissues is made possible by adhesion molecule interactions between the lymphocytes and activated endothelial cells in postcapillary venules described above. There are indications that specialized subsets of T cells home to different anatomical compartments, one of which is the skin. This is due to binding of specific adhesion molecules expressed on lymphocytes to matching ligands on the endothelial cells in a specific compartment such as the skin (Table 4.1). However, tissue specificity is relative. In the case of inflammation, the influx of T cells is increased in the tissue and the selectivity seen in normal homing is reduced. Also the migration of presumably naive T cells into lymph nodes is increased (Picker et al. 1991; Shimizu et al. 1991; Shimizu et al. 1992).

4.4.1 Lymphocytes in Normal Skin

Continuously recirculating lymphocytes homing to the skin are considered to be a part of the immune defense of the skin. Normal skin contains some T cells, but no B cells. The majority of the T cells are found around postcapillary venules in the upper dermis and close to adnexa. Only a few, about 2% of the total, are seen in the epidermis, and these are mainly T-suppressor cells expressing CD8 antigen. In the dermis the numbers of T-helper cells expressing CD4 antigen and $CD8^+$ cells are about equal (Bos et al. 1987). More lymphocytes and other cells important for defense, such as neutrophils, eosinophils, and macrophages, are recruited when needed.

4.4.2 Langerhans Cells

Langerhans cells, key cells in the skin immune system, are located in a network in the epidermis and may also be present in the dermis. They are bone marrow-derived and closely related to the interdigitating dendritic cells in the lymph nodes to which they present antigen (see below). In routinely stained sections, Langerhans cells are not visible in the epidermis and they cannot be differentiated from histiocytes in the dermis. However, they may be made visible by staining with S-100 or CD1a antibodies (Fig. 4.3). At the ultrastructural

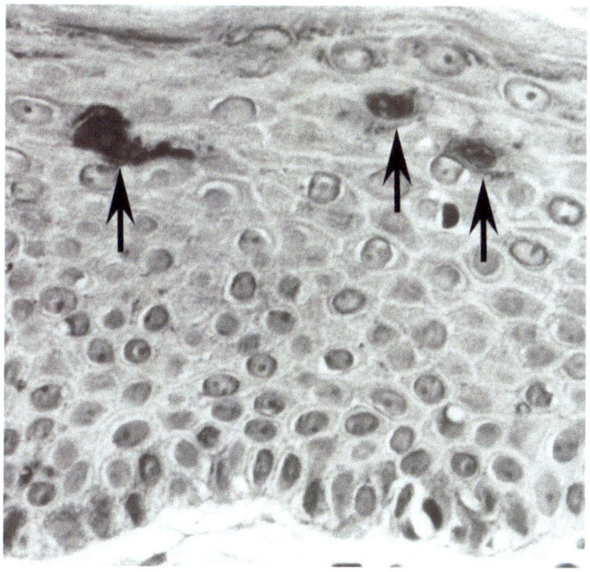

Fig. 4.3 Langerhans cells in the epidermis. *Arrows* Langerhans cells with more or less clearly visible dendrites; S-100

level they are identified by specific organelles in the cytoplasm, so-called Birbeck granules.

4.4.3 Keratinocytes

Keratinocytes also take part in the development of inflammation. They may be activated by cytokines and induced to express ICAM-1 and MHC class II antigen on the surface. They then become able to bind T cells. They may also produce cytokines (keratinocyte-derived cytokines).

4.5 The Immune Response and Skin Diseases

The mechanisms or the possible mechanisms involved in skin diseases are discussed in later chapters together with the related diseases. However, a simplified description of the supposed mechanism of one of the most common adverse immunologic reactions in the skin, allergic contact dermatitis, is presented below. It is a type IV delayed hypersensitivity reaction in which different kinds of cells, cytokines and CAMs take part.

As already mentioned, small molecules—haptens—may become antigenic by binding to a larger protein molecule (a carrier molecule). When haptens are introduced into the skin they bind to a protein component of the epidermis and are handled by the skin immune system, mostly without consequences (i.e., the individual is tolerant to the antigens). However, sometimes an individual becomes allergic to a protein-conjugated hapten antigen such as nickel, common in coins and clasps, or a component of a topical remedy. In the epidermis the antigen is taken up and processed by Langerhans cells. It is then expressed on the surface of the Langerhans cell together with MHC class II molecules. The antigen-bearing Langerhans cells migrate through the dermis and afferent lymphatics to the T cell area of the regional lymph nodes. They present the foreign antigen together with the MHC class II antigen to appropriate naive T cells and thereby activate and sensitize them. This gives rise to proliferation of effector T cells and memory T cells. Via efferent lymphatics and blood vessels these cells migrate to the antigen-affected skin and give rise to a transitory inflammatory reaction.

The next time the same antigen reaches the epidermis it is directly confronted with a small number of memory T cells present in the skin (Bos et al. 1989). These cells become activated, release cytokines and induce further recruitment and proliferation of sensitized T cells. The recruitment of sensitized T cells is made possible by activation also of the endothelial cells of dermal venules which become high and cuboidal (high endothelial venules). VCAM-1 is expressed on the high endothelial cells and bind to VLA-4 on activated sensitized T cells whereby the T cells get into transitory intimate contact with the activated endothelial cells enabling them to migrate into the surrounding tissue. By further adhesion molecule interactions and cytokine stimulation, lymphocytes may also invade the superficial part of dermis and the epidermis and cause a dermatitis which may be severe (Sect. 22.1.1). The provoked inflammatory reaction fades and disappears if the contact with the antigen stops, but flares up if the contact recommences.

References

1. Bos JD, Zonneveld I, Das PK, Krieg SR, Van der Loos CM, Kapsenberg ML (1987) The skin immune system (SIS): distribution and immunophenotype of lymphocyte subpopulations in normal human skin. J Invest Dermatol 88:569–573
2. Bos JD, Teunissen MBM, Kapsenberg ML (1989) Immunology of contact dermatitis. Acta Derm Venereol Suppl (Stockh) 151:84–87
3. Brehmer-Andersson E (1988) Allmän patologi—En introduktion. (in Swedish) Studentlitteratur, Lund, Sweden
4. Katz AM, Rosenthal D, Sauder DN (1991) Cell adhesion molecules. Structure, function, and implication in a variety of cutaneous and other pathologic conditions. Int J Dermatol 30:153–160

5. Nickoloff BJ (1988) Role of interferon gamma in cutaneous trafficking of lymphocytes with emphasis on molecular and cellular adhesion events. Arch Dermatol 124:1835–1843
6. Picker LJ, Kishimoto TK, Smith CW, Warnock RA, Butcher EC (1991) ELAM-1 is an adhesion molecule for skin-homing T cells. Nature 349:796–799
7. Shimizu Y, Shaw S, Graber N, Gopal TV, Horgan KJ, van Seventer GA, Newman W (1991) Activation-independent binding of human memory T cells to adhesion molecule ELAM-1. Nature 349:799–802
8. Shimizu Y, Newman W, Tanaka Y, Shaw S (1992) Lymphocyte interactions with endothelial cells. Immunol Today 13:106–112

Chapter 5

Cell and Vascular Response to Infection and Injury

5

Activation of the defense systems gives rise to inflammation which, if microbes are involved, is called infection. The reactions may be acute or chronic and involve different types of inflammatory cells together with lymphatics and blood vessels.

5.1 Inflammatory Cells

The types, number and proportion of inflammatory cells taking part in an inflammatory reaction depend on the type of inflammation/infection.

5.1.1 Neutrophils

Neutrophils or granulocytes (i.e., white blood cells with discreet granules in the cytoplasm) are continuously produced in the bone marrow and make up the main part of the white blood cells that normally circulate in the blood (40–75%). At need more neutrophils are recruited, which is followed by an increased number in the circulation. Neutrophils are end cells and thus cannot divide. Their life span is short (3–4 days). The nucleus of the cell is divided into two to five segments depending on the age of the cell (Fig. 12.1b). The cytoplasm carries two types of fine, inconspicuous, and enzyme-containing granules. Neutrophils engulf (phagocytose) microbes and kill them by means of the enzymes stored in the cytoplasm. When released into the tissue these enzymes also have the ability to degrade dead cells and tissue fragments. Neutrophils do not reside in the tissues under normal condition, but are called upon at need, and thus are the dominating cells in acute inflammation. In old multisegmented neutrophils the cytoplasm becomes eosinophilic and the cells may be mistaken for eosinophils.

5.1.2 Eosinophils

Like neutrophils, eosinophils are end cells, produced in the bone marrow. They circulate in the blood in small numbers (1–6%). Their life span is somewhat longer than that of the neutrophils. Under normal condition they migrate into the tissues and are found scattered everywhere, but especially in the mucosa of the gastrointestinal tract. In hypersensitivity reactions a high number of eosinophils may be present in tissues as well as in the circulating blood. Mostly the nucleus has no more than two segments and the cytoplasm carries large, bright, eosinophilic granules, which differentiate them from old neutrophils with eosinophilic cytoplasm. Eosinophilic granules contain cationic (positively charged) proteins, three of which are major basic protein (MBP), eosinophilic cationic protein (ECP), and eosinophilic derived neurotoxin (EDN) (Peters et al. 1986). These positively charged proteins make eosinophils able to bind to negatively charged molecules on other cells and make them toxic for worms and other large parasites.

5.1.3 Lymphocytes

As already mentioned, B cells originate in the bone marrow and T cells in the thymus. Together they make up 20–45% of the white cells circulating in the peripheral blood. Mature lymphocytes are small and have a round, compact and dark nucleus, and sparse cytoplasm (Fig. 15.1). In routinely stained sections, B and T cells look alike. However, it is possible to differentiate between them and also between their subgroups by means of immunohistochemical staining techniques using monoclonal antibodies directed against their surface antigens.

Stimulated lymphocytes are larger than mature lymphocytes. In routinely prepared sections stimulated B cells are easily identified in the fully developed germinal center of a lymphocytoma. They have large, light, and somewhat irregular nuclei, which contain one or two nucleoli (Fig. 18.2c). However, stimulated T cells, usually components of a mixed lymphocytic infiltrate, stand out because they have a slightly irregular form and are larger and seem more compact than the surrounding normal lymphocytes (Fig. 20.5c). The latter

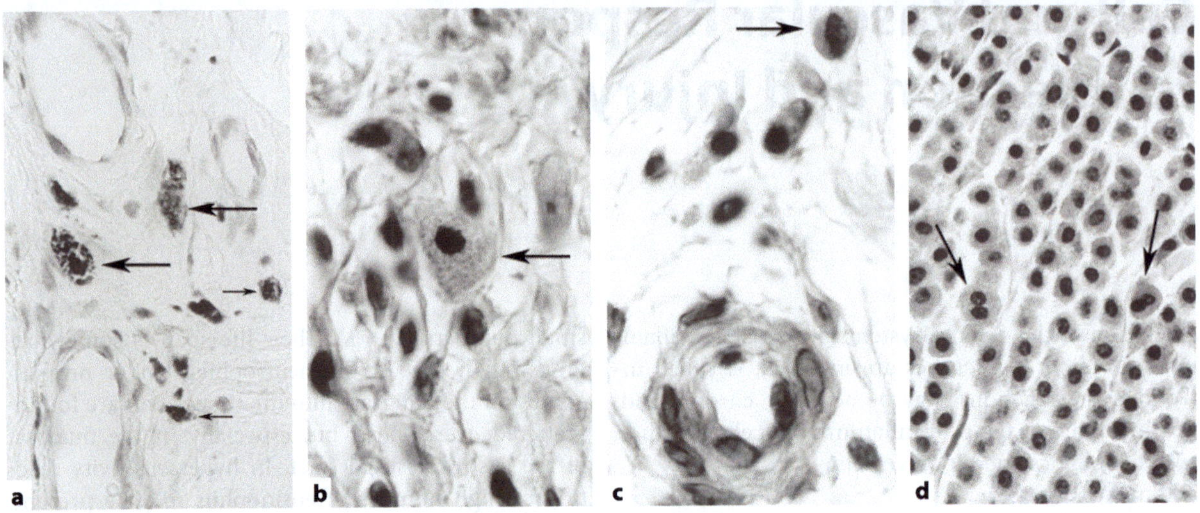

Fig. 5.1 Mast cells. **a** ACA. Between three dilated venules there are two large mast cells (*large arrows*) and two small heavily charged with granules (*small arrows*); toluidine blue, ×400. **b** ACA. A large mast cell stuffed with large granules in the center (*arrow*); H&E, ×1000. **c** ACA. A small mast cell with hazy cytoplasm (*arrow*). The vessel is an arteriole; H&E, ×1000. **d** Mastocytoma. *Arrows* binuclear cells; H&E, ×400

is an artifact probably due to too much stain and/or thick sections. The reason for this proposition is that in smears (Fig. 26.3c) and in sections, slightly faded after demonstration using a carbon arc lamp projector, these cells also reveal large nuclei containing one or two nucleoli and many mitotic figures (Fig. 26.3f). In routinely stained sections, stimulated T cells are impossible to differentiate from T cell lymphoma cells (Sect. 26.3.4).

5.1.4 Plasma Cells

Plasma cells, the effector cells of B cells, are larger than lymphocytes. They are oval and have a round and eccentrically located nucleus. In the cytoplasm close to the nucleus there is a typical crescent-like light area. In longstanding lesions binuclear plasma cells may be present (Figs. 18.1 and 18.4b). Plasma cells are common in chronic inflammation and are often numerous in infections caused by spirochetes and *Leishmania* protozoa. They develop and mature in the lymph nodes and migrate to the skin.

5.1.5 Mast Cells

Mast cells originate from the bone marrow and are able to divide. They do not normally circulate in the blood, but are present in connective tissue throughout the body. Morphologically there are two variants of mast cells, a larger and a smaller. The large cells are also called connective tissue mast cells, and the small cells mucosal mast cells. In spite of this, both variants may be present together in the skin as well as in the mucous membranes. The large mast cell is triangular, has a round nucleus and a rich cytoplasm stuffed with large granules. The small mast cell is round or slightly oval. It has a round nucleus and because of densely packed small granules the cytoplasm is hazy. Among other substances the granules contain histamine. In normal skin, mast cells are located around vessels in the papillary dermis and close to nerves and appendages.

A greatly increased number of mast cells are found in urticaria pigmentosa, mastocytoma, and related conditions. However, the number of mast cells is also increased in lesions of common dermatoses such as chronic dermatitis, psoriasis, and lichen planus (Tharp 2001). According to the experience of the author there is also an increase in mast cells in infectious diseases such as acrodermatitis chronica atrophicans (ACA), a kind of borreliosis, and secondary syphilis, and in amalgam tattoo. In acute inflammation/infection together with basophils they release histamine (Sect. 5.2.1).

Once recognized in H&E-stained sections, mast cells are not difficult to identify, but they are better

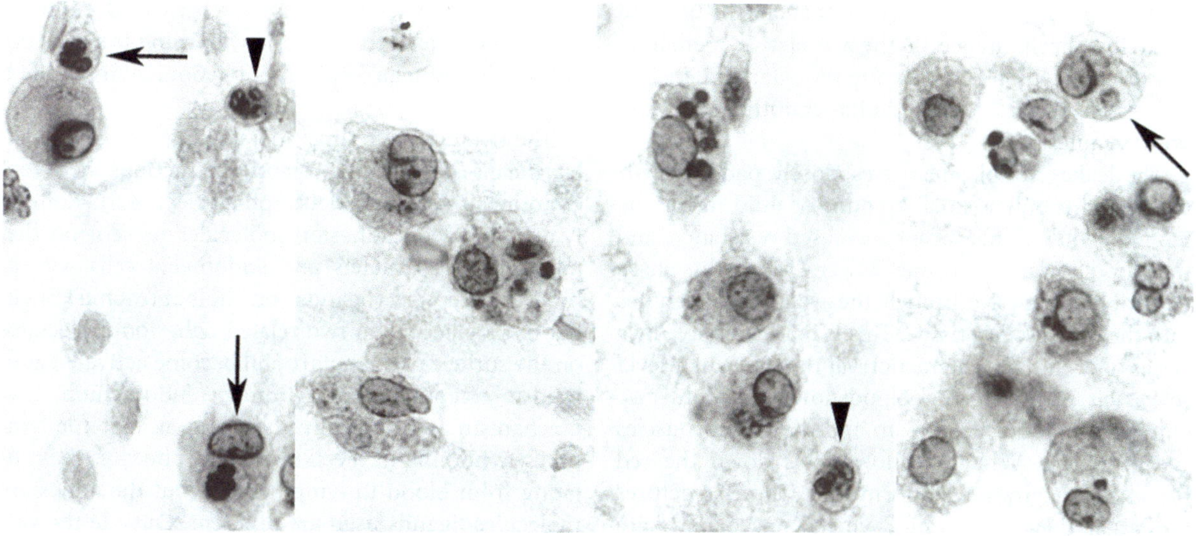

Fig. 5.2 Phagocytosis. Smear from a subepidermal vesicle. There are two old neutrophils with a multisegmented nucleus (*arrowheads*) and several macrophages. *Arrow, top left* macrophage in close contact with a neutrophil containing a disintegrating, swollen neutrophil; *arrow, bottom right* macrophage with a newly engulfed neutrophil. In the middle there is a group of macrophages which contain the remains of neutrophils in various stages of processing in the cytoplasm. In the macrophage in the top right corner the remains of a nucleus are lying in a vacuole (*arrow*). Mayer staining, ×1000

displayed by means of special stains such as toluidine blue or Giemsa stains, which accentuate the granules (Figs. 5.1 and 29.7b). In sections stained with toluidine and Giemsa, granules become blue and with May-Grünwald Giemsa metachromatically red.

5.1.6 Basophils

Basophils are bone marrow-derived granulocytes which circulate in the blood in small numbers (0–1%). They have a segmented nucleus and like mast cells carry basophilic granules containing histamine in the cytoplasm. They are not precursors of mast cells.

5.1.7 Monocytes/Macrophages

Monocytes have an abundant cytoplasm and a large bean-shaped nucleus. They originate from the bone marrow and circulate in the blood (2–10%). However, after a short time in the circulation they migrate into connective tissue where they become larger, acquire the capacity to phagocytose and when doing so become activated. Like neutrophils, macrophages recognize bacteria by surface receptors that are specific for bacterial products. On activation they become even larger, and their ability to phagocytose and kill bacteria increases. Tissue macrophages without signs of phagocytosis are often, as in this book, called histiocytes. Macrophages (histiocytes) are a common component of inflammatory cell infiltrates in chronic infections and in the healing stage of acute infections (Fig. 5.2).

5.2 Acute Inflammation

The histologic hallmarks of acute inflammation are exudation of plasma and migration of inflammatory cells, predominantly neutrophils, from postcapillary venules into the perivascular tissue.

5.2.1 Active Phase

In response to injury or bacterial infection, histamine and serotonin, short-lived vasoactive chemical mediators stored in the tissue (histamine in mast cells and basophils and serotonin in platelets) are released and start the inflammatory process. Histamine and serotonin cause dilatation of arterioles, which increases the blood flow and capillary pressure. Closed capillaries open up and become filled with blood. Due to the increased capillary flow and pressure, postcapillary venules become distended and gaps appear between the endothelial cells, through which plasma leaks out into the surrounding tissue. The gaps are the result of contraction of two adjacent endothelial cells brought about by the influence of the vasoactive mediators. Contracted cells bulge into the vascular lumen and the vessels become so-called high endothelial (epithelioid) venules.

The leakage of plasma leaves closely packed erythrocytes with only a small amount of fluid in the distended venules. This means increased resistance, and the blood flow now becomes slower. During this phase neutrophils migrate through the wall of the venules into the perivascular tissue. This is made possible by a series of events and interactions at the molecular level. In vessels with a normal blood flow, neutrophils occupy the center of the stream and the red corpuscles the periphery. When the flow slows down the red blood cells aggregate and form rolls. These structures are larger than neutrophils, which consequently are transposed to the periphery and get closer to the endothelial surface.

Neutrophils are attracted to the site of damage by chemotaxins which are molecular products released from injured tissue, extravasated blood and bacteria. Neutrophils, like other cells capable of phagocytosis, have membrane receptors for different kinds of chemotaxins. They also have a huge reserve of receptors stored in their cytoplasmic granules. When chemotactic molecules bind to appropriate receptors on the surface membrane of a neutrophil, the granule receptors fuse with the membrane and are then expressed on the cell surface, and in that way enhance the chemotactic response of the cell. Chemotaxin bound to neutrophils activates or turns on the neutrophils, which thereby make contact with the endothelium. At first the neutrophils are only loosely attached to the endothelium, which allows them to roll along the intima, but then they suddenly stop and stick to the intima before they sneak through the wall using the gaps between the epithelial cells. This phenomenon is called diapedesis.

The two events, rolling and sticking, are generated by means of receptor–ligand interactions between endothelial cells and neutrophils (Sect. 4.5). Rolling is dependent on adhesion molecules present on the membrane of platelets and endothelial cells, which bind to receptors (ligands) on the neutrophils. Sticking takes place when two related adhesion molecules on the surface of the neutrophil become activated and bind to receptors (ligands) on the endothelium. The mechanism is principally the same as that for lymphocyte homing in the skin and lymphocytes recirculating from blood to lymph nodes, but the adhesion molecules/ligands used are different. Outside the vessel, neutrophils phagocytose bacteria. Plasma that has leaked into the tissue provides antibodies and complement, which facilitate the phagocytosis, and even neutralize noxious agents.

An acute inflammatory process may heal without residue, give rise to an abscess, heal with fibrosis and scar formation, or change into a chronic inflammation.

5.2.2
Healing Without Residue

If the inflammation/infection has been slight and/or effectively controlled, the process starts to decline. The influx of neutrophils stops in favor of immigration of macrophages. The short-lived neutrophils die on the spot. When disintegrated they release the enzyme fibrinolysin which makes deposited fibrin soluble. In

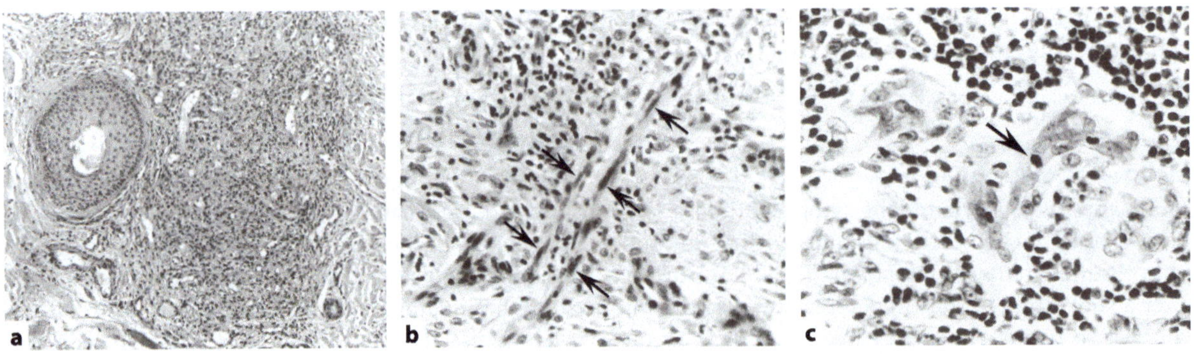

Fig. 5.3 Angiogenesis. **a** Bacillary epithelioid angiomatosis and AIDS. Close to a deep-seated hair follicle is a rather large area with proliferating vessels. **b** Granulation tissue at the margin of an abscess. In the middle there is a longitudinally cut newly formed vessel (*arrows*). **c** Close-up of another area shows proliferating endothelial cells containing a large light nucleus with a distinct nucleolus (*arrow* mitotic figure). H&E

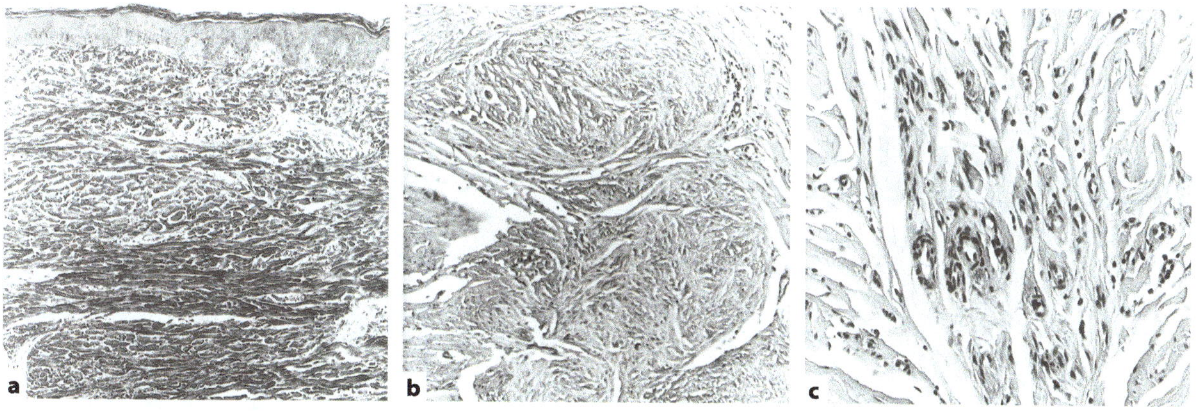

Fig. 5.4 Scar formation. **a** White scar on the back. In the mid-dermis there is a band of sclerotic collagen bundles arranged parallel to the epidermis; vG. **b** A small clinically keloid-like scar on the back. In the middle and deep dermis there are large nodules composed of sclerotic collagen bundles arranged in whirls. **c** Between some whirls there are strings of connective tissue and newly formed vessels; H&E

this form fibrin as well as accumulated exudate is removed from the tissue by the lymphatics. Macrophages phagocytose dead neutrophils (Fig. 5.2), necrotic tissue fragments, extravasated red blood cells, pigment, etc. They are also able to phagocytose and liquefy fibrin. Macrophages with engulfed material may be found in the sinuses of the regional lymph nodes. The result of these cleaning procedures is called resolution. If there is only a minimum of dead tissue it is replaced by regenerating new cells from the edge of the damaged zone. Provided the resolution and regeneration are complete, the pattern and function of the damaged area will be the same as before the injury.

5.2.3 Abscess Formation

Abscesses and pustules are local accumulations of pus (i.e., a large number of neutrophils, disintegrating neutrophils, and inflammatory exudate). The abscess is walled off by granulation tissue (Sect. 5.2.4). Boils, pimples and pustules caused by microbes such as bacteria and fungi are examples of abscesses (Figs. 12.1, 13.4c, 13.5, 14.1b and 29.2a and b).

5.2.4 Healing with Fibrosis and Scar Formation

If lost tissue cannot be replaced, or fibrin clots are not cleared rapidly enough, healing takes place by means of granulation tissue. Proliferation of new vessels and fibroblasts, promoted by macrophages, invade the damaged area (Fig. 5.3). Lymphocytes and plasma cells predominate in the inflammatory cell infiltrate. The newly formed vessels are leaky, and allow plasma and red blood cells to pass through the vessel wall, which makes the tissue edematous. Gradually the fibroblasts lay down collagen fibers, the vessels and edema disappear, and finally nonvascular fibrous tissue replaces the lost tissue; a scar is formed. Repair by granulation tissue and fibrosis is called organization (Figs. 7.12b,c and Fig. 10.1b).

Occasionally a scar becomes hypertrophic or develops into a keloid. Clinically a hypertrophic scar fades and flattens with time, while a keloid remains reddish and even becomes larger. Histologically it may be difficult to differentiate between the two. A spared papillary dermis, bands or whirls of sclerotic collagen in the reticular dermis are in favor of keloid (Lee et al. 2004).

5.2.4.1 Examples

Case 1. Scar

A 13-year-old girl over a period of 1.5 years had observed asymptomatic, white, papular lesions spreading over the trunk. The clinical suggestion was guttate lichen sclerosus et atrophicus.

A biopsy specimen from the back revealed scar tissue with a band of sclerotic collagen in the mid-dermis (Fig. 5.4a). In all probability the lesions were scars caused by varicella.

Case 2. Keloid

A 22-year-old man had a small keloid-like lesion on the back. It had developed without previous injury.

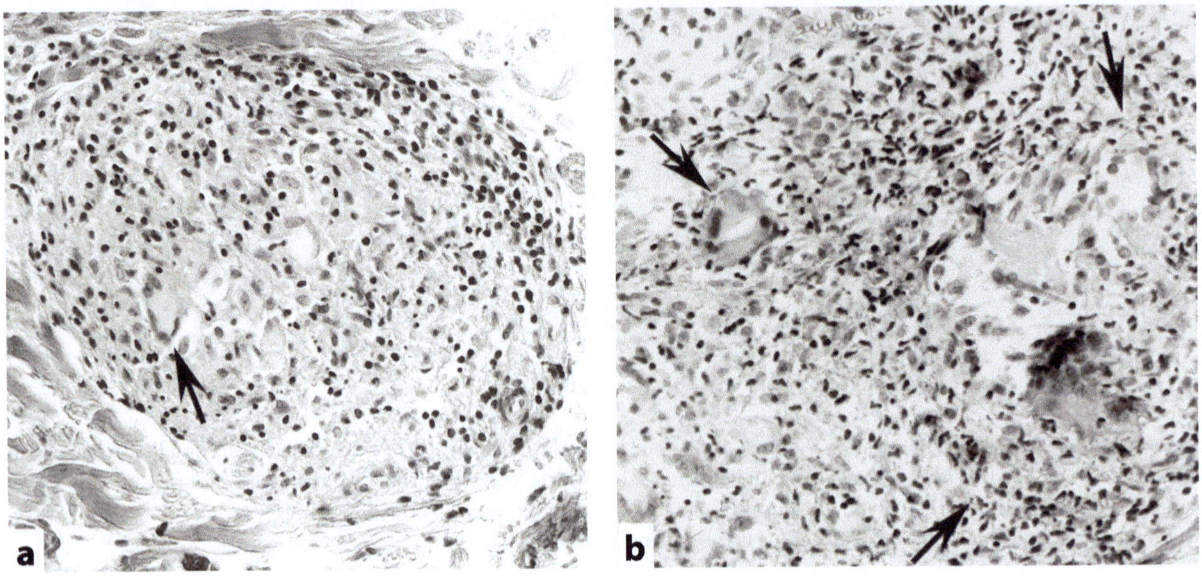

Fig. 5.5 Sarcoidosis. **a** Epithelioid cell granuloma with a giant cell of Langhans type (*arrow*). There are only a few lymphocytes. **b** Another granuloma in the same section contains a conglomeration of giant cells (*arrows*); the infiltrate of lymphocytes is more dense; H&E

Histologic investigation showed the typical picture of keloid (Fig. 5.4b,c). Keloid may be a complication in acne vulgaris. It is not known if this was the cause in this case.

5.3 Chronic Inflammation

As well as being the result of an acute process, chronic inflammation may start insidiously. The histologic hallmarks are infiltrates of macrophages, lymphocytes and plasma cells. Areas of tissue destruction alternate with areas of granulation tissue and fibrosis (healing).

Histiocytes/macrophages play a major role. Cytokines such as IFN-γ secreted by sensitized T cells, and bacterial endotoxins are examples of substances able to activate macrophages, which accumulate in the tissue by proliferation (cell division) and continued recruitment of monocytes from the blood. Also secretion of the cytokine migration inhibitor factor by sensitized lymphocytes restrains the macrophages from moving away from the area. In turn activated macrophages produce a wide variety of biologically active products, which are helpful in destroying persistent bacteria, but if not balanced also destroy the tissues. Promotion of new vessel formation, fibroblast proliferation, and collagen deposition finally lead to fibrosis. In longstanding conditions newly formed vessels become thick-walled due to edema and/or fibrosis, which may cause narrowing and even occlusion of the lumen (Figs. 7.17a–c and 7.18c).

Granulomatous inflammation is a type of chronic inflammation that develops in response to antigens or particles which are difficult to eliminate because they are poorly soluble or hard to disintegrate. The inflammatory tissue contains more or less well-circumscribed aggregates of inflammatory cells called granulomas. There are two main types of granuloma: immune granulomas and foreign body granulomas.

5.3.1 Immune Granulomas

Immune granulomas (hypersensitivity granulomas) are caused by antigenic particles or bacteria, which are difficult to eliminate, and are able to induce cell-mediated immunity. They are composed mainly of macrophages, epithelioid cells, and multinucleated giant cells, and are mostly surrounded by a moderately dense infiltrate of lymphocytes; older granulomas are encircled by fibroblasts. These types of granulomas are generally called epithelioid cell granulomas.

Epithelioid cells are derived from macrophages. Transitional cell forms exist, which sometimes makes it difficult to decide if an aggregate of cells is macrophages (histiocytes) or epithelioid cells. The latter have abundant, pale, poorly defined cytoplasm and a pale, rounded, oval or banana-like nucleus (Figs. 17.2d and 18.1).

With respect to morphology, there are two types of multinucleated giant cells: Langhans giant cells (LGC) and foreign body giant cells (FBGC) (Figs. 5.5 and 5.6, 15.1b and 15.2b). LGCs have several nuclei (up to 30) arranged at the cell membrane in a circular or horseshoe-like manner, and FBGCs contain numerous (more than than 30) disorderly spread nuclei (van der Rhee et al. 1978). It is likely that giant cells are formed by fusion of cells rather than by mitosis without cell division (Sect. 5.3.3).

Granulomas contain no or very few vessels. The central part may become necrotic. Occasionally a granuloma consists of a large area of necrosis surrounded by a brim or ring of epithelioid cells with scattered giant cells (Figs. 15.1c and 15.2). Microscopically, necrotic areas are usually composed of non-eosinophilic, amorphous and slightly granular material. Examples of immune granulomas are tuberculous granulomas (Sect. 15), syphilitic gummas (Sect. 17), and granulomas occurring in sarcoidosis (Sect. 5.3.1.2).

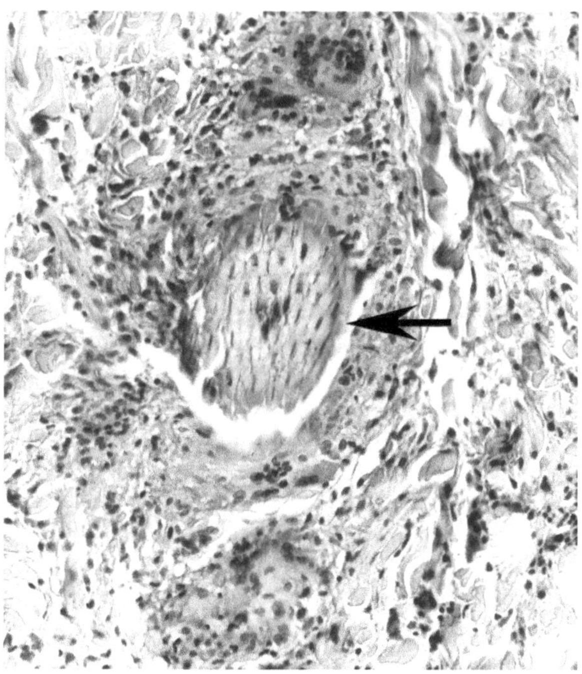

Fig. 5.6 Foreign body granuloma. A foreign body (*arrow*), probably a thorn, is surrounded by foreign body giant cells and lymphocytes; H&E

5.3.1.1 The Tuberculous Granuloma

The primary tuberculous granuloma of the lung is the prototype of infectious immune granulomas. Primary infection with *Mycobacterium tuberculosis* is usually contracted by inhalation of droplets dispersed in the air by an infected person coughing or sneezing. In the lungs the infected droplets give rise to usually only a single 10–20 mm large subpleural inflammatory focus. The first inflammatory cells to arrive are neutrophils, which engulf the mycobacteria and die without killing them. Macrophages phagocytosee the released bacteria and transport them to the regional lymph nodes at the hilus of the lung. At the first encounter with the mycobacteria, macrophages are not able to destroy them. They die and the freed bacteria infect other macrophages. In this way the regional lymph nodes also get infected and the cell-mediated immune response becomes activated. In contact with the bacterial antigen, naive $T4^+$ cells in the lymph nodes are stimulated and give rise to$T4^+$-1 cells. These produce the cytokine INF-γ, which in turn activates macrophages to kill intracellular bacteria. Furthermore, $T4^+$-1 cells induce the development of macrophages into epithelioid cells.

After a few weeks epithelioid cell granulomas occur both at the primary site of inoculation in the peripheral lung parenchyma and in the infected lymph nodes. As already mentioned, granulomas may be necrotic in the center. The necrosis is thought to be due to the toxic effect of the mycobacteria on macrophages in combination with lysis of macrophages by toxic lymphocytes; in the latter case living bacteria may be released into the tissue. However, mycobacteria cannot grow in the acid oxygen-deprived necrotic tissue and finally, in most cases, the infection is controlled and the lesions heal. The Ghon complex (i.e., a fibrotic scar in the parenchyma and enlarged and calcified lymph nodes at the hilus) is all that remains to the naked eye.

During the primary infection the patient becomes sensitized to tuberculin, a mycobacterial protein, and is said to be tuberculin positive. Intradermal injection of tuberculin leads to a local reaction with erythema and swelling which reaches its maximum after 48 h. This is a type IV hypersensitivity reaction, which, if moderate, is thought to be an indicator of a healed primary infection and a guarantee for at least some immunity to tuberculosis. Both the degree of sensitivity and the degree of immunity may vary, but do not parallel each other.

If the mycobacteria are not eliminated, the disease becomes chronic and gives rise to so-called secondary lung tuberculosis. Also an infection that is not 100%

eliminated can be reactivated later in life depending on the state of immunity of the individual. Even an exogenous reinfection may occur. In secondary lung tuberculosis the lesions are sometimes widespread and contain large areas of soft and yellowish-white necrosis, which macroscopically resembles curd cheese, and is therefore called caseation necrosis. Unfortunately this designation is also widely accepted in modern literature for necrosis in cutaneous epithelioid cell granulomas observed under the microscope (Sect. 15.3).

5.3.1.2 Sarcoidosis

Sarcoidosis is a systemic disease thought to be due to some unknown poorly degradable antigen, and may give rise to aggregates of epithelioid cell granulomas anywhere in the body. The organs most affected are the lungs, lymph nodes, liver, bone marrow, and skin. A typical granuloma consists of densely packed epithelioid cells and a variable number of giant cells of both types, and is surrounded by a sparse number of lymphocytes, and therefore is often called naked granuloma (Fig. 5.5). Necroses are not common, but, if present, are usually small and fibrinoid (i.e., have the same shiny eosinophilic appearance as fibrin deposited in the tissue). Plasma cells are sparse. Sometimes inclusions of laminated concretions (Schaumann bodies) or stellate (asteroid) bodies are observed in giant cells.

5.3.1.2.1 Example

Case 3. Sarcoidosis

A 48-year-old woman had a 7-year history of histologically verified lung sarcoidosis, later complicated with adenopathy and lacrimal gland enlargement. For several years she also had had progressing skin lesions suspected to be sarcoidosis. Biopsies were taken from lesions on the face and the forearm.

Both biopsies showed principally the same pattern. The whole dermis was permeated with different-sized epithelioid cell granulomas with a sparse number of lymphocytes and scattered LGC. A conglomeration of giant cells, mainly FBGC was located close to a hair follicle. Necrosis was not observed (Fig. 5.5).

5.3.2 Foreign Body Granuloma

Foreign body granulomas are caused by non-antigenic material such as silica and suture material. They consist mainly of macrophages and foreign body giant cells with admixture of lymphocytes. Sometimes epithelioid cells are also present (Fig. 5.6).

5.3.3 Relevant Investigations

Investigations performed on cultured human blood monocytes, to which were added different kinds of cytokines, indicated that giant cells are formed by fusion of differentiated monocytes (macrophages) and not directly from monocytes. It was found that the cytokine granulocyte-macrophage colony-stimulating factor (GM-CSF) promoted monocyte differentiation into macrophages, and that the cytokine IL-4 provoked the coalescence of histiocytes into large giant cells with many nuclei. If IL-4 is not added to the macrophage culture only a few giant cells, which rarely contained more than three nuclei, were observed (Dugast et al. 1997). Other investigations have shown that with the combination GM-CSF and IL-4 large giant cells with a high number of nuclei (FBGCs) were formed, whereas the combination GM-CSF and INF-γ, under otherwise identical conditions, gave rise to smaller giant cells with fewer than 30 nuclei (LGCs) (McNally and Anderson 1995).

5.4 Angiogenesis

Angiogenesis (neovascularization) implies formation of new blood vessels from already existing vessels both in the embryo and in the adult. In adult females angiogenesis normally occurs in the cyclic variations in the reproductive organs. It also plays an important role in wound healing and regeneration, and in many pathologic conditions such as chronic inflammation, organization of thrombi, and tumor growth (Figs. 5.3, 8.7c, and 22.5c,d).

The mechanism of angiogenesis is complicated and not all the details are clearly understood. The process may be induced by several angiogenic stimuli (cytokines), of which the two most important are vascular endothelial growth factor (VEGF) and TNF. It starts from small venules, which lack smooth muscle cells, and possibly also from capillaries. In the stimulated area endothelial cells and pericytes are activated. The activated endothelial cells produce proteolytic enzymes, which degrade the basal membrane of the parent vessel; this allows the endothelial cells to migrate (by means of pseudopodia) into the surrounding tissue and they then proliferate (by mitotic activity) towards the angiogenic stimulus. Thus, in the perivascular tissue, at first a sprout and then a cord of endothelial cells are formed. In general it is accepted that the lumen of

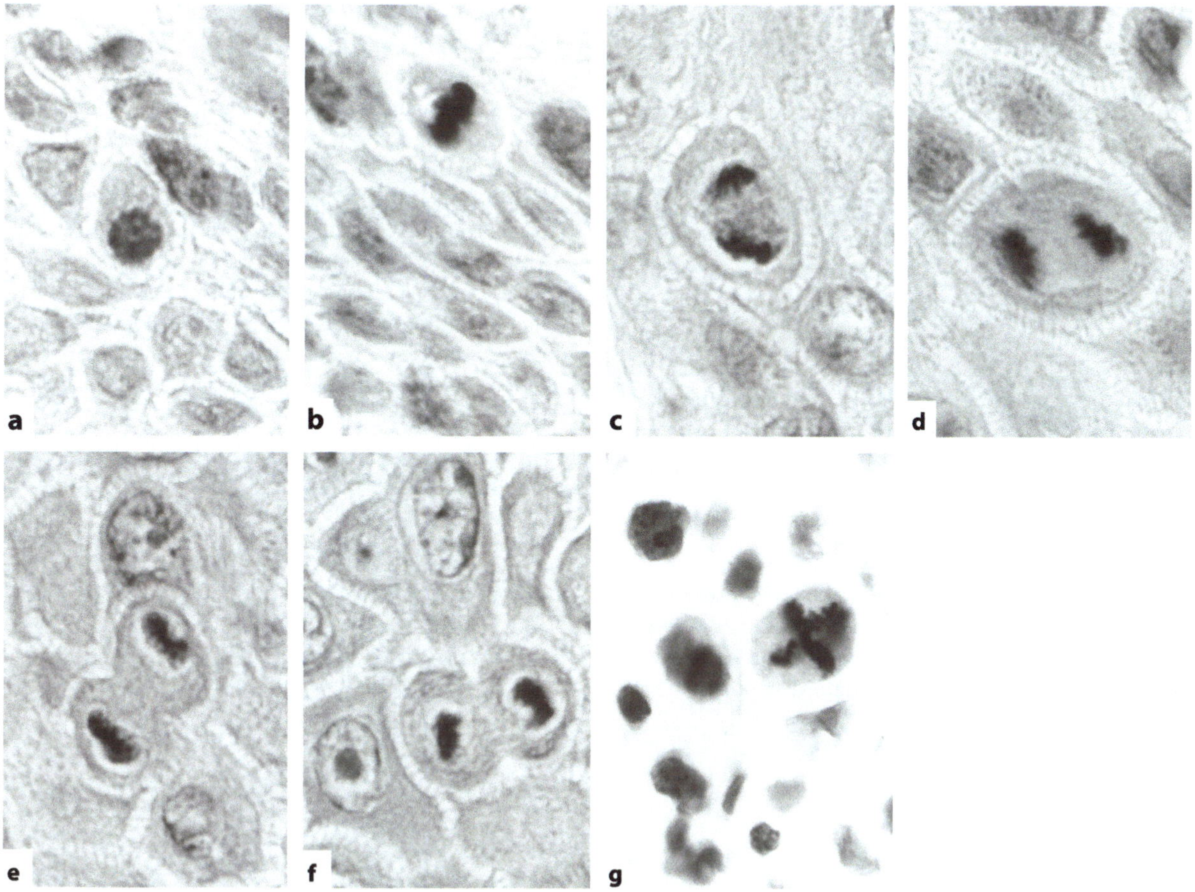

Fig. 5.7 Mitotic figures: **a** prophase; **b** metaphase; **c** anaphase; **d** anaphase; **e** telophase; **f** telophase, the cell to the left of the mitotic figure is in interphase; **g** atypical metaphase. H&E, ×1000

the vessel sprout is formed between two adjacent endothelial processes budding off the wall of the parent vessel, and thus is an elongation of the lumen of the parent vessel. When the angiogenic stimuli cease most of the newly formed vessels involute. Some capillaries may differentiate into arterioles and venules (Diaz-Flores et al. 1994).

5.5 Cell Division

Cells multiply, proliferate, by division in a process termed mitosis. This is a complicated process in which the cell and its chromosomes pass through four consecutive phases called prophase, anaphase, metaphase and telophase. In each phase the chromosomes form a different mitotic figure. Mitotic figures are rather common in inflammatory tissue and can be identified in routinely stained sections.

Interphase: The period when the cell is not in mitosis is called interphase. The chromatin, the carrier of the genes, is enclosed in the nucleus and is diffusely spread as a network of fine threads; individual chromosomes are not distinguishable under the light microscope.

Prophase: In prophase the cell is ready for mitosis and the chromatin is arranged in a long pleated thread, divided into chromosomes, the number of which is specific for each species. The chromosomes are longitudinally split up into two halves, which are made complete by building-stones (nucleic acids) already synthesized in the cell. There are now two identical sets of chromosomes in the cell and the nuclear membrane has dissolved (Fig. 5.7a).

Metaphase: In metaphase the two sets of chromosomes are situated close to each other at the equator of the cell and in routinely processed sections are seen as a single black band (Fig. 5.7b).

Anaphase: In anaphase the two sets slowly move away from each other towards the poles of the cell. At least at high magnification parts of individual chromosomes may be discerned (Figs. 5.7c,d).

Telophase: In telophase the cytoplasm starts to divide. At each pole the set of chromosomes becomes surrounded by a nuclear membrane and once more becomes dispersed as chromatin. Telophase completed, the dividing cell has become two cells with exactly the same set of chromosomes (Fig. 5.7e,f).

In routinely processed specimens it is rare to find cells in prophase and telophase, but mitotic figures of the metaphase and anaphase are often observed (Figs. 7.5a, 7.17c, 18.2c, 21.3a and 26.3f). Atypical mitotic figures contain either too many or too few chromosomes, and may be seen in malignant tumors and sometimes even in benign conditions. The mitotic figures in Fig. 5.7a–f were observed in a carcinoma in situ of the preputium penis. It is not possible to decide if they or some of them are atypical. In tissue, the only reliable signs indicating atypia are the presence of tri- or multipolar mitotic figures. The figure shown in Fig. 5.7g is quadripolar and occurred in a dermal cell infiltrate in a lesion of lymphomatoid papulosis (Sect. 26.3.4).

References

1. Diaz-Flores L, Gutiérrez R, Varela H (1994) Angiogenesis. An update. Histol Histopathol 9:807–843
2. Dugast C, Gaudin A, Toujas L (1997) Generation of multinucleated giant cells by culture of monocyte-derived macrophages with IL-4. J Leukoc Biol 61:517–521
3. Lee JY-Y, Yang C-C, Chao S-C, Wong T-W (2004) Histopathologic differential diagnosis of keloid and hypertrophic scar. Am J Dermatopathol 26:379–384
4. McNally AK, Anderson JM (1995) Interleukin-4 induces foreign body giant cells from human monocytes/macrophages. Differential lymphokine regulation of macrophage fusion leads to morphological variants of multinucleated giant cells. Am J Pathol 147:1487–1499
5. Peters MS, Rodriguez M, Gleich GJ (1986) Localization of human eosinophil granule major basic protein, eosinophil cationic protein, and eosinophil-derived neurotoxin by immunoelectron microscopy. Lab Invest 54:656–662
6. Tharp MD (2001) Skin mast cells. In: Freinkel RK, Woodley DT (eds) The biology of the skin. Parthenon, New York, pp 265–279
7. van der Rhee HJ, Hillebrands W, Daems WT (1978) Are Langhans giant cells precursors of foreign-body giant cells? Arch Dermatol Res 263:13–21

Chapter 6

Cell Death in the Living Body

In the cells of the dead body hydrolytic enzymes are released from lysosomes in the cell cytoplasm and rapidly degrade organelles and membrane systems of all cells throughout the body. This is called *autolysis.* All structures gradually fade and disappear mainly by means of this autolytic process, which is diffuse, but develops more rapidly in tissues and organs rich in hydrolytic enzymes such as the gastric mucosa and brain than in those containing lower levels of hydrolytic enzymes, for example heart and kidneys. Autolysis of normal tissue in the dead body is called post-mortem change. It does not give rise to an inflammatory response. In the living body, cell death may appear due to different causes and develop in different ways. There are two main kinds of cell death: *accidental cell death* and *apoptosis* (Majno and Joris 1995).

6.1 Accidental Cell Death

Lack of oxygen (ischemia) or exposure to injurious agents may be followed by massive cell death in a circumscribed area of an organ or tissue, and is referred to as *necrosis*. In contrast to post-mortem change, an area of necrosis evokes an inflammatory response in the surrounding tissue. Myocardial infarction is an instructive example of ischemic necrosis. In myocardial infarction the flow of blood is suddenly stopped by, for example, a thrombus in a coronary artery or in one of its branches. The muscle cells are deprived of oxygen in an area as large as the supplying zone of the vessel peripherally to the obstruction and die after a short time. Two important processes, denaturation of proteins (see Glossary) and autolysis begin the disintegration of the damaged tissue. These processes are progressive and continue for several hours after the cells have died. First, after about 12 h, signs of disintegration of the dead muscle cells become visible under the microscope as a necrotic area. If the patient survives, this area will be converted into a fibrotic scar after about 2 months. The myocardial infarction is a coagulative necrosis (i.e., the denaturation process prevails over the autolytic one), and gives the necrotic area a firm texture. This is in contrast to ischemic infarction in the brain, in which the tissue becomes soft due to a rich content of hydrolytic enzymes and in the end turns into a fluid-filled cavity (liquefaction necrosis). Majno and Joris (1995) have referred to this kind of cell death as oncosis, which means swelling.

6.2 Apoptosis

Apoptosis is a type of cell death in the living body that, in contrast to ischemic, toxic, or traumatic cell death, befalls scattered single cells or small groups of cells and does not cause an inflammatory response. It was first noticed in 1885, by Walter Flemming as a physiological phenomenon in the involution of rabbit ovarian follicles, and at the same time independently by Franz Nissen in the lactating mammary gland (Majno and Joris 1995). In the early 1970s, Kerr (1971) and Kerr et al. (1972) highlighted the phenomenon, which until then had received very little attention from pathologists. They had studied acidophilic round bodies, Councilman bodies, observed in the liver in yellow fever, viral hepatitis and other liver diseases, chemically and by means of electron microscopy. They concluded that these bodies were derived from condensed and irrevocably damaged liver cells in spite of seemingly preserved organelles. They called the phenomenon shrinkage necrosis.

Kerr and coworkers even investigated the damage caused to the rat liver by ligation of the portal vein branches at different levels. They found that, if the veins were tied close to the liver, massive necrosis developed in the liver parenchyma, while if the main branches to the left and median lobes were ligated, extensive formation of Councilman bodies and consequently atrophy of these lobes developed instead of necrosis. The first alternative was considered to evoke spasm in the nearby hepatic artery thus giving rise to a more severe ischemia than did ligation of the two main branches located at a distance from the artery. By means of light and electron microscopy they realized that changes in and the fate of cells undergoing what

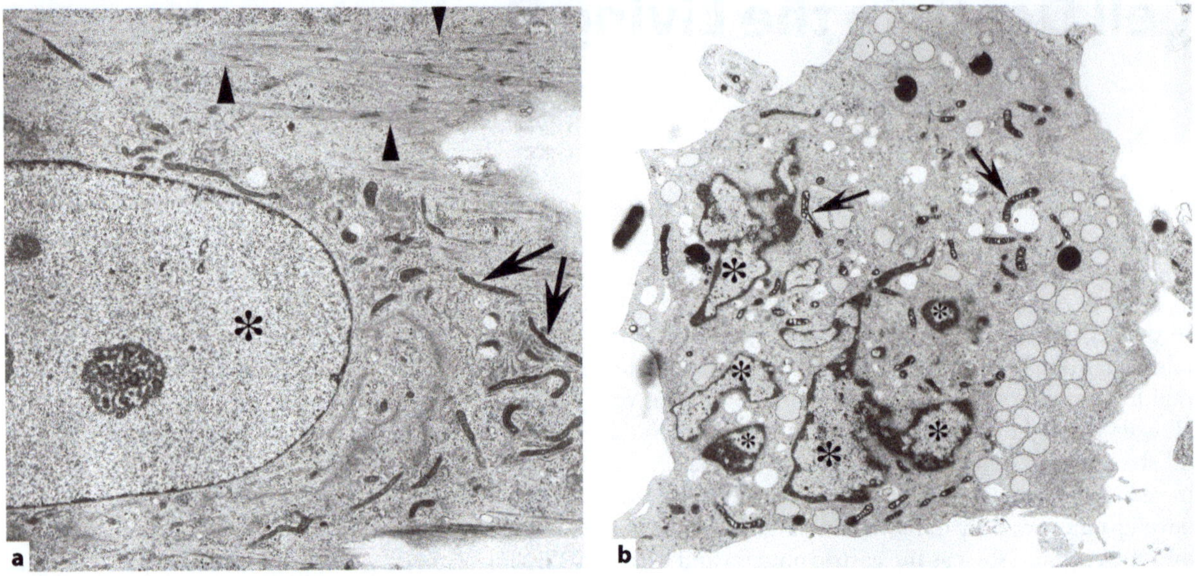

Fig. 6.1 Apoptosis in a cultured prostate stroma cell. Transmission electron micrographs. **a** Normal cell. The nucleus (*asterisk*) has a regular cell membrane and normally distributed chromatin. In the cytoplasm there are mitochondria (*arrows*); *arrowheads* a group of myofilaments. Original magnification ×2500. **b** A cell after heat-induced apoptosis. The apoptotic cell is markedly shrunken in comparison with the normal cell in a; it was not possible to catch the whole normal cell in spite of a lower magnification. The nucleus is broken up into many fragments surrounded by nuclear membrane, to which clumps of chromatin are aggregated (*asterisks*). The mitochondria are condensed (*arrows*). The vacuoles represent cross sections through dilated endoplasmic reticulum. Original magnification ×3000. Courtesy of Dr. Marianne Brehmer, Karolinska University Hospital, Stockholm, Sweden

they called shrinkage necrosis and cells taking part in massive circumscribed cell death leading to necrosis, were essentially different. They therefore renamed the "shrinkage necrosis" apoptosis (see Glossary) and its end products apoptotic bodies. Since the 1970s investigations on apoptosis have exploded resulting the discovery of its great regulatory importance in body functions. The differences between changes in dying and dead cells in the two processes observed by light and electron microscopy can be summarized as follows (Majno and Joris 1995; Kerr et al. 1995):

- *Oncosis*: The cell and its organelles swell, and the membrane permeability increases. Superficial membrane-covered "blebs" appear on the cell surface; the largest may burst, which is probably a deadly blow to the cell. Finally, all structures including the nucleus fade and the cell disintegrates as described above in myocardial infarction. The fading and disintegration of the nucleus is called karyolysis. In this process the leakage through the cell membrane gives rise to an inflammatory response in the tissue around the necrotic area.
- *Apoptosis*: The shrinking cell is detached from the surrounding epithelial or parenchymal cells. It has a condensed and conspicuously budding cytoplasm with tightly packed organelles, which at least in the early stage of the process are preserved and membrane-bound. The small and dark (pyknotic) nucleus has condensed chromatin, typically aggregated in clumps at the nuclear membrane. It breaks up into several fragments, a process referred to as karyorrhexis (Fig. 6.1b). Finally, the whole cell falls apart giving rise to rounded and membrane-covered apoptotic bodies of various sizes, some of which contain nuclear fragments and/or organelles. The apoptotic bodies are then rapidly (in minutes) phagocytosed and digested by nearby normal epithelial or parenchymal cells, or by macrophages. There is no leakage of intracellular substances and no inflammatory response in the surrounding tissue.

6.2.1 Apoptosis in Embryonic Development

During embryonic development apoptosis is the tool in some of the programmed and time-scheduled deletions of tissues necessary for the design of the final organism. Examples are regression of the pronephros in the development of the kidney, the tadpole tale in the development of frogs, shaping of fingers and toes in humans and animals, and wings in birds.

6.2.2 Apoptosis in Postnatal Life

In the postnatal life apoptosis occurs as:

- *Physiologic events*: Examples are involution of ovarian follicles and uterus after childbirth.
- *Defense and control of tissues and organs*: Sensitized cytotoxic T cells are able to kill virus-infected cells and probably also malignant and potentially malignant cells, which they recognize as non-self (Sect. 4.1.2.2). Attacked cells die by apoptosis. There is also a type of programmed cell death that befalls white blood cells, which normally have a restricted life span. For example, neutrophils are programmed to die by apoptosis after a life span of only a few days.
- *Response to injuring agents not strong enough to cause oncosis*: Early investigations (Kerr 1971; Kerr et al. 1972) showed that a severe degree of ischemia gives rise to massive tissue necrosis, but to a less-severe degree to apoptotic bodies. The same difference was later found in tissue exposed to strong or mild heating (Harmon et al. 1990) or radiation (Cohen 1993). This seems contradictory, but possibly it is not—it could be that all cells in the right context and at the right time, such as lymphocytes (see below), have an inherent instruction to commit apoptotic suicide.

6.2.3 Relevant Investigations

Knowing that thymus cells exposed to adequate concentrations of steroids will die, Cohen (1993) submitted thymocytes to lethal concentrations of steroids and at the same time to drugs that blocked either RNA synthesis or protein synthesis. Under these conditions the cells did not die. They concluded that steroids were not directly toxic to the cells, but induced gene expressions leading to cell death through apoptosis. By blocking either the transcription or the translation stage of the signal(s), apoptosis did not occur.

The same experiment was carried out using γ irradiation and lymphocytes, and gave the same result. This initiated the idea that perhaps, at least in lymphocytes (with a high potential for proliferation), gene expressions for apoptosis could be induced by any, even small, unfavorable environmental change (i.e., acting as a defense mechanism against tumor proliferation). To test this hypothesis fibroblast and lymphocytes were heated to 43°C for an hour. Both cell populations were inactivated, but the fibroblasts recovered, while the lymphocytes died through apoptosis.

To activate a $CD4^+$ T cell and initiate the formation of a clone of this T cell, two requirements must be fulfilled. One is that an antigen binds to its specific antigen receptor (TCR) and the other that its $C4^+$ receptor binds to a MHC class II molecule on the surface of the antigen-presenting cell (Sect. 4.1.2.2). Experiments carried out with $CD4^+$ cells in culture showed that if these two events occurred at the same time, the $CD4^+$ cells started to proliferate, but if they occurred at an interval of 30 minutes, the lymphocytes died via apoptosis. This behavior could explain the continual depletion of $CD4^+$ cells in the blood in patients with HIV infection. In these patients the $CD4^+$ receptors of the circulating $CD4^+$ cells are blocked by an HIV antigen–antibody complex. This is not enough to induce proliferation or apoptosis. However, if the patient acquires another infection, for example a "flu" virus infection, the T cell receptors become engaged leading to delay and apoptosis is triggered. This mechanism may explain the depletion of T-helper lymphocytes seen in patients with advanced HIV infection.

The investigations described above indicate that lymphocytes have an inherent instruction to commit apoptotic suicide when necessary (i.e., when the cell has become damaged, or has wrongly developed antibodies against the organism itself). Also, it is possible that prolonged and uncontrolled activation of lymphocytes is stopped by means of apoptosis (Cohen 1993). Investigations also indicate the possibility that inability to carry out apoptosis may trigger widespread autoimmune disease (Cohen 1993; Raskin 1997).

6.2.4 Apoptosis and the Skin

Weedon et al. (1979) introduced the concept of apoptosis in dermatopathology. They claimed that eosinophilic bodies observed in the epidermis and in the subepidermal area in certain skin diseases and given many different names such as colloid bodies, Civatte bodies, Councilman bodies, single-cell necrobiosis, sunburn cells, and dyskeratotic cells, are apoptotic bodies. Also by means of electron microscopy they were able to differentiate between apoptotic bodies and real dyskeratotic cells (i.e., premature keratinization of individual keratinocytes). Scattered apoptotic bodies may be seen in the healthy epidermis and in many skin diseases. In lesions of lichen ruber, lichenoid eruptions, and in some drug eruptions they may be present in abundance (Figs. 24.1, 24.3, 28.4 and 28.5).

References

1. Cohen JJ (1993) Apoptosis: the physiologic pathway of cell death. Hosp Pract 28:35–43
2. Harmon BV, Corder AM, Collins RJ, Gobé GC, Allen J, Allan DJ, Kerr JFR (1990) Cell death induced in a murine mastocytoma by 42-47°C heating in vitro. Evidence that the form of death changes from apoptosis to necrosis above a critical heat load. Int J Radiat Biol 58:845–858
3. Kerr JFR (1971) Shrinkage necrosis. A distinct mode of cellular death. J Pathol 105:13–20
4. Kerr JFR, Wyllie AH, Currie AR (1972) Apoptosis. A basic biological phenomenon with wideranging implications in tissue kinetics. Br J Cancer 26:239–257
5. Kerr JFR, Gobé GC, Winterford CM, Harmon BV (1995) Anatomical methods in cell death. Methods Cell Biol 46:1–27
6. Majno G, Joris I (1995) Apoptosis, oncosis, and necrosis. An overview of cell death. Am J Pathol 146:3–15
7. Raskin CA (1997) Apoptosis and cutaneous biology. J Am Acad Dermatol 36:885–896
8. Weedon D, Searle J, Kerr JFR (1979) Apoptosis. Its nature and implications for dermatopathology. Am J Dermatopathol 1:133–144

Chapter 7

Vasculitis

As already mentioned, the dermis normally contains only a sparse amount of lymphocytes, mainly located around postcapillary venules. There are no neutrophils or eosinophils (Bos et al. 1987). In response to inflammatory stimuli, a variable number of one or several kinds of inflammatory cells migrate through the walls of venules and accumulate in the tissue. Even though these vessels take part in an inflammatory process, we do not talk about vasculitis if there are no signs of vascular damage. To call it vasculitis there should be, in addition to perivascular cell infiltrates, injury to the vessels visible under the light microscope and expressed as thrombi and/or fibrinoid (i.e., eosinophilic and glossy) necrosis of the wall. The lesions (whether few or numerous) are always segmental (i.e., focal), and engage only a very small part of the length of the vessel. In the engaged segment the whole or only a part of the vessel's circumference may be involved. Fibrin thrombi and wall necrosis are fresh lesions that indicate an acute vascular injury or acute vasculitis. There is also deposition in the tissue outside the vessel of eosinophilic fibrinous (protein-rich) exudate and extravasation of erythrocytes. This is the result of necrosis of the vessel wall including the basement membrane. However, extravasation of erythrocytes is not per se a sign of acute vasculitis. It may occur without visible signs of damage to the wall, as is the case in scurvy, where the production of the collagen, supporting the vessel wall is impaired, in senile, atrophic skin, and in the tissue around newly formed vessels, which are leaky (Fig. 22.5).

While scrutinizing material comprising vascular skin lesions collected since the 1960s, the author found that with respect to the histopathologic pattern, it is possible to discriminate six distinct categories of vasculitis, which the author has tried to anchor in the literature. In a further category (category VII), a group of vasculitis is discussed, which includes entities and cases, which clinically are widely different, but histopathologically show some similarities (Fig. 7.1):

- *I. Neutrophilic venular vasculitis*: venules in the dermis and the dermal–subcutaneous interface are affected. The inflammatory cell infiltrate consists mainly of neutrophils. The presence of nuclear fragments from disintegrating neutrophils (leukocytoclasis) is a conspicuous phenomenon.
- *II. Lymphocytic venular vasculitis*: venules in the dermis and the dermal–subcutaneous interface are affected. The perivascular cell infiltrates consist of lymphocytes.
- *III. Granulomatous venular vasculitis*: venules in the dermis and the dermal–subcutaneous interface are affected and surrounded by small areas of necrotic tissue, in turn encircled by epithelioid cell granulomas and a sparse number of lymphocytes.
- *IV. Neutrophilic arterial vasculitis*: arterioles in the deep dermis and arterioles and small arteries in the subcutis are affected. The inflammatory cell infiltrate is strictly perivascular and mainly composed of neutrophils. Leukocytoclasis is prominent.
- *V. Lymphocytic/monocytic arterial vasculitis*: arterioles in the deep dermis and arterioles and small arteries in the subcutis are affected and surrounded by a well-demarcated mononuclear inflammatory cell infiltrate.
- *VI. Granulomatous neutrophilic arterial vasculitis*: small arteries in the subcutis and ascending arterioles show neutrophilic leukocytoclastic vasculitis. In the surrounding tissue there are large necrotic areas surrounded by epithelioid cell granulomas and sometimes abscesses.
- *VII. Mixed group*: venules in the dermis and at the dermal–subcutaneous interface are affected. In a dense inflammatory cell infiltrate of mixed type there are dilated venules with protruding endothelial cells and/or conspicuously thick-walled venules, and in some cases simultaneously venules showing fibrinoid necrosis and/or thrombosis.

7.1 Category I: Neutrophilic Venular Vasculitis

This kind of vasculitis is generally called *leukocytoclastic vasculitis* (synonyms are, among others: necrotiz-

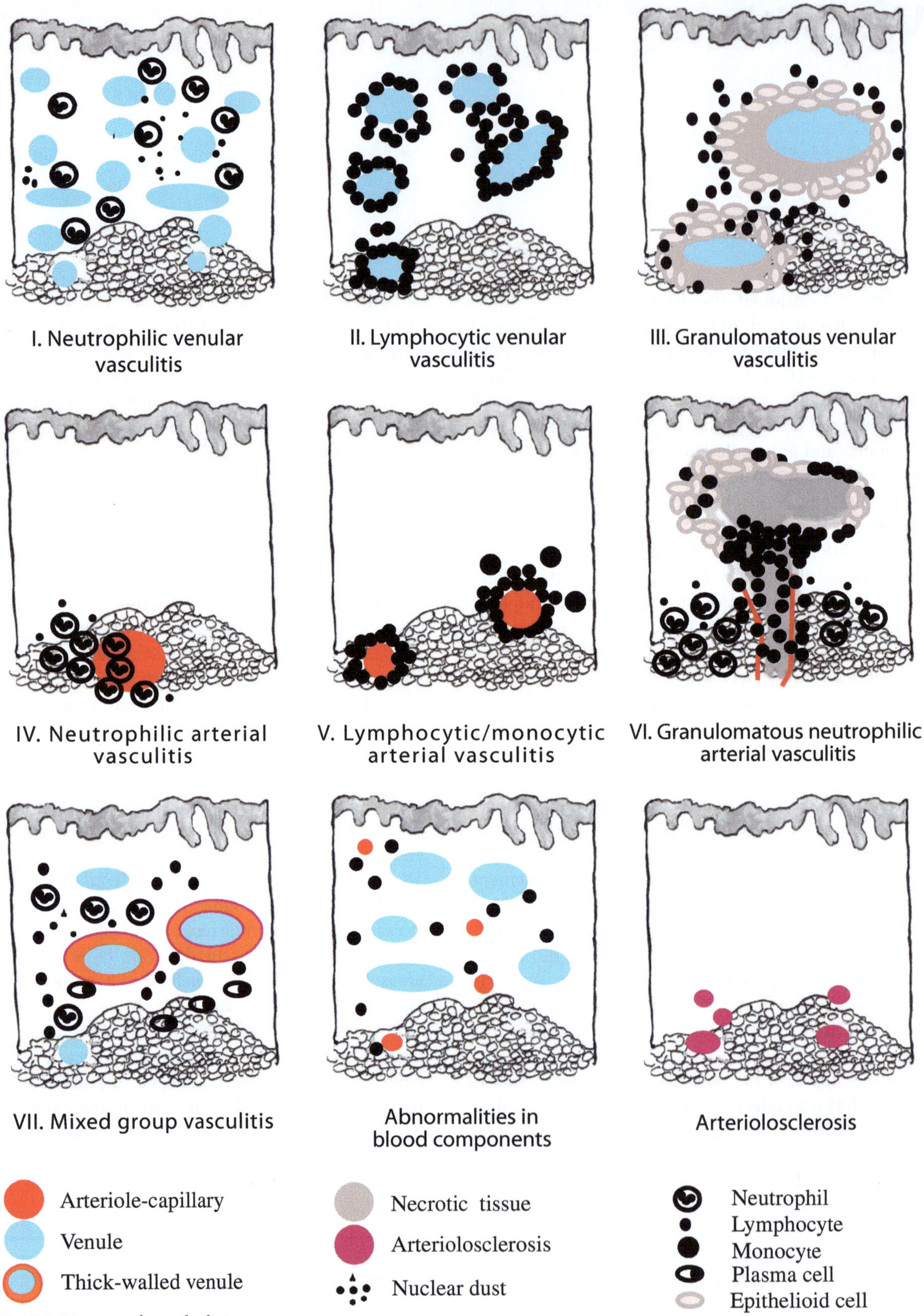

Fig. 7.1 Diagram of vascular lesions

ing vasculitis, hypersensitivity vasculitis, hypersensitivity angiitis, allergic vasculitis, and anaphylactoid purpura). Spells of leukocytoclastic vasculitis may be triggered by bacterial and viral infections and drugs. Sometimes an eruption appears shortly after an incident of sore throat due to streptococcal infection or after a spell of gastrointestinal malaise. It may appear without any other symptoms, but can be accompanied by fever and increased erythrocyte sedimentation rate (ESR), or hematuria indicating renal involvement.

Also leukocytoclastic vasculitis may be an expression of systemic diseases such as classic systemic polyarteritis nodosa, systemic lupus erythematosus and rheumatoid arthritis (Weedon 1997).

7.1.1 Clinical Appearance

The patient exhibits one or several spells of a polymorphic, widespread, or localized rash. This includes different-sized reddish papules (sometimes coalescing to plaques), petechiae and ecchymoses. Some papules are markedly edematous and have a central vesicle/bulla or are ulcerated/crusted. If the outbreak is localized, the most common areas affected are the lower legs. The rash is called "palpable purpura", a term often used by dermatologists as synonymous with leukocytoclastic vasculitis. However, sometimes purpura is the only manifestation of leukocytoclastic vasculitis. In patients with palpable lesions, petechiae are common in areas exposed to pressure and may be found under the elastic bands of underwear, or arise in normal-appearing skin after a blood pressure check. The rash usually vanishes spontaneously in a few weeks with hyperpigmentation or atrophic scars, or without any residue. Ulcerations on the lower legs may remain and enlarge, and thus imitate varicose ulcers.

7.1.2 Histopathologic Appearance

Different-sized venules at all levels of the dermis are affected, but the most conspicuous changes are often seen in the upper half. If the only clinical sign is purpura, the vasculitis is discreet and confined to the subepidermal area. The pattern is variegated. There are fibrinoid necrosis of vessel walls with or without thrombosis, and a fibrinous exudate and red blood cells in the perivascular tissue. In fresh lesions the inflammatory cell infiltrates consist mainly of neutrophils, but there also are some lymphocytes, and sometimes a substantial number of eosinophils. The presence of nuclear dust due to disintegration of neutrophils is a typical phenomenon and often striking. Serious injury to vessels in the subepidermal region gives rise to areas of spongiosis and vesicles/bullae in the epidermis, and sometimes to ulceration. When the acute phase declines the histopathologic pattern becomes nonspecific and neutrophils are replaced by macrophages and lymphocytes.

7.1.3 Pathogenesis

Investigations have shown that leukocytoclastic vasculitis, which is not caused by direct invasion of bacteria or virus, is an expression of the hypersensitivity reaction type III. In the blood, soluble antigens from bacteria, virus or drugs bind to antibodies and form antigen–antibody complexes (immune complexes). The size of the immune complexes, which is critical, depends on the concentration of the two components antigen and antibody. A high excess of antibody gives rise to large complexes. These are rapidly trapped and phagocytosed by macrophages lining the sinusoids of the liver, spleen and bone marrow, and consequently are put out of action. A high excess of antigen gives rise to small and harmless complexes. However, a moderately high excess of antibody forms medium-sized complexes which are small enough to circulate for a long time but large enough to be caught in small vessels and cause damage. Antibody in the immune complexes is mainly IgG and IgM.

It has been shown by means of electron microscopy and immunofluorescence that these complexes are taken up focally by the endothelial cells and are stored in the wall of the venules and in the perivascular tissue before any damage appears in the vessel. The inflammatory process leading to tissue destruction is triggered when complement binds to IgG or IgM antibodies in the complexes and becomes activated. The three activated components of complement C3a, C4a and C5a (also called anaphylatoxins) cause direct injury to tissue cells. Like histamine and serotonin they induce venular leakage, and attract neutrophils (Sect. 5.2.1). Neutrophils phagocytose the immune complexes. When the neutrophils die and disintegrate they release hydrolytic enzymes which contribute to the tissue damage. The consumption of complement gives rise to hypocomplementemia (Braverman and Yen 1975; Lawley and Kubota 1990).

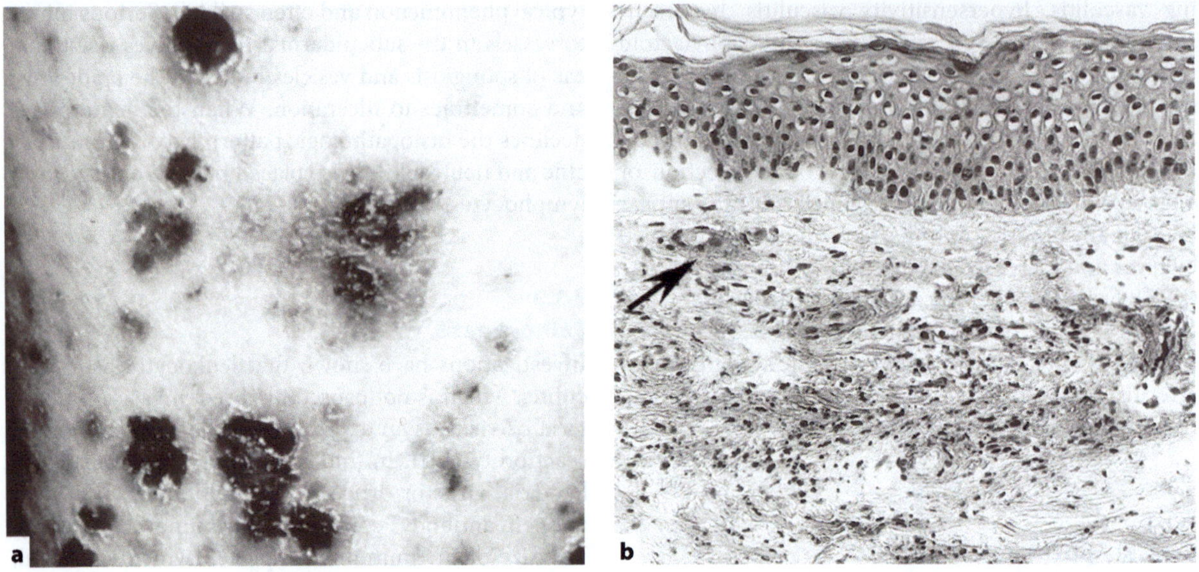

Fig. 7.2 Neutrophilic venular vasculitis. **a** Lower leg with densely set different-sized papules and plaques. The plaques are covered with crusts, some of which are encircled by tiny scales. **b** Only one unaffected venule is clearly discernible (*arrow*). The rest of them are more or less obscured by nuclear fragments and fibrinous exudate. The tissue is edematous and in the left upper corner there is a subepidermal vesicle in the making. Note also the many keratinocytes with intracellular edema. H&E, ×200

7.1.4 Examples

Case 1. Neutrophilic Venular Vasculitis

A 36-year-old woman presented with a striking eruption of erythematous and edematous papules and plaques, mainly located on the lower legs. Some plaques showed a regressing bulla, others were crusted; also most papules had a small vesicle, a superficial ulceration or a crust on the top (Fig. 7.2a). The eruption appeared suddenly 2 weeks after an infection of the upper respiratory tract. Histopathologic investigation revealed typical leukocytoclastic vasculitis.

Case 2. Neutrophilic Venular Vasculitis

A 77-year-old man suffered from colicky abdominal pain for 2 months. Shortly after the beginning of this distress he experienced two spells of hemorrhagic, vesicular efflorescences on the lower legs. The ESR increased to 68 mm/h. The urine contained albumin and many red blood cells.

Histologic investigation revealed typical leukocytoclastic vasculitis with marked wall necrosis, extravasation of red blood cells, dense infiltrates of neutrophils, and a conspicuous number of nuclear fragments (Fig. 7.2b).

Case 3. Neutrophilic Venular Vasculitis

This 66-year-old woman had had tonsillitis 8 years previously followed by glomerulonephritis that healed. Thereafter vasculitis-like or bullous lesions now and then appeared on the ankles. Also some lesions ulcerated.

Investigation of a clinically non-bullous lesion revealed marked leukocytoclastic vasculitis affecting venules in the dermis and upper subcutis. Neutrophils and nuclear fragments dominated the cell infiltrates, but there were also a fair number of eosinophils and histiocytes. The epidermis contained rather large, vesiculopustules filled with exudate, neutrophils and erythrocytes (Fig. 7.3).

7.1.5 Variants of Leukocytoclastic Vasculitis

This group includes Henoch-Schönlein purpura, infantile acute hemorrhagic edema of the skin, urticarial vasculitis, and recurrent cutaneous necrotizing eosinophilic vasculitis.

7.1.5.1 Henoch-Schönlein Purpura

Henoch-Schönlein purpura has a predilection for children aged 2 to 4 years, but can also affect older children and adults. The rash is most prominent on the

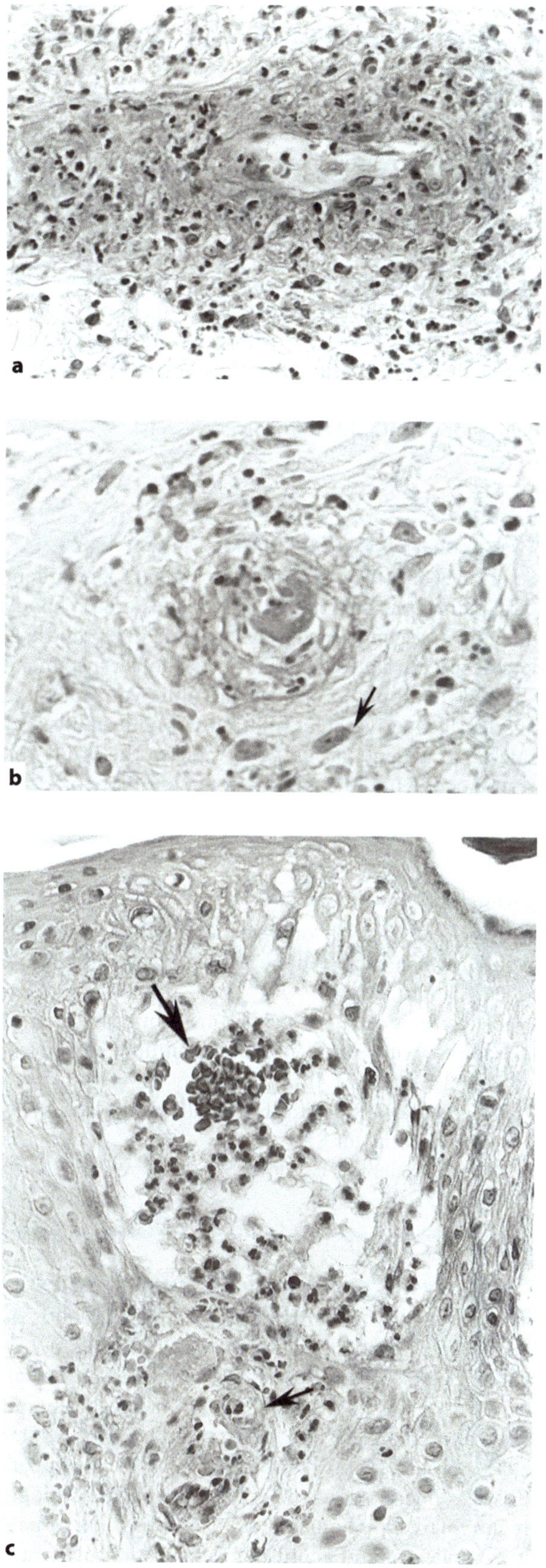

Fig. 7.3 Neutrophilic venular vasculitis. **a** Totally necrotic venule. The wall is massively permeated and surrounded by nuclear fragments and erythrocytes. **b** Another thrombotic and necrotic venule is surrounded by nuclear fragments, a few leukocytes, and a fair number of histiocytes (macrophages), one of which is indicated (*arrow*). **c** There is a mainly intraepidermal vesicle containing neutrophils and a conglomerate of erythrocytes (*arrow*). At the base the vesicle is connected with a papilla comprising a necrotic vessel (*small arrow*), fibrinous exudate, and erythrocytes. H&E, ×400

lower legs and buttocks and is accompanied by arthritis and/or gastrointestinal symptoms, and sometimes nephritis. Histologic investigation shows leukocytoclastic vasculitis. Antibodies in the complexes are IgA, which are activated by the alternative pathway (Sect. 4.3.1) (Lawley and Kubota 1990; Reinauer et al. 1995).

7.1.5.2 Infantile Acute Hemorrhagic Edema of the Skin

Infantile acute hemorrhagic edema of the skin is seen in children less than 2 years old. The children have one or several spells of hemorrhagic efflorescences together with edema, mainly localized to the limbs and face. Often there is a history of a recent infection and/or medication. There could be slight fever, but visceral involvement is uncommon. The rash spontaneously vanishes within 1 to 3 weeks. Histologic investigation displays leukocytoclastic vasculitis (Legrain et al. 1991).

7.1.5.3 Urticarial Vasculitis

Painful, non-pruritic, urticaria-like wheals that remain longer than ordinary urticaria efflorescences and histologically show leukocytoclastic vasculitis are called urticarial vasculitis. Some lesions are purpuric. Reported associated symptoms are angioedema, arthralgia, and abdominal pain. Infrequently these patients may suffer from a connective tissue disease. Probably urticarial vasculitis is only a milder variant of leukocytoclastic vasculitis. However, the definition of urticarial vasculitis is not always as clear-cut, and some authors do not include fibrinoid necrosis and leukocytoclasis as a requirement (Lawley and Kubota 1990; Mehregan et al. 1992).

7.1.5.4
Recurrent Cutaneous Necrotizing Eosinophilic Vasculitis

In many cases of leukocytoclastic vasculitis there is a more or less massive admixture of eosinophils. There is probably no reason to discriminate these cases from other cases of leukocytoclastic vasculitis. However, Chen et al. (1994) described three patients with recurrent episodes of pruritic, erythematous, purpuric papules, and angioedema associated with peripheral blood eosinophilia. Histologic investigation revealed leukocytoclastic vasculitis with cell infiltrates consisting exclusively of eosinophils. In one of the patients it was possible to prove the presence of adhesion molecules for eosinophils in involved vessels.

7.1.5.5
Pustular Vasculitis of the Hands

Strutton et al. (1995) described six patients, all women, with painful sterile nodules and plaques on the hands and fingers accompanied by fever and neutrophilic leukocytosis. The cause was unknown. Biopsy specimens showed neutrophilic venular vasculitis with massive, abscess-like perivascular infiltrates of neutrophils and nuclear fragments around the vessels. The eruptions responded to prednisone, but not to antibiotics.

7.1.6
Differential Diagnosis

- Pyogenic bacteria or virus, locally invading the tissue, may cause leukocytoclastic vasculitis (Sect. 20.1.5; Fig. 20.2d).
- Langerhans cell histiocytosis may contain scattered venules with neutrophilic vasculitis (Sect. 21.4; Figs. 21.3c and 21.4b).
- Vascular lesions due to abnormalities in blood components (Chapter 8).
- Arteriolosclerosis (Chapter 9).

7.2
Category II: Lymphocytic Venular Vasculitis

The existence of a lymphocytic venular vasculitis as a specific clinicopathologic entity comparable to leukocytoclastic vasculitis was described by Soter et al. (1976), but was later the subject of much debate and was called into question (Massa and Su 1984; Jones 1985; Smoller et al. 1990; Carlson et al. 1996). In part this was due to disagreement on the histopathologic requirements for lymphocytic vasculitis, and in part to complicated and confusing classification proposals (Carlson et al. 1996).

However, lymphocytic venular vasculitis certainly exists. The most common cause is drugs (Soter et al. 1976; Massa and Su 1984). Investigations have revealed that lymphocytic vasculitis is associated with normocomplementemia, while leukocytoclastic vasculitis often shows hypocomplementemia (Soter et al. 1976; Massa and Su 1984). Soter et al. even observed stimulated lymphocytes in several of their patients.

7.2.1
Clinical Appearance

The skin eruptions are episodic and variable and may show papules, nodules and plaques, which are sometimes vesicular and/or purpuric. The clinical appearance can be indistinguishable from that of leukocytoclastic vasculitis (Soter et al. 1976; Massa and Su 1984; Smoller et al. 1990).

7.2.2
Histopathologic Appearance

As in category I, venules in the dermis and superficial subcutaneous tissue are affected and show thrombosis and/or fibrinoid wall necrosis, but the perivascular cell infiltrates are composed of lymphocytes, sometimes with an admixture of eosinophils. There are no neutrophils.

7.2.3
Pathogenesis

The underlying mechanism in lymphocytic venular vasculitis is not as well understood as that in leukocytoclastic vasculitis. Some kind of cell-mediated hypersensitivity reaction has been suggested (Carlson et al. 1996). The possibility that the lymphocytic vasculitis may represent a declining leukocytoclastic vasculitis has also been suggested (Smoller et al. 1990). However, in lymphocytic vasculitis there are venules with fresh thrombi and wall necrosis surrounded by infiltrates composed only of lymphocytes. In resolving lesions of leukocytoclastic vasculitis there is a mixed cell infiltrate consisting of macrophages, lymphocytes and neutrophils, while foci of acute vasculitis are lacking.

7.2.4
Examples

Case 4. Lymphocytic Venular Vasculitis

A 39-year-old woman had over several years now and then experienced single erythematous swellings on different sites of the body. She presented with a

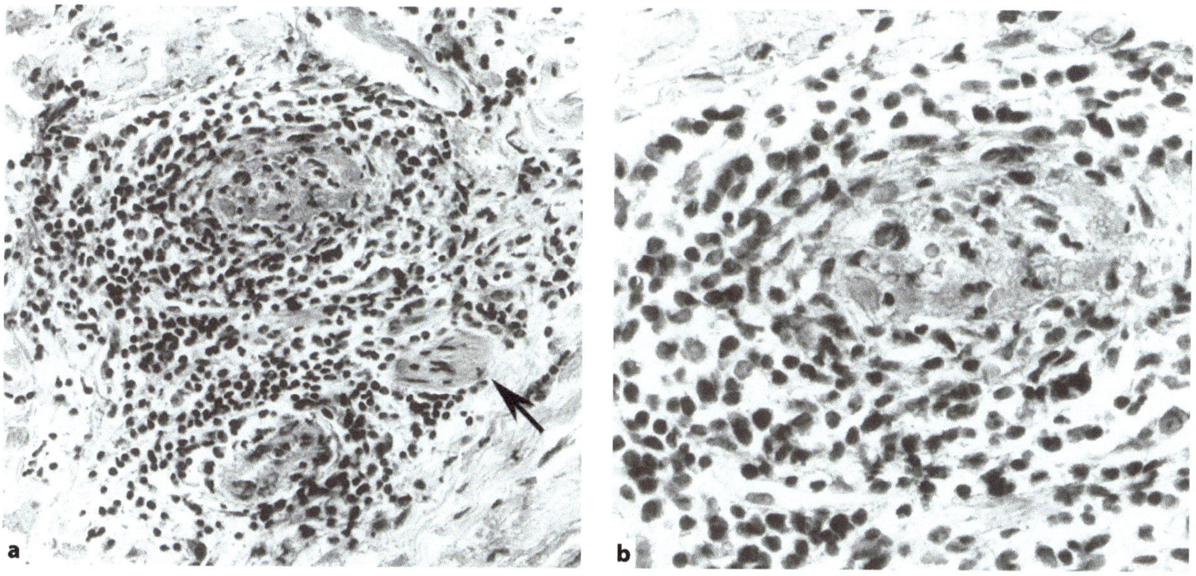

Fig. 7.4 Lymphocytic venular vasculitis. **a** Two venules in the middle of the dermis are surrounded by a dense infiltrate of lymphocytes. The small structure to the right is a nerve (*arrow*); ×250. **b** Close-up of the larger vessel shows fibrinoid wall necrosis. The lumen is occluded by a thrombus of erythrocytes, mononuclear cells and nuclear fragments. H&E, ×400

circumscribed erythematous and edematous lesion, about 50 mm in diameter, on the dorsal aspect of the left thigh. The lesion was very painful to the touch. A drug reaction was suspected, but the cause of the lesion was never determined.

The biopsy specimen comprised dermis and a substantial part of subcutaneous tissue. At all levels of the dermis and at the dermal–subcutaneous interface there were medium-sized or small, well-defined, dense infiltrates of lymphocytes. In the center of several of these infiltrates there was a necrotic venule occluded by a thrombus. The wall of the vessel was necrotic and there were many extravasated erythrocytes. The epidermis was normal (Fig. 7.4).

Case 5. Lymphocytic Venular Vasculitis

A 41-year-old man was receiving treatment with the β-receptor blocking drug atenolol for hypertension when he suddenly developed an itchy, erythematous, vesicular, and purpuric eruption on the hands and feet. Atenolol, suspected to be the cause, was withdrawn and the exanthema subsided. As a test he was then given one tablet of the drug and reacted with fever and a new eruption.

A biopsy specimen was taken from the thenar region. In the papillae and upper dermis within a rather well-demarcated area there were dense, mainly perivascular cell infiltrates. These were composed of ordinary small lymphocytes and larger slightly atypical lymphocytes (stimulated lymphocytes) with a light nucleus, distinct chromatin and a nucleolus. Scattered vessels contained a fibrin thrombus and showed wall necrosis. Extravasation of erythrocytes was conspicuous. Inflammatory cells had invaded the epidermis, which was spongiotic and edematous (Fig. 7.5).

7.2.5 Differential Diagnosis

- Vascular lesions due to abnormalities in blood components (Chapter 8).
- Pityriasis lichenoides et varioliformis (Sect. 26.3.2).
- Direct invasion of the vessel by bacteria, which is probably the case in the lesions demonstrated in Figs. 12.2c and 18.4e.

7.3 Category III: Granulomatous Venular Vasculitis

Case 6 discussed below is one of only two cases the author has observed; unfortunately the other one was not documented. The course, and the clinical and histopathologic patterns are notable, but difficult to identify in the literature. Winkelmann (1980) described a rare non-infectious necrotizing granulomatous disease in the dermis that, according to him, had no other name or description and only rarely was investigated. He did not describe the clinical appearance, but the photomicrographs show necrotic venules surrounded

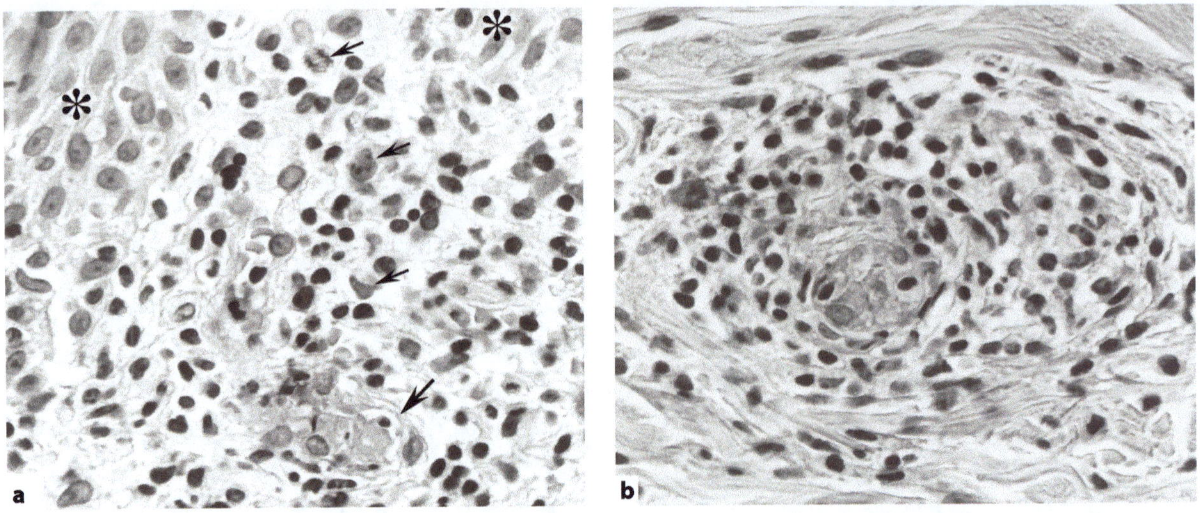

Fig. 7.5 Lymphocytic venular vasculitis. **a** In the upper dermis, partly between two edematous rete pegs (*asterisks*), there is a dense cell infiltrate surrounding a necrotic thrombotic venule (*large arrow*). The cell infiltrate is slightly atypical and contains scattered irregular and different-sized lymphocytes and a mitotic figure in anaphase (*small arrows*). **b** Another infiltrate contains a partly necrotic vessel filled with disintegrating erythrocytes. H&E, ×600

by epithelioid cell granulomas and a slight admixture of lymphocytes in the dermis, a pattern very like that observed in Case 6.

The triggering cause in Case 6 was never identified. The epithelioid cell granulomas indicate a cell-mediated immunologic reaction.

7.3.1 Example

Case 6. Granulomatous Venular Vasculitis

A 56-year-old alcoholic man, who for a long time had been treated with the β-receptor blocker alprenolol and the diuretic amiloride, presented with an itching eruption that had developed during the previous 4 days. On the dorsal aspect of the hands, forearms and the nape of the neck there were closely set small, slightly scaling, brownish-red papules and petechiae. On the dorsal aspect of the right hand the papules coalesced and nearly covered the area. The palms were not affected. The eruption disappeared completely after a short time, and did not return. Only topical treatment was given.

With the exception of a markedly elevated serum γ-glutamyl-transpeptidase, indicating impaired liver function (probably due to over-consumption of alcohol) all routine laboratory values were normal. Cryoglobulins were not found. Direct immunofluorescence was negative and the complement value was normal. Biopsy specimens were taken from the wrist and forearm.

Both specimens included the whole dermis and showed the same pattern. At all levels of the dermis there were several scattered small epithelioid cell granulomas, which embraced a necrotic venule and a hemorrhagic necrosis. There was a slight admixture of lymphocytes. The epidermis was normal (Fig. 7.6).

7.4 Category IV: Neutrophilic Arterial Vasculitis

This pattern of vasculitis was first described more distinctly by Diaz-Perez and Winkelmann (1974) as benign cutaneous polyarteritis nodosa. Their series included 23 patients with a prolonged and benign disease course. Later Daoud et al. (1997) analyzed 79 cases with the diagnosis of cutaneous periarteritis nodosa seen at the Mayo Clinic between 1973 and 1995, which did not include the series of Diaz-Peres and Winkelmann. They generally verified the findings of Diaz-Peres and Winkelmann. The disease course was prolonged, but systemic periarteritis nodosa did not occur. In these two series, at least four patients were children. A further four children suffering from cutaneous periarteritis nodosa with a benign course have been described by Sheth et al. (1994).

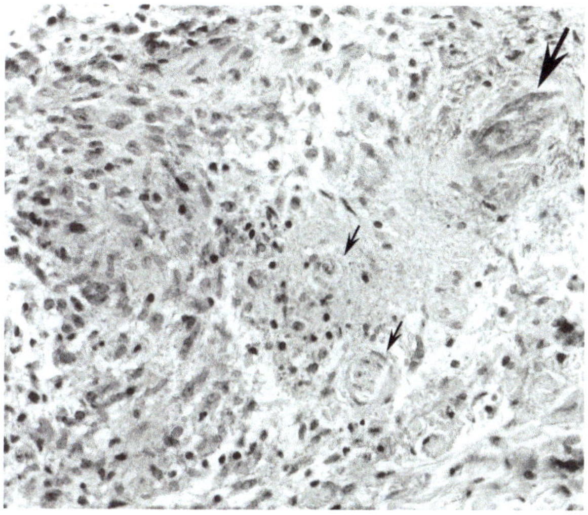

Fig. 7.6 Granulomatous venular vasculitis. Lesion in the upper half of the dermis. There is an elongated hemorrhagic necrosis, at the top of which is a necrotic venule (*large arrow*). The necrotic area includes two smaller vessels (*small arrows*) and is encircled by a wide brim of epithelioid cells and a sparse number of lymphocytes. H&E, ×250

7.4.1 Clinical Appearance

Most patients have spells of painful and slowly regressing nodules. The location could be anywhere, but the lower extremities are the most common sites. In the series of Diaz-Perez and Winkelmann, livedo reticularis (see Glossary) was observed in 78% of the patients and ulcerations were noted during the course in 39%. Corresponding figures in the series of Daoud et al. were 56% and 50%. The only consistent laboratory finding described was an elevated ESR (Diaz-Perez and Winkelmann 1974; Daoud et al. 1997).

7.4.2 Histopathologic Appearance

Histopathologic investigation shows vasculitis in arterioles in the lower dermis and/or small arteries in the superficial subcutaneous tissue. Usually only a single affected vessel is seen in a punch biopsy specimen (Sect. 2.2; Figs. 2.1 and 2.2). The specimen shows fibrinoid wall necrosis with infiltrates of neutrophils and nuclear fragments with an admixture of eosinophils. The inflammatory reaction is confined to the area around the vessel (Diaz-Perez and Winkelmann 1974; Daoud et al. 1997).

7.4.3 Pathogenesis

In many cases it is not possible to determine the triggering cause of this kind of vasculitis. However, previous or concurrent acute infections, especially with streptococci, have been noted (Daoud et al. 1997; Sheth et al. 1994). The disease has also been linked to hepatitis B and C virus infections, but this could not be verified in the series of Daoud et al. Notably, in the series of Daoud et al., five patients had inflammatory bowel disease (four had Crohn disease, and one had ulcerative colitis). Provided the lesions in these patients really did meet the histopathologic inclusion criteria of neutrophilic arterial vasculitis, inflammatory bowel diseases may give rise to different kinds of nodular vasculitis (Sect. 7.6).

7.4.4 Examples

Case 7. Neutrophilic Arterial Vasculitis

A 35-year-old-man had an infiltrated area on the leg. The ESR was 104 mm/h. A biopsy specimen was taken; the question at issue was collagenosis.

Histologic investigation revealed a single affected small artery located in the subcutaneous tissue. A fresh thrombus with fibrinoid wall necrosis and breakthrough into the surrounding tissue was observed. The perivascular tissue was edematous and permeated with neutrophils and a fair number of eosinophils. The lesion was circumscribed; no other changes of importance were seen in the specimen (Fig. 7.7).

Case 8. Neutrophilic Arterial Vasculitis

A 5-year-old boy from the age of 18 months had had spells of fever and painful nodules on the arms and legs including the soles.

A biopsy specimen showed a single affected small artery in the subcutis. The vessel was partly thrombotic and surrounded by a circumscribed large and dense perivascular infiltrate of neutrophils with a slight admixture of eosinophils. There was a small rupture in the wall (Fig. 7.8).

7.4.5 Differential Diagnosis

- Classic systemic polyarteritis nodosa. The histopathologic pattern in affected vessels is the same as in so-called benign periarteritis nodosa, but larger vessels than those in the skin and upper subcutis (i.e., medium-sized arteries of different organs such

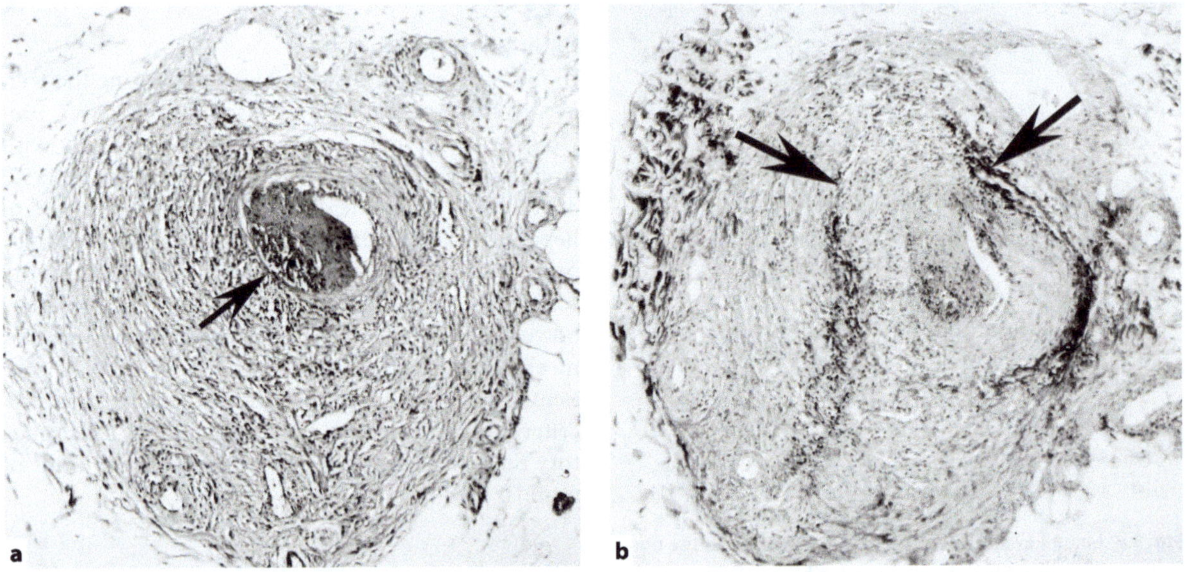

Fig. 7.7 Neutrophilic arterial vasculitis. **a** A single small artery in the subcutaneous tissue contains a fresh thrombus and is surrounded by a well-circumscribed neutrophilic cell infiltrate. At the *arrow* the vessel wall is very thin and close to disruption. **b** At this level the breakthrough of the wall is evident (*arrows*). H&E

as heart, liver, kidney and gastrointestinal tract) are affected. Hypertension, fever and weight loss are common symptoms in the systemic disease, but are not seen in so-called benign periarteritis nodosa. However, sometimes leukocytoclastic venular vasculitis in the dermis is a symptom in systemic polyarteritis nodosa.

- Microscopic polyarteritis (polyangiitis) nodosa refers to a variant of systemic polyarteritis, which engages small arterial vessels, primarily in the kidneys, and gives rise to rapidly progressing glomerulonephritis (Lhote et al. 1996).

7.5 Category V: Lymphocytic/Monocytic Arterial Vasculitis

7.5.1 Clinical Appearance

The lesions are located on the lower legs and appear as spells of painful erythematous infiltrates or nodules with or without livedo reticularis. However, in some cases the only symptom is livedo reticularis. The disease is chronic and benign, but during the course some lesions may ulcerate. Thus the clinical pattern is very similar to that described in Category IV.

7.5.2 Histopathologic Appearance

One or two vessels (Sect. 2.2; Figs. 2.1 and 2.2) show thrombosis and wall necrosis and are surrounded by a well-demarcated infiltrate of mononuclear cells composed of lymphocytes or monocytes, or by a mixture of both.

7.5.3 Examples

Case 9. Lymphocytic Arterial Vasculitis

A 35-year-old man for about 2 years had experienced spells of skin lesions with scattered small ulcerations on the lower legs and feet associated with nocturnal pains in the feet and ankles. The initial investigation revealed marked livedo reticularis on the lower legs and feet and on the medial side of the lower legs also purpura and slight infiltration (Fig. 7a). During the subsequent observation, about 2 years later, he had had two more spells and presented with scattered infiltrations up to 10 mm in diameter, minute superficial ulcerations and shallow scars. Laboratory investigations showed no evidences of autoimmune disease and all routine blood tests including electrophoresis were normal.

A biopsy specimen was taken from the knee region

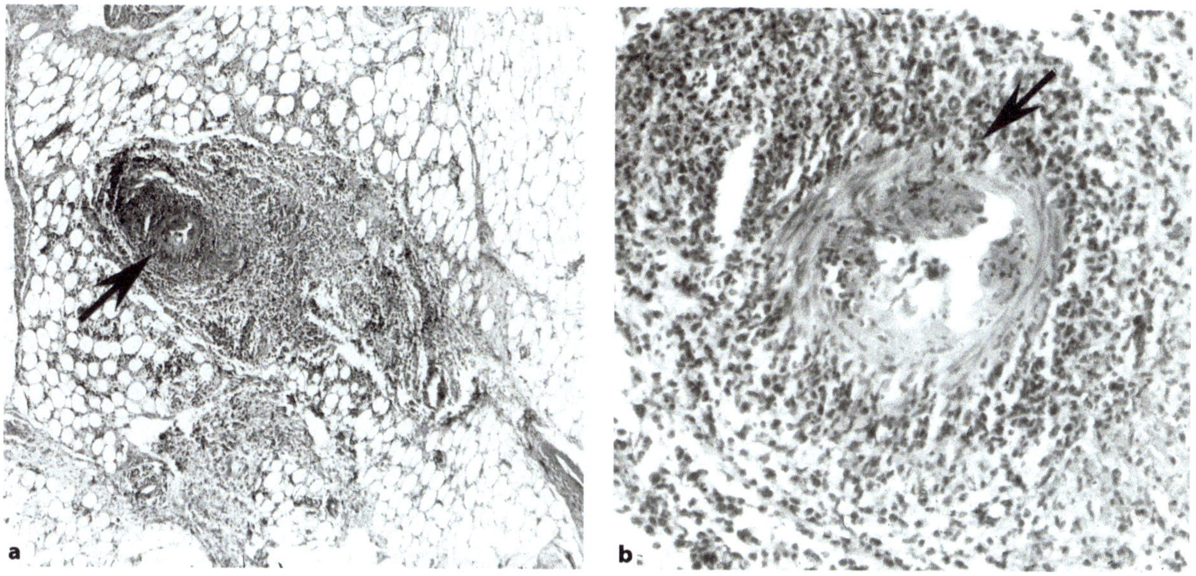

Fig. 7.8 Neutrophilic arterial vasculitis. **a** A single small artery (*arrow*) in the subcutaneous tissue is affected and surrounded by a well-circumscribed inflammatory cell infiltrate. **b** Close-up shows a small rupture in the wall (*arrow*). The cell infiltrate consists of neutrophils. H&E

at the first visit. The changes were confined to a single arteriole located close to a group of sweat glands at the dermal–subcutaneous border. The vessel was occluded by a thrombus of disintegrating red blood cells and fibrin. A part of the wall was edematous and penetrated by erythrocytes and some inflammatory cells. The surrounding small, dense, well-demarcated infiltrate consisted of lymphocytes with a slight admixture of cells with a rounded nucleus and a small distinct nucleolus. There were no eosinophils or neutrophils (Fig. 7.9).

Case 10. Monocytic/Lymphocytic Arterial Vasculitis

A 38-year-old woman had since about two years noticed a livedo reticularis pattern on the lower legs without nodules or ulcerations. The results of the laboratory investigations and follow up are lacking.

A biopsy specimen was taken from the cyanotic net on the frontal aspect of the lower leg. It comprised dermis, but no subcutaneous tissue. In the deep dermis at the lower limit of the specimen a single affected arteriole was observed. It could be followed only in a few sections. The wall of the vessel was necrotic and surrounded by a well-circumscribed ring of inflammatory cells. Close to the vessel, the cell infiltrate consisted of mononuclear cells larger than ordinary lymphocytes, and at the periphery mainly of small lymphocytes. There were no eosinophils or neutrophils. The lumen of the vessel was filled with disintegrating cells. The dermis was otherwise normal. The epidermis was also normal (Fig. 7.10).

Case 11. Presumably Monocytic Arterial Vasculitis

The patient, a 41-year-old previously healthy woman, had for 7 months experienced a painful infiltrate on the medial aspect of the left lower leg, and for a month a smaller one above the medial right malleolus. The overlying skin was erythematous, but there was no ulceration.

A biopsy specimen was taken from the infiltrated area on the left leg and 2 weeks later another specimen from the lesion on the right leg. The material was cut into several sections at different levels and included dermis and superficial subcutaneous tissue. Investigation disclosed scattered and similarly affected arterioles at the dermal–subcutaneous interface. In one of the specimens two engaged arterioles were observed. In one of these there was total wall necrosis with perforation into the surrounding tissue. A well-demarcated broad band of large and closely packed mononuclear cells surrounded the necrotic wall and was in turn encircled by a ring of loose connective tissue and lymphocytes. The mononuclear cells had a large, oval or round, and somewhat irregular nucleus, some of which contained a distinct nucleolus. In a single section two giant cells with a few clustered nuclei were observed. In another section there was a single mitotic

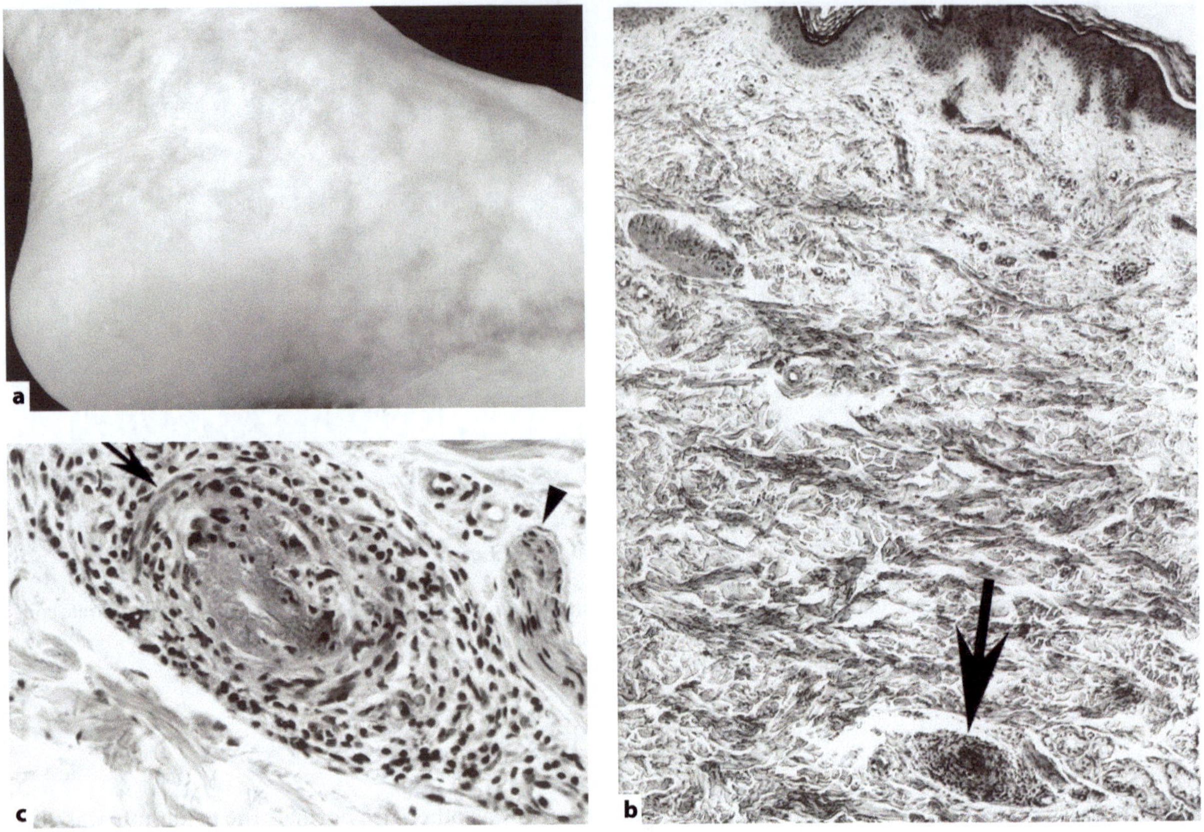

Fig. 7.9 Lymphocytic arterial vasculitis. a Livedo reticularis. b The *arrow* indicates the affected vessel, an arteriole, located close to a sweat gland group at the dermal–subcutaneous interface; ×125. c Close-up shows the thrombotic vessel which is surrounded by a circumscribed infiltrate of small lymphocytes. At the *arrow*, smooth muscle cells of the wall are discernible. To the right there is a small peripheral nerve (*arrowhead*) situated between the vessel and the sweat gland group seen in b. H&E, ×250

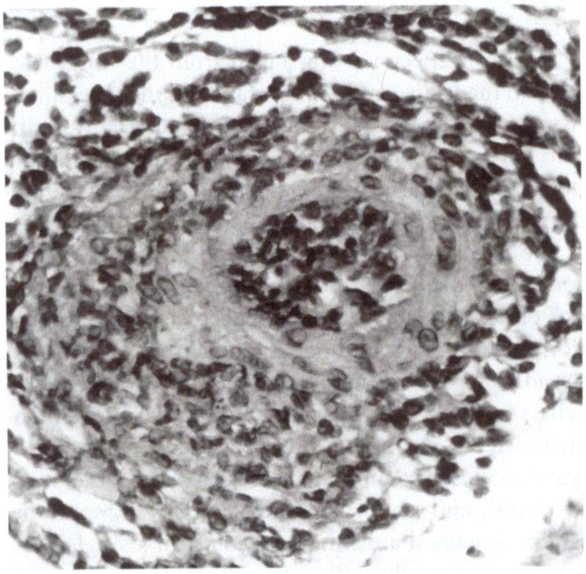

Fig. 7.10 Monocytic/lymphocytic vasculitis. Arteriole in the deep dermis. The wall of the vessel is necrotic and the lumen is filled with disintegrating cells. A dense and well-circumscribed band of mononuclear cells, larger than ordinary lymphocytes, surrounds the vessel. H&E, ×400

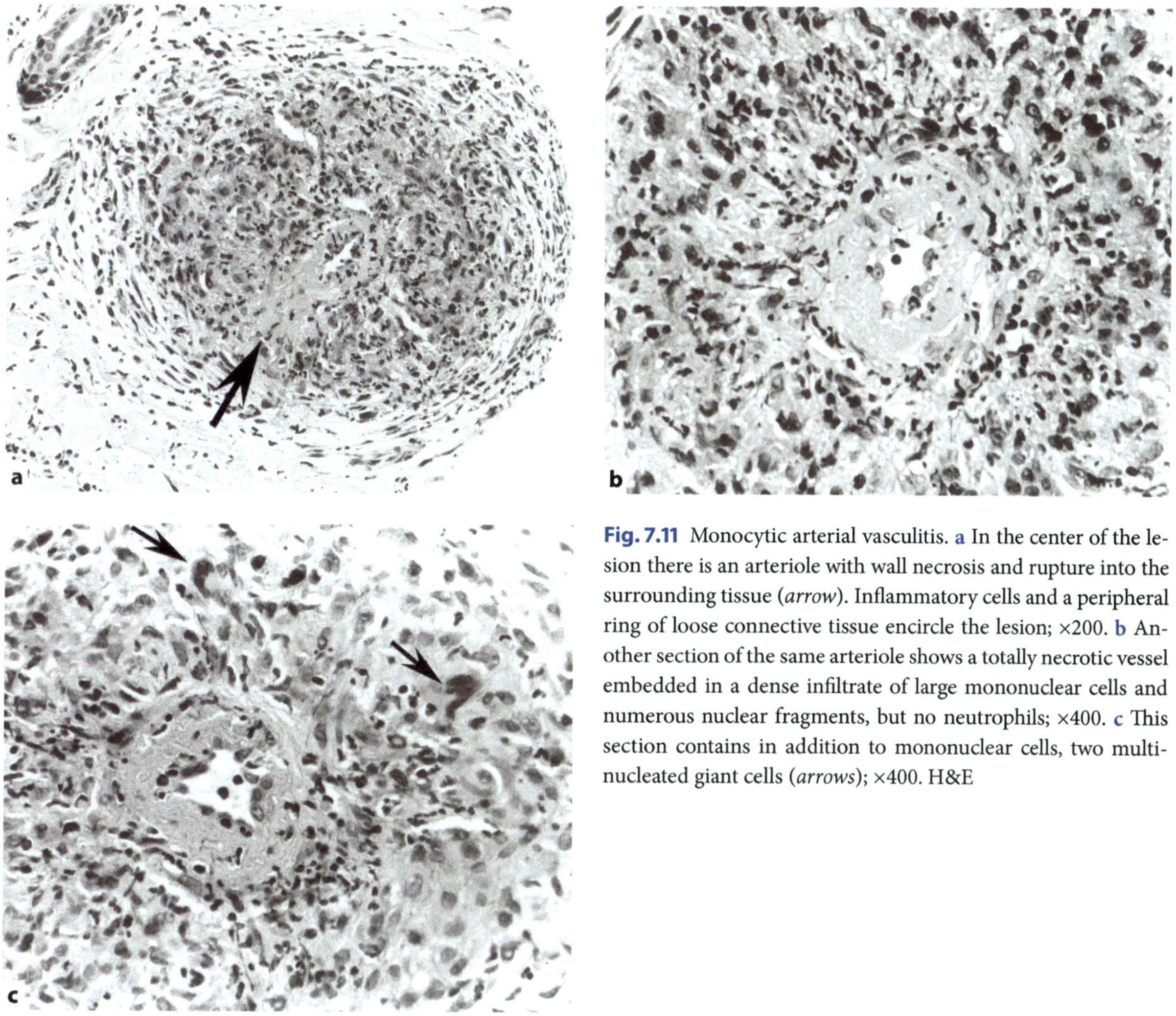

Fig. 7.11 Monocytic arterial vasculitis. **a** In the center of the lesion there is an arteriole with wall necrosis and rupture into the surrounding tissue (*arrow*). Inflammatory cells and a peripheral ring of loose connective tissue encircle the lesion; ×200. **b** Another section of the same arteriole shows a totally necrotic vessel embedded in a dense infiltrate of large mononuclear cells and numerous nuclear fragments, but no neutrophils; ×400. **c** This section contains in addition to mononuclear cells, two multinucleated giant cells (*arrows*); ×400. H&E

figure. Nuclear fragments were conspicuous around the necrotic vessel wall. At another level detached endothelial cells and nuclear fragments occluded the lumen. Eosinophils and neutrophils were not seen in the core of the lesion. In the immediate surroundings there were dilated venules and scattered inflammatory cells of different types. The epidermis was essentially normal (s. Figs 2.2 and Fig. 7.11).

Two months later the lesion on the left lower leg had ulcerated and the patient was referred to the dermatology department at the university hospital. On admission there was a 30×15 mm large, fibrin-covered ulceration with irregular borders on the medial aspect of the left lower leg. On the right medial malleolus an erythematous patch, 20 mm in diameter, was noted. Laboratory investigation revealed moderately elevated ESR, markedly increased serum IgA, and antineutrophilic cytoplasmic antibodies (c-ANCA). Wegener granulomatosis was suspected, but could not be verified (biopsy specimen from the nasal mucosa was negative). No other autoantibodies were detected; thus systemic disease could not be proved. There was no evidence of hepatitis A, B or C virus infection, or of borreliosis. No circulating antigen–antibody complexes or cryoglobulins were found; complement analysis was normal and no deposition of IgM, IgG, IgA, or C3 was found in the tissue.

At the time of writing the patient was still regularly monitored at the hospital. The first ulceration healed, but over the years new lesions developed, some of which ulcerated. She has mainly been treated with oral corticosteroids. At a check-up about 8 years after her first consultation she had been free from ulcerations for a year by means of a small maintenance dose. She was in good condition, had no symptoms, and was at work.

Case 12. Arterial Vasculitis in Organization

A 64-year-old woodwork teacher was hospitalized for investigation. For about a year he had had erythematous nodules on the lower legs. He was otherwise healthy and did not use drugs. On both lower legs there were scattered erythematous or bluish red infiltrates up to 20 mm in diameter without ulcerations. There was also a slight edema, but no livedo reticularis pattern. Laboratory investigation was normal. Thus, there was no evidence for autoimmune diseases or heart disease. Virus serology was negative. There were no cryoglobulins, and the platelet aggregation test was negative. He was given sulfasalazine and a diuretic, and healed.

A biopsy specimen was taken from an infiltrated area and included a fair part of the subcutis. Close to the deep margin there was a small artery occluded by a thrombus in organization. In some sections there

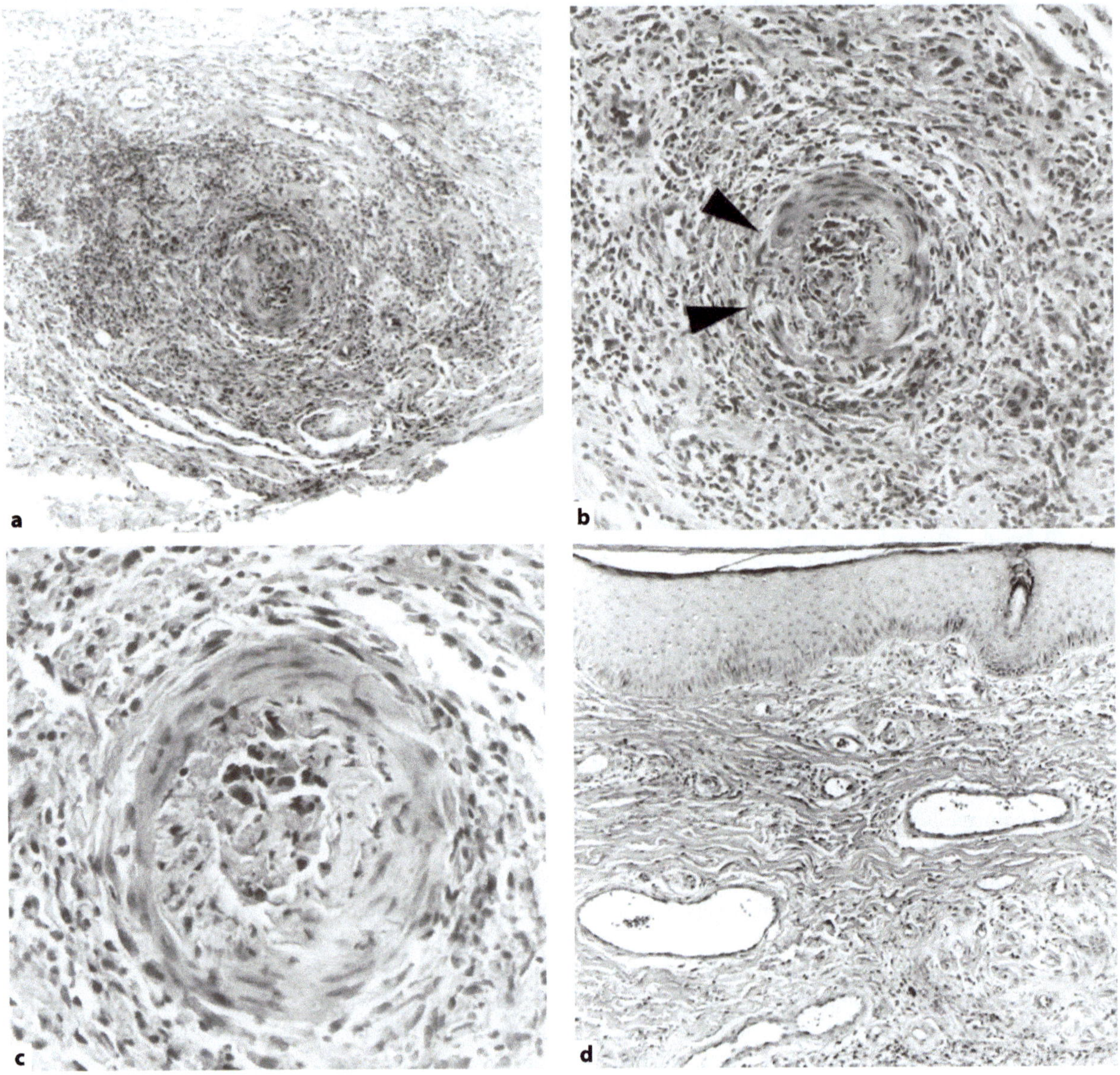

Fig. 7.12 Arterial vasculitis in organization. **a** A small artery in the subcutis is occluded by a thrombus in organization and surrounded by granulation tissue; ×100. **b** Close-up shows a gap in the vessel wall (*arrowheads*). Both the gap and the lumen are filled with granulation tissue. The area around the vessel is richly vascularized and densely infiltrated by inflammatory cells; ×200. **c** Close-up of another section displays the smooth muscle cells of the vessel wall; ×400. **d** Markedly dilated thin-walled vessels in the upper half of the dermis indicate stasis. In the right lower corner there is a group of proliferating capillaries; ×100. H&E

was a gap in the vessel wall plugged with fibrous tissue, testimony to a previous rupture. There was a wide area of richly vascularized granulation tissue (Sect. 5.2.4) permeated with inflammatory cells of different kinds including many eosinophils and neutrophils; however, close to the vessel most cells were lymphocytes. Also, there were a conspicuous extravasation of erythrocytes and a massive deposition of hemosiderin. No epithelioid cell granulomas or abscesses were noted. The middle and upper parts of the dermis contained several markedly dilated thin-walled vessels, indicating stasis. The epidermis was flat, but otherwise normal (Fig. 7.12).

7.5.4 Comment

As in category IV, arterial vessels are affected and the lesions are circumscribed, but the inflammatory cell infiltrate is composed of mononuclear cells. Lymphocytic/monocytic arterial vasculitis is difficult to anchor in the literature because of incomplete and confusing histopathologic description and confusing nomenclature. Feldaker et al. (1955) compared two clinical groups called "livedo reticularis with summer ulcerations" and "livedo reticularis with ulcerations during the fall and winter". They found that the patterns were generally the same in the two groups, but in some patients arteries and in some veins were affected. Bard and Winkelmann (1967) discussed the histopathologic pattern in lesions they called livedo vasculitis, though none of the nine patients displayed livedo reticularis. The involved vessels were described as arterioles and were located at the sweat gland level. The perivascular cell infiltrate was circumscribed and composed of lymphocytes, a pattern in accordance with that found in Case 9.

The histopathologic pattern displayed in Case 9, a thrombosed arteriole surrounded by a discreet infiltrate of small lymphocytes, is in the author's experience rather common and mostly accompanied by livedo reticularis. For the author it symbolizes a distinct and seemingly rather benign vasculitis, and is called here livedo reticularis vasculitis. However, livedo reticularis is not always present and may even be a symptom in category IV vasculitis and in arteriolosclerosis. Furthermore, Case 11 with the protracted course and the histopathologic pattern with large mononuclear cells and giant cells with a few nuclei, provokes thought. Are the patterns demonstrated in cases 9–11 expressions of different kinds of mononuclear vasculitis with different genesis or do they represent different ages or grades of severity of lesion caused by the same mechanism? Presumably the large cells observed in Case 10 and Case 11 are monocytes which when stimulated become macrophages with the ability to form giant cells and, if not further stimulated, give rise to giant cells with only a few nuclei (Dugast et al. 1997) (Sect. 5.3.3.1). Investigations at the molecular level (at that time not possible to perform) could have been of great value.

Case 12 demonstrates arterial vasculitis in healing. In this stage it is not possible to distinguish with certainty between a neutrophilic and a mononuclear arterial vasculitis.

In most cases of livedo reticularis and livedo reticularis with vasculitis the triggering cause cannot be determined. It is known that some drugs may give rise to livedo reticularis, the most common of which is amantidine used for Parkinson disease (Litt 2001).

7.6 Category VI: Granulomatous Neutrophilic Arterial Vasculitis

7.6.1 Clinical Appearance

As in categories IV and V, the patients suffer spells of painful, erythematous infiltrates or bluish-red nodules on the lower legs, which may ulcerate.

7.6.2 Histopathologic Appearance

Usually only one affected artery is observed and shows thrombosis and wall necrosis with dense infiltrates of neutrophils and nuclear fragments in and around the vessel wall, which may develop into an abscess. There are also widespread areas of necrosis both in the subcutaneous tissue and in the dermis. Necrotic areas are surrounded by a brim of histiocytes and epithelioid cells with an admixture of giant cells of Langhans or foreign-body type. Even small epithelioid cell granulomas without necrosis may be seen in the upper dermis.

Necrotic areas sometimes include one or several necrotic venules. These are an integral part of the necrotic tissue and thus secondary to the arterial thrombosis, and not the cause of the lesion. Also abscesses, if present, may be surrounded by richly vascularized granulation tissue. Altogether the pattern may be highly variegated and confusing if the biopsy specimen contains only a part of the lesion.

7.6.3 Examples

Case 13. Granulomatous Neutrophilic Arterial Vasculitis

This 60-year-old man suffered from Crohn disease. For 5–6 years he had experienced erythematous lesions with petechiae and a small central ulceration on the lower leg in association with acute spells of the intestinal disease. Now over 1 week a new lesion had developed on the ventral aspect of the right lower leg. He used paracetamol, codeine, and temporarily sulfasalazine.

A biopsy specimen that included a large part of subcutaneous tissue was taken. It was investigated at several levels and stained with H&E, vG and PAS. In the subcutaneous tissue, close to the dermal–subcutaneous interface there was a large irregular abscess, which merged into a vast and likewise irregular granular necrotic area. The latter mainly involved the subcutis, but in some places reached into the dermis as long narrow strips. In several consecutive sections a "shadow" vessel with a totally necrotic wall was seen in the abscess. Below the abscess a small artery, another part of the "shadow" vessel, was observed. In this segment the lumen was obliterated by an erythrocyte thrombus, and the partly necrotic wall was permeated with disintegrating neutrophils. In further sections the same vessel displayed a wall with well-preserved smooth muscle cells and only a partially occluded lumen. The necrotic areas in the dermis were surrounded by a rim of histiocytes and epithelioid cells. Scattered small epithelioid cell granulomas without necrosis were observed high in the dermis (Fig. 7.13).

Case 14. Granulomatous Arterial Vasculitis

A 47-year-old master-builder was admitted because of recurrent vasculitis-like lesions on the lower legs which had been present for about 4 years. The lesions remained for weeks or months, but never ulcerated. On admission he had some slightly reddened and tender nodules, 10-mm in diameter, located on the right lateral malleolus. Also, on both lower legs there were areas of brownish pigmentation, remnants of earlier nodules. On four occasions he had had gastrointestinal hemorrhage, probably due to duodenal ulcers. Routine laboratory values were normal. There was no evidence of systemic disease. The values for serum complement factors were normal. Hepatitis B antigen (Au antigen) was negative. Cryoglobulins were not found. Direct immunofluorescence showed the presence of IgG, IgA, IgM and C3 in material from both normal and affected skin.

A biopsy specimen taken from the lower leg included dermis and the dermal–subcutaneous interface. The epidermis was normal. In several sections a single, severely affected ascending arteriole could be followed from the dermal–subcutaneous interface to the mid-dermis. Epithelioid cells, scattered multinucleated giant cells and lymphocytes surrounded the vessel. The infiltrate was mixed up with mononuclear cells somewhat larger than ordinary lymphocytes and endowed with a large round nucleus and distinct nucleoli; these were probably stimulated lymphocytes. Adjacent to the affected vessel there was a vast granular necrosis in the dermis walled off by epithelioid cells, a few giant cells, and lymphocytes (Fig. 14).

7.6.4 Comment

The histopathologic pattern described in Case 13 (Fig. 7.13) was very much like that seen in subcutaneous vasculitis called erythema induratum when associated with tuberculosis and nodular vasculitis when tuberculosis cannot be proved. The biopsy specimen in this case probably displayed an unusually complete picture of a lesion of granulomatous neutrophilic arterial vasculitis with widespread changes both in the subcutis and dermis. In Case 14 (Fig. 7.14) only a part of an ascending arteriole tightly surrounded by epithelioid cells and lymphocytes was seen. The deep part of the lesion, which presumably contained a neutrophilic arterial vasculitis, was missing.

In recent years several case reports focusing on a possible correlation between Crohn disease and granulomatous skin lesions with or without vasculitis have appeared (Shum and Guenther 1990; Peltz et al. 1993; Hackzell-Bradley et al. 1996). Also the vasculitis described in Category IV, neutrophilic arterial vasculitis (so-called benign cutaneous periarteritis nodosa), has been associated with Crohn disease (Daoud et al. 1997; Gudbjörnsson and Hällgren 1990). However, if the investigated material is not complete or if the lesion is in regression the histopathologic diagnosis may be difficult. Probably not all cases described as benign periarteritis nodosa or nodular vasculitis are what they are said to be.

7.7 Category VII: Mixed Group

In this heterogeneous group are included: erythema elevatum diutinum, granuloma faciale, angiolymphoid hyperplasia with eosinophilia (all three of unknown genesis), bacillary angiomatosis caused by Bartonella

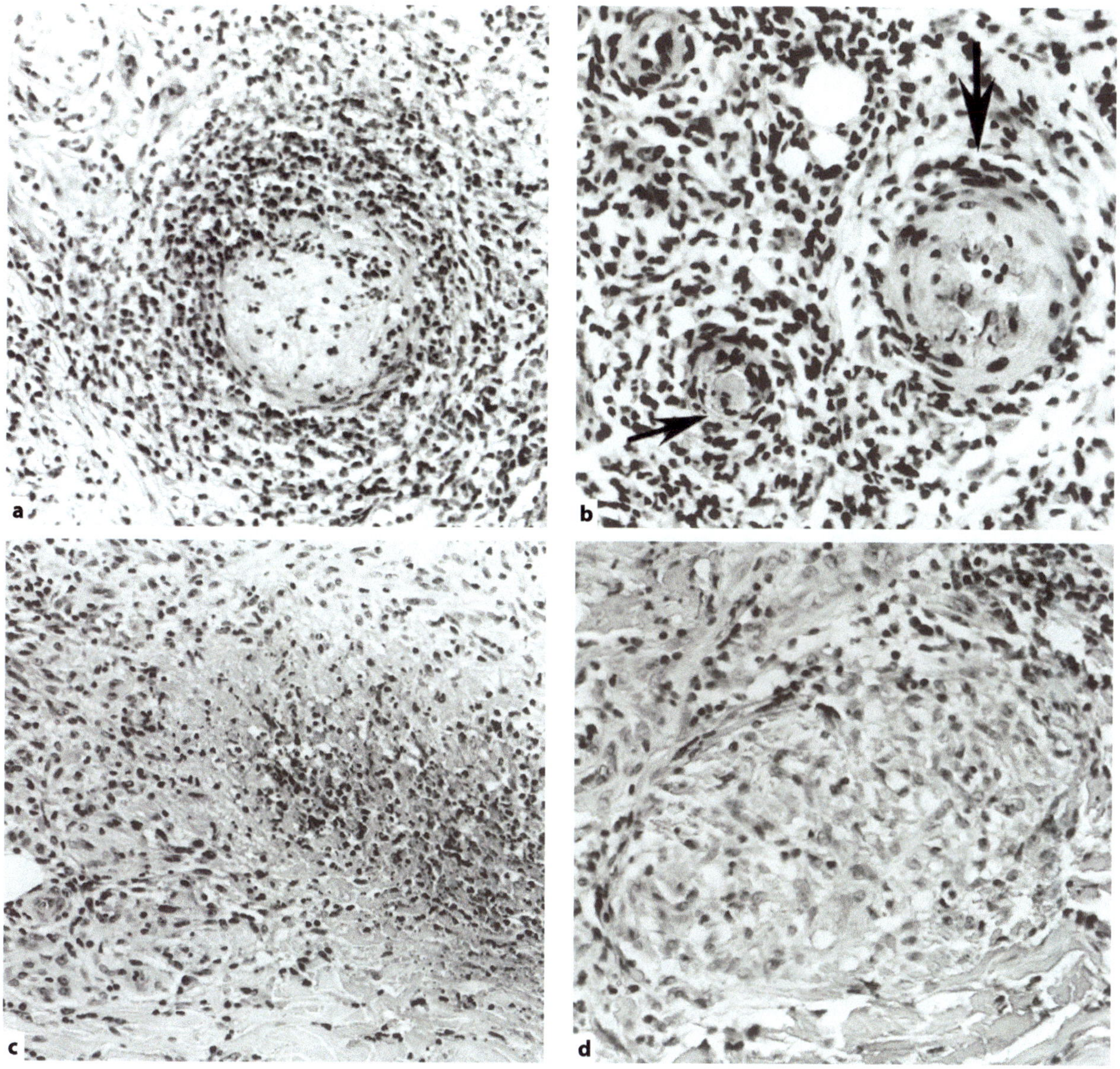

Fig. 7.13 Granulomatous neutrophilic arterial vasculitis. **a** A thrombotic small artery is located in a severely inflamed area in the subcutis. The vessel wall is densely infiltrated by disintegrating neutrophils; PAS, ×250. **b** The same vessel at another level. The wall of the vessel is preserved, but the lumen is obliterated (*large arrow*). In the left lower corner there is a small thrombotic branch (*small arrow*); H&E, ×300. **c** A necrotic area in the dermis is densely permeated by disintegrating neutrophils and walled off by a brim of histiocytes and epithelioid cells; H&E, ×200. **d** A small epithelioid cell granuloma without necrosis located in the upper half of the dermis; vG, ×300

(Rochalimeae) henselae and a further case suspected to be caused by an infectious agent.

7.7.1 Erythema Elevatum Diutinum

Erythema elevatum diutinum (EED), which means protracted elevated erythema, is a rare disease, described and named by Radcliffe-Crocker and Williams in 1894 (Laymon 1962). In the 1960s, case reports with reviews of the old literature were presented by among others Laymon (1962) and Mraz and Newcomer (1967). The following sections are in accordance with their descriptions of the disease and its natural course.

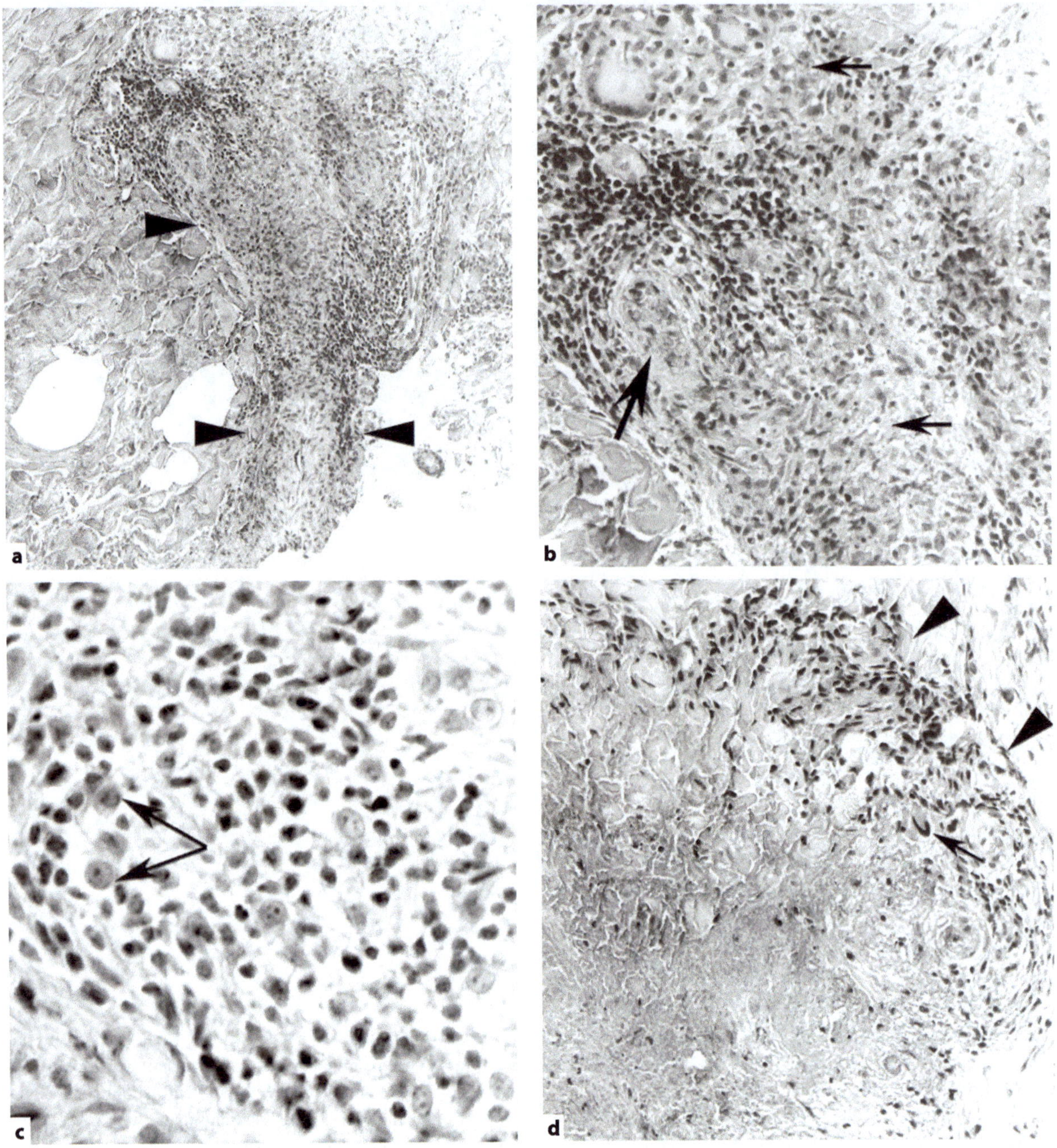

Fig. 7.14 Granulomatous arterial vasculitis. **a** The micrograph shows an ascending arteriole, which can be followed from the dermal–subcutaneous interface into the dermis (*arrow heads*); vG, ×100. **b** Close-up of the upper part of the vessel in **a**. The vessel is embedded in a dense inflammatory cell infiltrate which consists of epithelioid cell granulomas with scattered giant cells of Langhans type and lymphocytes (*small arrows*). At the *large arrow* a part of the thrombotic vessel is revealed; H&E, ×200. **c** Close-up of the lower part of the vessel in **a**. Lymphocytic cell infiltrate that, in addition to small lymphocytes, contains larger cells with a light nucleus and one or several nucleoli (stimulated lymphocytes). *One arrow* indicates one such cell, the *other arrow* a mitotic figure in anaphase; PAS, ×600. **d** Part of the large necrotic area, which to the right is walled off by a granulomatous cell infiltrate (*arrowheads*) including a giant cell of Langhans type (*arrow*); H&E, ×200

7.7.1.1 Clinical Appearance

Both children and adults were affected, and, as the name indicates, the disease was chronic and the course protracted. Histories of up to 10 years or more were described. Typically bluish-red or reddish-brown, infiltrated papules and plaques were located symmetrically on the dorsal aspect of the hands, fingers, toes, heels, knees, elbows and buttocks. Also the face could be involved. The trunk and mucous membranes were rarely affected and vesicular and ulcerated lesions were unusual. New lesions appeared continuously. There could be remissions and lesions could disappear, but at the same time new papules poped up. Fibrotic tumor-like nodules could develop in patients with a long disease duration. Usually patients did not complain of other symptoms than those from the skin.

7.7.1.2 Histopathologic Appearance

Generally the tissue was profusely vascularized and contained thick-walled venules with protruding endothelial cells. However, some vessels were thrombotic and/or displayed fibrinoid wall necrosis. There were perivascular and dense patchy or confluent interstitial inflammatory cell infiltrates composed of lymphocytes, histiocytes and neutrophils together with nuclear fragments. In some areas lymphocytes and histiocytes dominated, in others neutrophils. In some specimens the number of neutrophils was conspicuous. Also, some eosinophils and plasma cells were noted. In tumor-like lesions the normal dermal architecture was replaced by fibrotic tissue and contained patchy inflammatory cell infiltrates of neutrophils, sometimes with nuclear fragments, but only a few vessels. The investigators were surprised to find acute vasculitis in such a chronic disease as EED.

7.7.1.3 Example

Case 15. Erythema Elevatum Diutinum

A 62-year-old male patient had suffered for a year from gradually enlarging and coalescent, reddish-blue and rather thick, asymptomatic infiltrates on the dorsal aspect of the hands, fingers and toes, and on the chin and upper lip. He had no other complaints. At a check-up 2 years later the described lesions were mainly stationary, but brownish-blue, large, elongated infiltrates had developed on the extensor area of the elbows and forearms.

Two biopsy specimens were taken, one from the dorsal aspect of the hand and one from the face. They showed principally the same changes. The epidermis was slightly hyperkeratotic but otherwise normal. In the dermis dense patchy and partially coalescent inflammatory cell infiltrates composed mainly of lymphocytes and histiocytes with admixture of plasma cells and neutrophils were seen. There were many dilated vessels, both lymphatics and venules, and the latter often had protruding endothelial cells. In addition there were scattered venules, some of which were thrombotic, other necrotic and permeated with nuclear fragments. The cell infiltrates around these vessels consisted mainly of lymphocytes and histiocytes. Eosinophils were not observed. There were also many extravasated erythrocytes and a massive deposition of hemosiderin pigment (Fig. 7.15).

7.7.1.4 Comment

In Case 15, both the clinical picture with chronic infiltrates in acral areas and the histopathologic pattern with the notable mixture of marked chronic inflammation and acute vascular damage are in accordance with those described as typical of EED in the old literature.

However during more recent years the criteria for the diagnosis EED have changed. Katz et al. (1977) reported on five cases believed to be EED and thereby changed the criteria for the diagnosis. Thus they declared that all early and most late lesions showed leukocytoclastic angiitis associated with a dense dermal infiltrate composed primarily of neutrophils and occasionally monocytes, though some late lesions showed a "fibrocytic" replacement of normal dermal structures. They found the histopathologic pattern of EED difficult to differentiate from that of leukocytoclastic vasculitis. They based the diagnosis on the combination of the presence of leukocytoclastic vasculitis and the clinical pattern (i.e., efflorescences distributed acrally and symmetrically over extensor surfaces). However, this distribution is characteristic also of leukocytoclastic vasculitis. Furthermore, these patients differed from those in other reported series by having long histories of recurrent bacterial infections (prominently streptococcal) or by having other associated diseases (rheumatic fever, IgA monoclonal gammopathy). The lesions disappeared dramatically when the patients were treated with dapsone, but reappeared promptly after withdrawal of the drug.

During the 1990s, there were an abundance of articles on this rare disease associated with disorders such

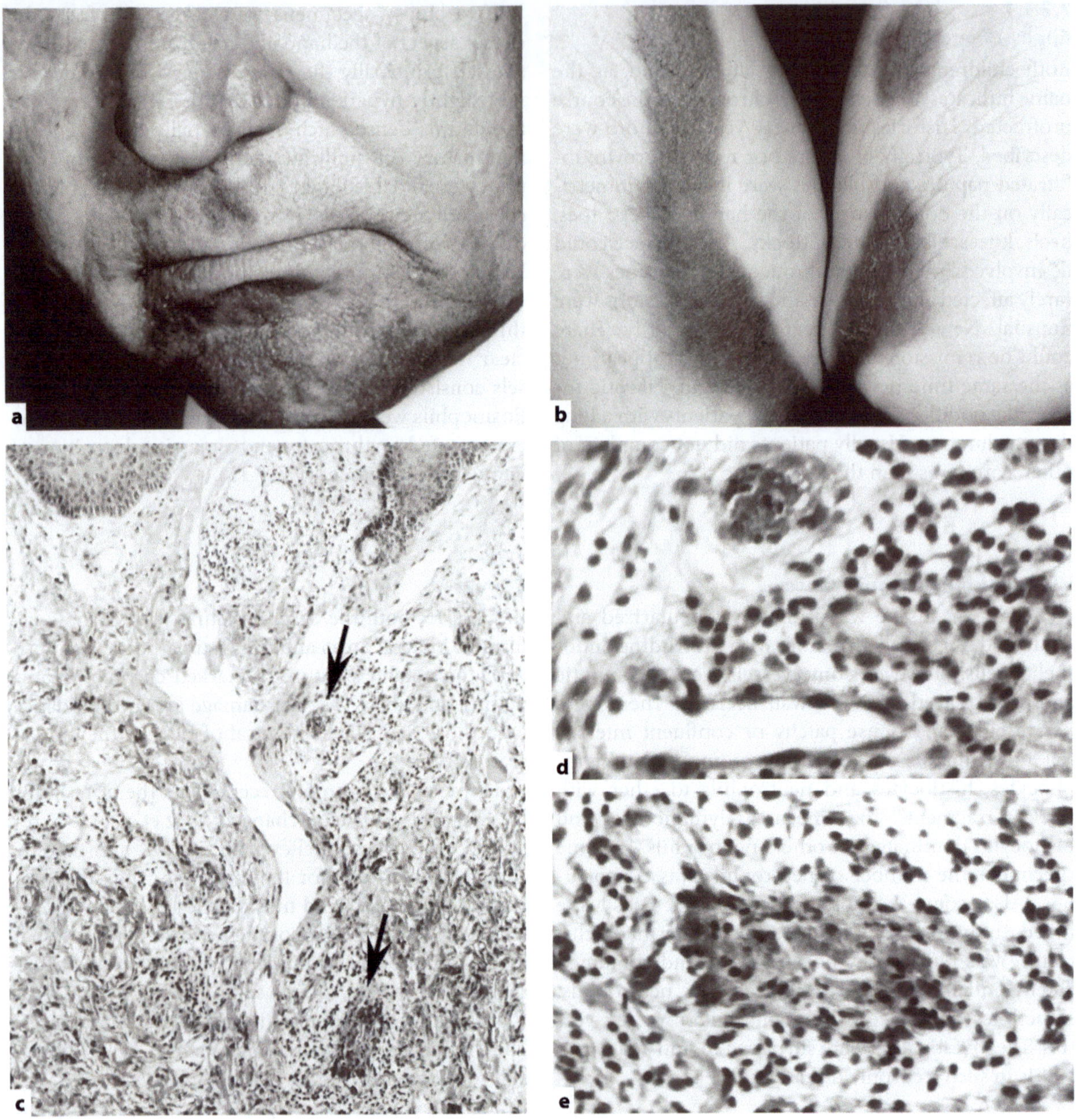

Fig. 7.15 Erythema elevatum diutinum. **a, b** Lesions on the chin, upper lip and elbows. **c** In the dermis there are dense and confluent cell infiltrates and dilated thin-walled vessels. The *arrows* indicate two affected venules. **d** Close-up of the area indicated by the upper arrow in **c** shows that the vessel is thrombotic. The perivascular cell infiltrate consists mainly of lymphocytes. The dilated venule at the base has protruding endothelial cells. **e** Close-up of the lower vessel. It is totally necrotic and permeated by a mixed cell infiltrate and nuclear fragments. H&E

as IgA paraproteinemia, relapsing polychondritis, Wegener granulomatosis, celiac disease, and herpes virus 6 infection (Yiannias et al. 1992; Bernard et al. 1992; Kavanagh et al. 1993; Chow et al. 1996; Tasanen et al. 1997; Drago et al. 1999). In these cases, the diagnosis of EED was based on one or several spells of symmetrically dispersed efflorescences on prominent parts of the body. Mostly only a single biopsy specimen showing unmitigated leukocytoclastic vasculitis was taken before treatment. It follows that in these patients the only proved diagnosis was leukocytoclastic vasculitis. However, it is interesting to note that in several of these patients there was an association with IgA just as in Henoch-Schönlein purpura (Sect. 7.1.5.1).

The cause of EED is not known, but it is thought to be a variant of classic leukocytoclastic vasculitis and thus presumably caused by circulating antigen–antibody complexes (Lawley and Kubota 1990; Weedon 1997). However, there are important differences, clinically as well as histopathologically, between these two diseases. Leukocytoclastic vasculitis presents as an acute spell of lesions, which reaches a maximum and then declines and heals. As described in the old literature, EED starts insidiously and gives rise to remaining infiltrated papules and plaques, which at the same time reveal conspicuous chronic inflammation and acute vasculitis with thrombotic/necrotic venules and nuclear fragments.

7.7.2 Granuloma Faciale

Granuloma faciale is a rare disease, but much more common than EED.

7.7.2.1 Clinical Appearance

It presents as one or several well-circumscribed, brown, brownish-red, or bluish-red plaques localized to the face. The lesion slowly enlarges and can become several centimeters in diameter. It is a chronic, usually asymptomatic and non-ulcerating condition. If excised, it usually recurs. Extrafacial lesions have been described (Roustan et al. 1999). Usually, the patient is middle aged. Males predominate.

7.7.2.2 Histopathologic Appearance

The histopathologic pattern is highly characteristic. Below the essentially normal epidermis there is a distinct narrow zone that is free of inflammatory cells. In the rest of the dermis and sometimes even in the superficial subcutaneous tissue there are dense, patchy, or confluent cell infiltrates, which encircle sebaceous glands and hair follicles without invading them. The cell infiltrates are polymorphic and composed mainly of lymphocytes and histiocytes with a rich admixture of eosinophils and neutrophils. There are also some plasma cells and mast cells. Macrophages stored with hemosiderin pigment are found at all levels. Eosinophils are diffusely scattered, while neutrophils and nuclear dust more often are found in aggregates and close to dilated venules with protruding endothelial cells. Occasionally, fibrin deposition outside the vessel wall and even wall necrosis are noted. Extravasation of red blood cells is conspicuous.

7.7.2.3 Pathogenesis

The cause is unknown. Like EED, it is thought to be a variant of leukocytoclastic vasculitis, although there are important clinical as well as histopathologic differences.

7.7.2.4 Example

Case 16. Granuloma Faciale

A 39-year-old woman had noted for more than a year a light-brown lesion in the right temporal area. It was excised for cosmetic reasons.

Histologic investigation revealed the above-described pattern typical for granuloma faciale. There also were dilated venules with marginal vacuoles and numerous dilated lymphatics (Fig. 7.16).

7.7.2.5 Comment

In this case several vessels with wall necrosis and deposition of fibrin were observed. In the author's experience these findings are rare, and may even be missing in otherwise clinically as well as histopathologically typical cases.

7.7.3 Angiolymphoid Hyperplasia with Eosinophilia

The concept angiolymphoid hyperplasia with eosinophilia, also called histiocytic hemangioma by Rosai et al. (1979) and Rosai (1982), and epithelioid hemangioma by Fetsch and Weiss (1991), is confusing, and a review of the literature is necessary.

Wells and Whimster (1969) described nine patients with subcutaneous nodules in the head and neck region. Histologic investigation of early lesions showed diffusely demarcated proliferation of vessels with protruding and vacuolated endothelial cells and inflammatory cell infiltrates with many eosinophils, while in older lesions lymphoid follicles with germinal centers dominated. Other than blood eosinophilia, systemic symptoms were not observed. The course was benign, but often protracted and excised lesions had a tendency to recur. It was regarded as a distinct

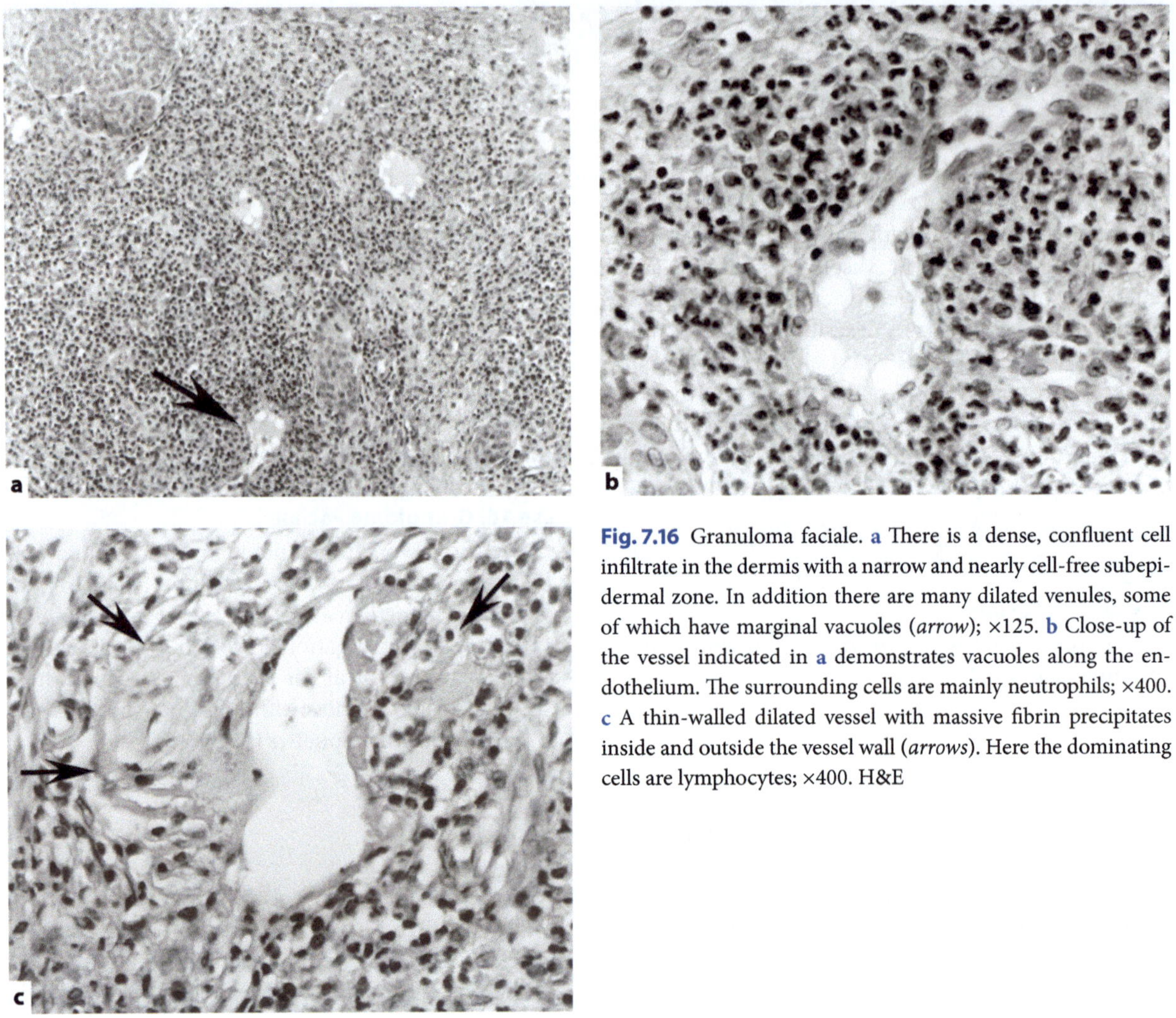

Fig. 7.16 Granuloma faciale. **a** There is a dense, confluent cell infiltrate in the dermis with a narrow and nearly cell-free subepidermal zone. In addition there are many dilated venules, some of which have marginal vacuoles (*arrow*); ×125. **b** Close-up of the vessel indicated in **a** demonstrates vacuoles along the endothelium. The surrounding cells are mainly neutrophils; ×400. **c** A thin-walled dilated vessel with massive fibrin precipitates inside and outside the vessel wall (*arrows*). Here the dominating cells are lymphocytes; ×400. H&E

pathologic entity and named subcutaneous angiolymphoid hyperplasia with eosinophilia (ALHE). Because of the presence of lymphoid follicles in older lesions of ALHE, the authors suggested an association with Kimura disease, described in Japan in the 1940s (see Glossary). This is why Kimura disease and ALHE were thought to be related diseases. Kandil (1970) reported a patient with dermal nodules on the ear with a similar histopathologic pattern as described by Wells and Whimster (1969). The author thought his case to be a cutaneous counterpart to subcutaneous ALHE, included similar previously reported cases (Peterson et al. 1964; Jones and Bleehen 1969), and called the condition dermal ALHE. Thereafter the designation became ALHE and included subcutaneous as well as dermal lesions (Mehregan and Shapiro 1971). Rosai et al. (1979) reported on ALHE and stressed that the peculiar kind of vascular changes could also be found in mucous membranes and bone and may affect large veins and arteries as well as small vessels. Also in the investigation of Fetsch and Weiss (1991), including 96 patients with ALHE, most of the lesions were located in subcutaneous fat tissue, in which a medium-sized artery or vein was affected. There is no agreement as to whether ALHE is a kind of benign tumor or a reactive process, but the latter view prevails. A possible relationship between Kimura disease and ALHE has been strongly opposed by Rosai (1982) and Chun and Ji (1992).

7.7.3.1 Example

Case 17. Angiolymphoid Hyperplasia with Eosinophilia

A 73-year-old woman presented with an erythematous nodule which had been present for a month and was located on the forehead; it was rounded and about 10 mm in diameter. After 4 months of watching the lesion, which had remained stationary, was excised. In a telephone interview two and a half years later the patient said that she was well and that the lesion had not returned.

The specimen was covered with a moderately acanthotic but otherwise normal epidermis. The dermis was thickened and composed of loose, edematous connective tissue, which contained dispersed collagen bundles and different-sized, bizarre-looking, thick-walled venules. In a fully developed vascular lesion the endothelium was prominent and composed of large cells with condensed eosinophilic cytoplasm, and a large vesicular nucleus with a distinct nucleolus. In scattered vessels one or two mitotic figures were observed seemingly in the layer of cells just below the endothelium. Many lumina were more or less filled up with large, empty PAS-negative vacuoles. Some of these vacuoles were without any doubt situated in the cytoplasm of endothelial cells, which had a signet-ring appearance with a peripheral crescent-like nucleus. The layer below the endothelium contained dispersed cells with vesicular nucleus and light indistinct cytoplasm. This core was surrounded by several loosely arranged rings of thin collagen threads. Also thin-walled vessels had protruding endothelial cells, some of which were more or less filled with vacuoles. In longitudinally cut vessels of this type there were also small areas where endothelial cells were missing or appeared damaged and collapsed. Vascular wall necrosis and thrombosis were not seen. Engaged vessels were surrounded by different-sized, circumscribed, dense inflammatory cell infiltrates composed mainly of eosinophils and lymphocytes with an admixture of histiocytes, and plasma cells. Neutrophils were not seen. Lymphocytoma or lymphocytoma-like formations were not seen. The lesion was not sharply defined and was not completely excised (Fig. 7.17).

7.7.3.2 Comment

The conspicuous vascular pattern with highly vacuolated endothelial cells demonstrated in this case is well in accordance with what in the modern literature is described as ALHE in the skin and elsewhere. However, the significance of the vacuolated endothelial cells is unclear. Rosai et al. (1979) postulated that the protruding and sometimes vacuolated endothelial cells could represent primitive endothelial cells and referred to embryonal angiogenesis, a view also supported in some of the modern literature (Requena and Sangueza 1997). The background is a hypothesis that during angiogenesis a new lumen is formed in the proliferating string of endothelial cells due to intracellular vacuolization followed by fusion of vacuoles in adjacent cells. However, today it is generally accepted that the new lumen is formed between two abutting endothelial outgrowths from the wall of the parent vessel and is probably an elongation of the parent vessel lumen (Diaz-Flores et al. 1994). Investigations made by Jones and Bleehen (1969) and Eady and Jones (1977) by light microscopy and enzyme histochemistry, correlated with electron microscopy, indicated that the vacuoles are empty (i.e., do not contain lipids or glycogen) and that involved vessels are postcapillary venules with a highly stimulated endothelium. The vacuolated endothelial cells are considered to be cells undergoing liquefaction degeneration (i.e. cells with intracellular edema; compare intracellular edema in keratinocytes in Fig. 22.1a with those in Fig. 7.17b–d).

In plain words, it seems likely that the vacuoles in the endothelial cells represent intracellular edema that focally ends up in disintegration of the cells, which in turn stimulates subendothelial cell proliferation and results in thickening of the wall. This hypothesis favors the view that ALHE is a protracted reactive process in response to some kind of continuous endothelial injury, which may appear in different settings (Rosai 1982; Fetsch and Weiss 1991). One possibility is infection caused by a so-far-unknown agent. It may be considered as a kind of chronic vasculitis.

7.7.4 Bacillary Epithelioid Angiomatosis

Bacillary epithelioid angiomatosis (BEA) was first described only in patients with advanced HIV infection and was connected with cat-scratch disease. However, intensive investigation has shown that the causative agent is *Bartonella (Rochalimeae) henselae*. This is a small rod-shaped organism which can be cultured and may be visualized in tissue by the silver staining technique (Warthin-Starry, Steiner, and variants of Steiner staining) (Cockerell 1995). BEA has also been observed in patients not infected with HIV (Requena and Sangueza 1997).

Clinically small lesions could be taken for early Kaposi sarcoma because of their bluish tint. Also histopathologically the two disorders share some features. They are both richly vascularized and have groups of proliferating vessels, often located close to hair follicles and sweat glands, structures that are normally surrounded with a dense capillary network (Fig. 5.3a). In both, the so-called promontory sign, a dilated lym-

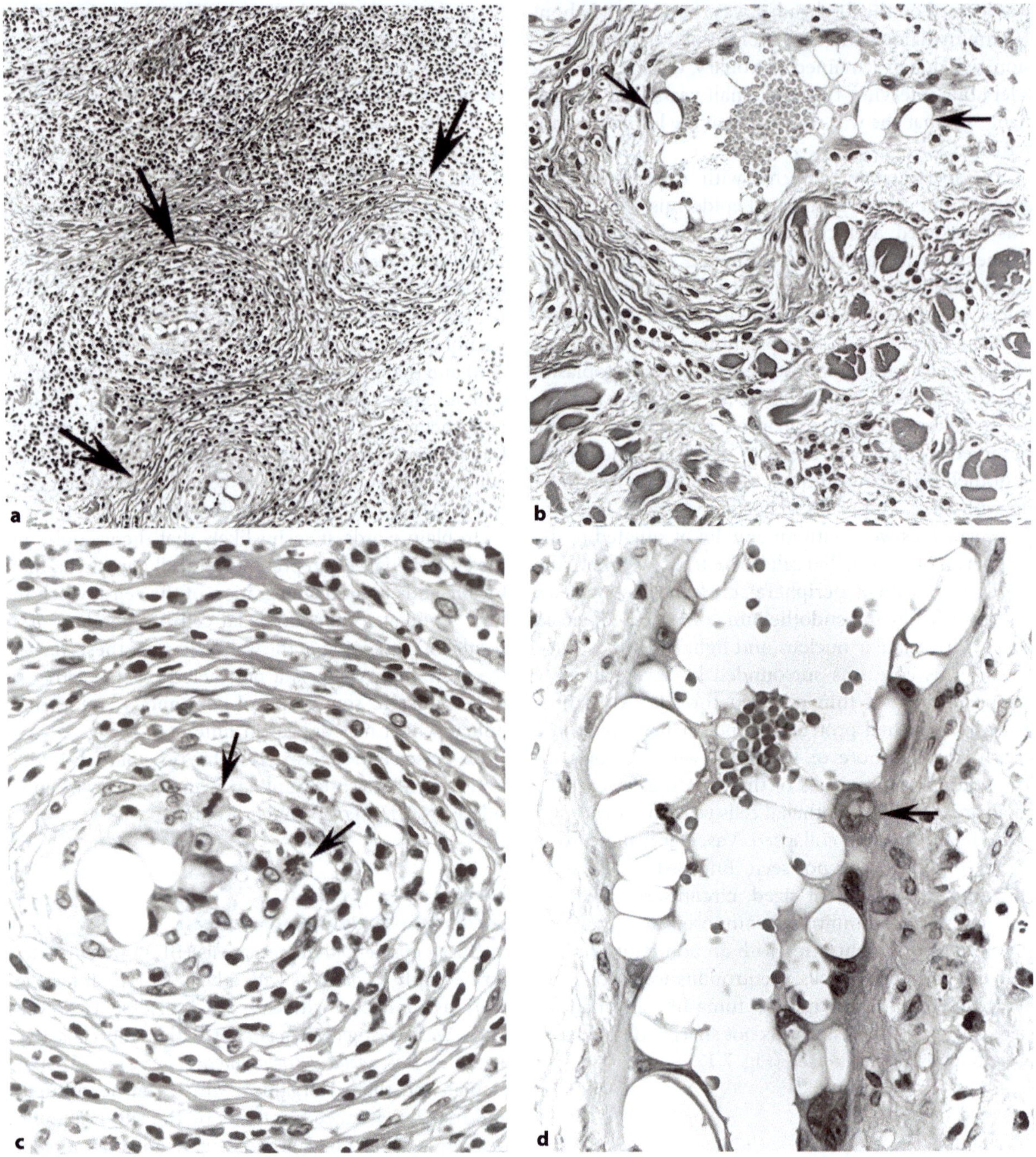

Fig. 7.17 Angiolymphoid hyperplasia with eosinophilia. **a** A dense inflammatory cell infiltrate obscures the dermis, in the middle of which there are three affected vessels (*arrows*); ×100. **b** The thick-walled vessels are embedded in a conspicuously edematous tissue that contains dispersed irregular collagen bundles. The vessel wall consists of three layers: endothelium, a markedly edematous subendothelial layer, and an outer ring of thin collagen threads. At least two endothelial cells have large intracytoplasmic vacuoles and the signet-ring appearance (*arrows*). There are large marginal vacuoles in the lumen, some of which seem to originate from burst vacuoles; ×200. **c** Close-up of the vessel indicated in **a**. The lumen is obliterated by vacuolated endothelial cells with the signet-ring appearance. In the subendothelial layer there are scattered large cells with a large clear nucleus and a distinct nucleolus and two cells in mitosis, one in metaphase and one in prophase (*arrows*). The collagen ring is diffusely penetrated by inflammatory cells; ×400. **d** A longitudinally cut, thin-walled vessel with vacuolated and partly fused endothelial cells. The *arrow* indicates an endothelial cell containing small intracytoplasmic vacuoles; ×400. vG

phatic vessel containing a bud of connective tissue which often contains one or several capillaries, may be observed (see Glossary). However, in BEA in the dermis there are densely packed thick-walled vessels with epithelioid-like endothelium and dense infiltrates of neutrophils, while in nodular Kaposi sarcoma there are densely packed bundles of spindle cells arranged in whirls.

It is possible that an unknown infectious agent is the joker in other kinds of unusual skin lesions combined with mixed inflammatory cell infiltrates and mixed vascular changes. Case 19 may be such a case.

7.7.4.1 Examples

Case 18. Bacillary Epithelioid Angiomatosis

A 45-year-old man who suffered from AIDS with spells of *Pneumocystis carinii* pneumonia had over 4 weeks developed 10 to 15 bluish-red, 2–3 mm elevated and slightly scaling papules on the abdomen and thighs. During the following 14 days the efflorescences diminished, apparently spontaneously. However, over the following months the eruption became generalized and some of the lesions enlarged. The latter had a central crust or pustule encircled by a scale, which in turn was surrounded by an erythematous zone. The patient also had fever and an increased ESR.

Biopsy specimens from the early lesion and the later general eruption showed principally the same pattern and included the dermal–subcutaneous interface. The tissue was highly vascularized and contained large conglomerates of thick-walled venules with very high epithelioid endothelial cells with scattered mitotic figures. Some of these cells contained marginal empty PAS-negative vacuoles. Scattered venules were thrombotic. In addition many thin-walled dilated venules and lymphatics were observed. Between the thick-walled vessels especially there were dense aggregates of neutrophils and nuclear fragments. In the surrounding tissue lymphocytes and fibroblasts dominated. Mast cells, but no plasma cells, were noted. There was no evidence of fungal infection. Unfortunately, the material was cut in series for a seminar; silver staining of the poor material remaining in the blocks showed the tissue to be negative for bacteria.

The clinical appearance and the histopathologic characteristics, as well as the disappearance of skin lesions and general symptoms after treatment with erythromycin, verified the diagnosis bacillary epithelioid angiomatosis. In retrospect it was found that the period of seemingly spontaneous amelioration coincided with doxycycline treatment for a spell of *Pneumocystis carinii* pneumonia (Fig. 7.18).

Case 19. Mixed Venular Vasculitis of Unknown Cause

A 35-year-old woman discovered a small insect-bite-like patch at the dorsal aspect of the left wrist on the way home to Sweden from a visit to Portugal. The lesion slowly increased in size and she attended an outpatient clinic for infectious diseases. Treatment with oral penicillin was unsuccessful and she was referred to the Department of Dermatology. On the left forearm there was then a 50×70 mm well-demarcated lesion with some central clearing and a slightly raised erythematous margin and just inside the border zone a scale collar. There were no pustules or vesicles. A similar 10 mm patch without central clearing was seen on her left shoulder. She was given topical treatment. For some time the lesion continued to slowly enlarge and scattered small new lesions appeared on the left arm and also on the right forearm. However, about 7 weeks after the first patch was noted the two oldest lesions begun to regress spontaneously and finally all lesions disappeared without further treatment.

A biopsy specimen taken from the left wrist included the whole dermis and showed prominent changes. In the upper and middle part of the dermis there were widespread coalescent inflammatory cell infiltrates which mainly consisted of neutrophils with conspicuous leukocytoclasis. There also were many eosinophils. In spite of the many nuclear fragments only scattered small venules with fibrinoid wall necrosis were observed. However, there were many dilated venules with protruding endothelial cells, some of which were filled with vacuoles and often surrounded mainly by lymphocytes. The epidermis was normal. There were no signs of folliculitis. Fungal structures were not found.

Laboratory investigations, including the blood, liver, urine, and electrophoresis, were normal with the exception of a slightly increased ESR, and increased polyclonal IgG. Direct microscopy and culture for fungus were negative (Fig. 7.19).

7.7.5 Comment

In four of five of the cases described in Category VII, the occurrence of marginal vacuoles in vessel lumina was a prominent feature. Scattered marginal vacuoles in the lumen of both veins and arteries are now and then observed in seemingly normal vessels and are thought to be artifacts due to poor fixation (Majno

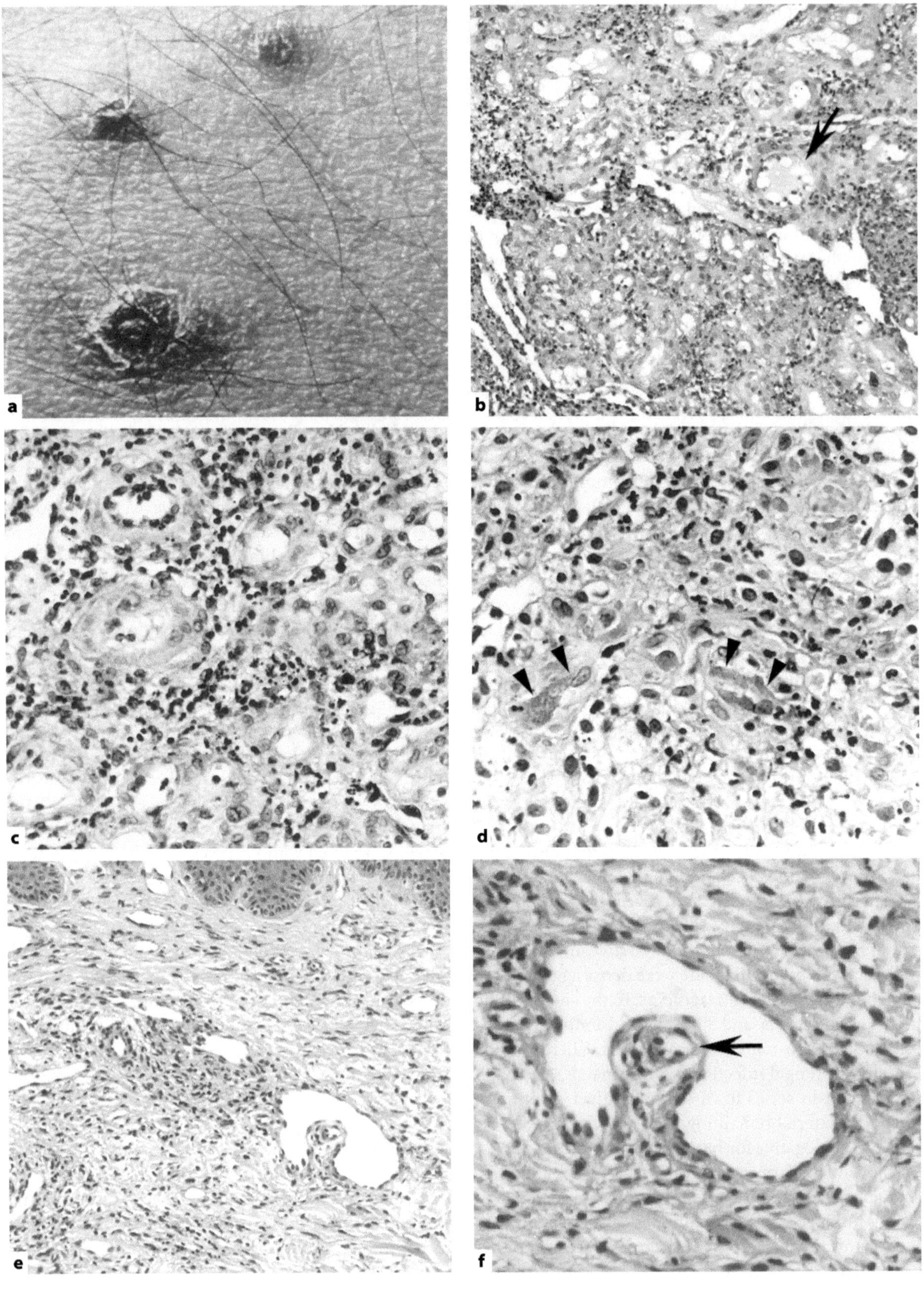

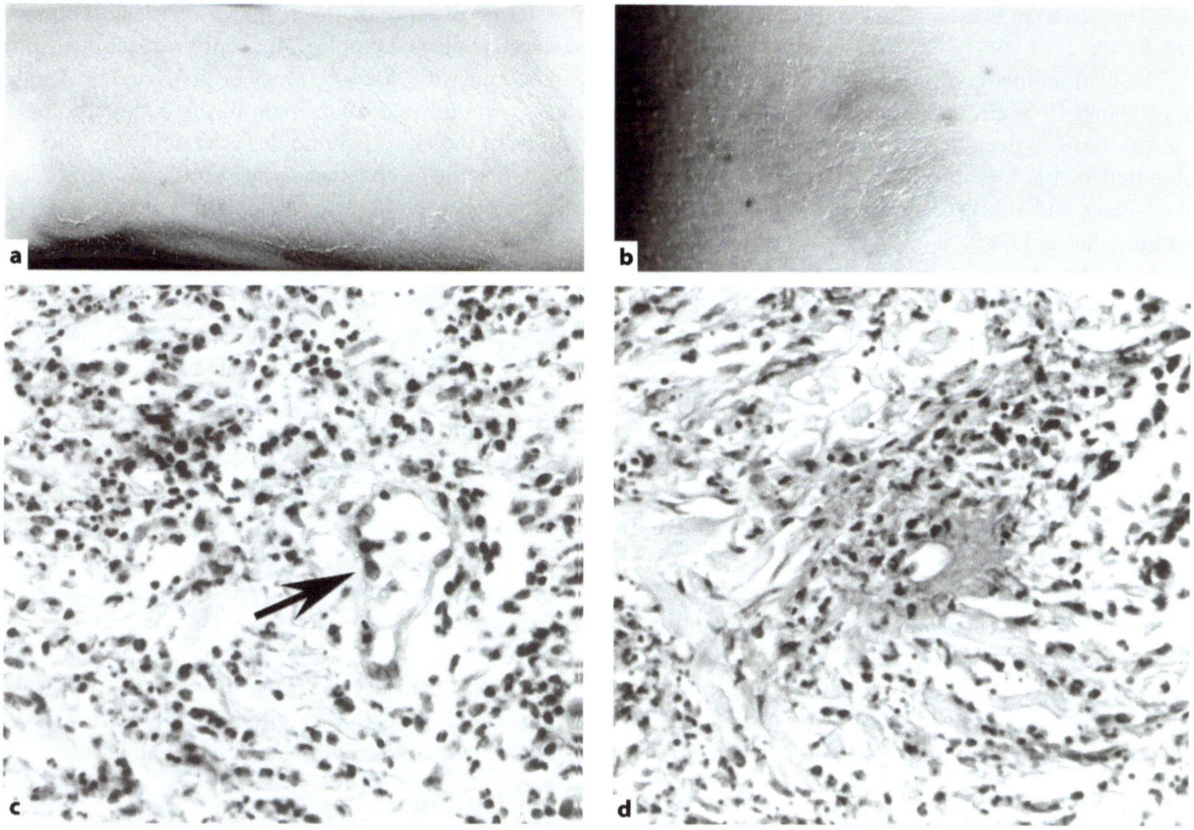

Fig. 7.19 Lesion, probably due to infection. **a** Well-circumscribed, erythematous lesion on the left forearm with active margin and inside this a scale collar. **b** Fresh satellite lesion on the left upper arm. **c** A dilated venule with protruding endothelial cells and vacuoles (*arrow*) is surrounded by edematous tissue with a dense inflammatory cell infiltrate composed of a mixture of disintegrating neutrophils and lymphocytes. **d** A necrotic venule with perivascular fibrinous exudate and disintegrating neutrophils. H&E, ×400

Fig. 7.18 Bacillary epithelioid angiomatosis. **a** Three typical papular lesions. The papules have a scale collar and are surrounded by an erythematous zone. **b** In the dermis there are densely packed epithelioid venules, separated by thin-walled and irregular vascular spaces (lymphatics). The *arrow* indicates a venule with marginal vacuoles; PAS, ×150. **c** Close-up shows thick-walled venules surrounded by dense aggregates of neutrophils and nuclear fragments; H&E, ×400. **d** *Arrowheads* indicate two parts of a horizontally running necrotic venule. The cell infiltrate is mixed, but neutrophils and nuclear dust predominate; H&E, ×400. **e** The richly vascularized upper dermis in the right lower corner shows a promontory sign; H&E, ×150. **f** Close-up of the promontory sign. The *arrow* indicates a capillary

and Joris 1996). However, the high number of both vacuolated endothelial cells and vacuoles in the vessel lumina in Case 17 give rise to the audacious thought that the vacuoles may be tombstones over disintegrated endothelial cells and not artifacts.

7.8 Nomenclature

A big problem concerning vasculitis is the synonym-rich and bewildering nomenclature. Sometimes the designation is based on a clinical symptom, which is not present in all cases with the same kind of histopathologic pattern, or also occurs in vasculitis with distinctly different histopathology. Some names are illusory, such as benign cutaneous polyarteritis nodosa and metastatic Crohn disease. Also a given designation may have different meanings to different authorities. The situation is exemplified in the following paragraphs.

The distinct histopathologic pattern described here in Category IV as circumscribed leukocytoclastic arterial vasculitis in deep dermis and subcutis is well documented in the literature and by authorities such as Diaz-Peres and Winkelmann (1974), Lever and Schaumburg-Lever (1990), and Weedon (1997) is called benign cutaneous poly- or periarteritis nodosa. However, Ryan (1992), wanting to preserve the designation polyarteritis nodosa for the systemic disease, called it livedo with nodules, even though livedo is missing in many cases and ulceration is common in this type of vasculitis (Daoud et al. 1997). Furthermore, livedo vasculitis is used synonymously with livedo with ulceration, livedo reticularis with summer ulceration, segmental hyalinizing vasculitis, and *atrophie blanche* (Ryan 1992).

The clinical pattern *atrophie blanche* is applied by most authorities to spells of purpura and small ulcerations on the lower legs, ankles and dorsal aspects of the feet followed by whitish atrophic scars, pigmentation, and sometimes livedo reticularis (Fig. 8.7a). The lesions are due to fibrinoid necrosis and/or thrombosis of venules and capillaries in the dermis. In some cases, where the lesions have been called *atrophie blanche* or livedo vasculitis, hypercoagulability has been proved (Pizzo et al. 1986; McCalmont et al. 1992).

It is obvious that symptoms, such as livedo reticularis and the designation *atrophie blanche*, common to vascular lesions with a distinctly different histopathologic pattern should not be used as diagnoses. Also, the acceptance of designations such as benign cutaneous polyarteritis nodosa and metastatic Crohn disease impedes one's mind and prevents further development. There are strong indications that systemic polyarteritis nodosa and so-called benign cutaneous polyarteritis nodosa are two different diseases. The mechanism behind cutaneous manifestations of Crohn disease is not clear. The word metastatic implies vascular or lymphatic spreading of either infectious agents or tumor cells and therefore should be avoided.

7.9 Conclusion

The different kinds of vasculitis described above may each be provoked by several different antigens, and may be expressed by different mechanisms (pathways). This means that one type of vasculitis could be a part of various skin diseases. For example, neutrophilic venular vasculitis (leukocytoclastic vasculitis) can be a hypersensitivity reaction type III, a component in a systemic disease, or the result of direct invasion of bacteria or virus. Lymphocytic venular vasculitis (like leukocytoclastic vasculitis) may be provoked by drugs, and is sometimes a component in the histopathologic pattern of pityriasis lichenoides et varioliformis acuta. Crohn disease has been associated both with granulomatous neutrophilic arterial vasculitis (Category VI) and with arterial neutrophilic vasculitis (Category IV). The clinical pattern *atrophie blanche* may be caused by different types of diseases. Furthermore, histologic investigations of nodules on the lower legs with or without livedo reticularis or ulcerations may reveal Category IV, V or VI vasculitis. It is therefore difficult to make sensible classifications of vasculitis based on causes, symptoms, or associated diseases.

It seems logical that the histopathologic features should be the backbone in the labeling and classification of different types of vascular lesions. To be of value the investigation has to fulfill the following requirements:

- A fresh and non-ulcerated lesion should be chosen. An ulcerated lesion could be in organization (healing) and therefore lack significant characteristics or could be secondarily infected, which gives rise to a variegated and confusing pattern.
- The biopsy must include the whole dermis and a fair part of the subcutaneous tissue. The latter is mandatory if the lesion is deep-seated.
- The type of affected vessels and their location should be specified: small artery (subcutis), ascending arteriole (subcutis, dermis), capillaries (dermis), postcapillary venules (dermis), or a vein (dermal/subcutaneous interface, subcutis). Designations such as medium-sized vessels and muscular vessels do not give adequate information and are deceptive (Chapter 2).
- The type of inflammatory cells taking part and their extension should be specified.
- The presence of abscesses, necrotic areas and epithelioid reactions should be noted.

However, from a histopathologic point of view the capacity of the tissue to respond to different kinds of stimuli is restricted. Therefore classification based on histopathology must be completed with investigations at the molecular level. With few exceptions, knowledge concerning mechanisms and pathways in vasculitis is incomplete. Presumably systematic, prospective investigations of vascular lesions based on the histopathologic mapping described above, in combination with immunohistochemical stainings designed to disclose involved inflammatory cells (including subtypes), cytokines and CAMs will give further information. To be complete these basic investigations have to be matched with the history, clinical appearance, a wide laboratory investigation (with respect to infections, systemic diseases, abnormal blood components) and the course of the disease. It may then be possible to obtain answers to the following questions:

- What are the mechanisms behind the different kinds of arterial/arteriolar vasculitis and the basic differences between arterial/arteriolar and venular vasculitis?
- Could Crohn disease give rise to both Category IV and Category VI vasculitis or only Category VI vasculitis?
- Are lymphocytic and monocytic arterial/arteriolar vasculitis variants of the same disease or different diseases?

References

1. Bard JW, Winkelmann RK (1967) Livedo vasculitis. Segmental hyalinizing vasculitis of the dermis. Arch Dermatol 96:489–499
2. Bernard P, Bedane C, Delrous J-L, Catanzano G, Bonnetblanc J-M (1992) Erythema elevatum diutinum in a patient with relapsing polychondritis. J Am Acad Dermatol 26:312–315
3. Bos JD, Zonneveld I, Das PK, Krieg SR, Van der Loos CM, Kapsenberg ML (1987) The skin Immune system (SIS): distribution and immunophenotype of lymphocyte subpopulations in normal human skin. J Invest Dermatol 88:569–573
4. Braverman IM, Yen A (1975) Demonstration of immune complexes in spontaneous and histamine-induced lesions and in normal skin of patients with leukocytoclastic angiitis. J Invest Dermatol 64:105–112
5. Carlson JA, Mihm MC Jr, LeBoit PE (1996) Cutaneous lymphocytic vasculitis. A definition, a review, and a proposed classification. Semin Diagn Pathol 13:72–90
6. Chen K-R, Pittelkow MR, Su WPD, Gleich GJ, Newman W, Leiferman KM (1994) Recurrent cutaneous necrotizing eosinophilic vasculitis. A novel eosinophil-mediated syndrome. Arch Dermatol 130:1159–1166
7. Chow RKP, Benny WB, Coupe RL, Dodd WA, Ongley RC (1996) Erythema elevatum diutinum associated with IgA paraproteinemia successfully controlled with intermittent plasma exchange. Arch Dermatol 132:1360–1364
8. Chun SI, Ji HG (1992) Kimura's disease and angiolymphoid hyperplasia with eosinophilia. Clinical and histopathologic differences. J Am Acad Dermatol 27:954–958
9. Cockerell CJ (1995) Bacillary angiomatosis and related diseases caused by Rochalimaea. J Am Acad Dermatol 32:783–790
10. Daoud MS, Hutton KP, Gibson LE (1997) Cutaneous periarteritis nodosa. A clinicopathological study of 79 cases. Br J Dermatol 136:706–713
11. Diaz-Perez JL, Winkelmann RK (1974) Cutaneous periarteritis nodosa. Arch Dermatol 110:407–414
12. Diaz-Flores L, Gutiérrez R, Varela H (1994) Angiogenesis. An update. Histol Histopathol 9:807–843
13. Drago F, Semino M, Rampini P, Lugani C, Rebora A (1999) Erythema elevatum diutinum in a patient with human herpesvirus 6 infection. Acta Derm Venereol 79:91–92
14. Dugast C, Gaudin A, Toujas L (1997) Generation of multinucleated giant cells by culture of monocyte-derived macrophages with IL-4. J Leukoc Biol 61:517–521
15. Eady RA, Jones EW (1977) Pseudopyogenic granuloma. Enzyme histochemical and ultrastructural study. Hum Pathol 8:653–668
16. Feldaker M, Hines EA Jr, Kierland RR (1955) Livedo reticularis with summer ulcerations. Arch Dermatol Syph 72:31–42
17. Fetsch JF, Weiss SW (1991) Observations concerning the pathogenesis of epithelioid hemangioma (angiolymphoid hyperplasia). Mod Pathol 4:449–455
18. Gudbjörnsson B, Hällgren R (1990) Cutaneous polyarteritis nodosa associated with Crohn's disease. Report and review of the literature. J Rheumatol 17:386–390
19. Hackzell-Bradley M, Hedblad M-A, Stephansson EA (1996) Metastatic Crohn's disease. Report of 3 cases with special reference to histopathologic findings. Arch Dermatol 132:928–932
20. Wilson Jones E, Bleehen SS (1969) Inflammatory angiomatous nodules with abnormal blood vessels occurring about the ears and scalp (pseudo or atypical pyogenic granuloma). Br J Dermatol 81:804–816
21. Jones REJ (1985) Questions to the editorial board and other authorities. What are your criteria for identifying vasculitis of small blood vessels by conventional microscopy. Am J Dermatopathol 7:181–187
22. Kandil E (1970) Dermal angiolymphoid hyperplasia with eosinophilia versus pseudopyogenic granuloma. Br J Dermatol 83:405–408
23. Katz SI, Gallin JI, Hertz KC, Fauci AS, Lawley TJ (1977) Erythema elevatum diutinum: skin and systemic manifestations, immunologic studies, and successful treatment with dapsone. Medicine 56:443–455
24. Kavanagh GM, Colaco CB, Bradfield JW, Archer CB (1993) Erythema elevatum diutinum associated with Wegener's granulomatosis and IgA paraproteinemia. J Am Acad Dermatol 28:846–849
25. Lawley TJ, Kubota Y (1990) Vasculitis. Dermatol Clin 8:681–687
26. Laymon CW (1962) Erythema elevatum diutinum. A type of allergic vasculitis. Arch Dermatol 85:62–68
27. Legrain V, Lejean S, Taïeb A, Guillard J-M, Battin J, Maleville J (1991) Infantile acute hemorrhagic edema of the skin. Study of ten cases. J Am Acad Dermatol 24:17–22
28. Lever WF, Schaumburg-Lever G (1990) Histopathology of the skin. JB Lippincott, Philadelphia

29. Lhote F, Cohen P, Généreau T, Gayraud M, Guillevin L (1996) Microscopic polyangiitis. Clinical aspects and treatment. Ann Med Interne 147:165–177
30. Litt JZ (2001) The pocketbook of drug eruptions and interactions. Parthenon, New York
31. Majno G, Joris I (1996) Cells, tissues and disease: principles of general pathology. Blackwell Science, Cambridge
32. Massa MC, Su WPD (1984) Lymphocytic vasculitis: is it a specific clinicopathologic entity? J Cutan Pathol 11:132–139
33. McCalmont CS, McCalmont TH, Jorizzo JL, White WL, Leshin B, Rothberger H (1992) Livedo vasculitis. Vasculitis or thrombotic vasculopathy? Clin Exp Dermatol 17:4–8
34. Mehregan AH, Shapiro L (1971) Angiolymphoid hyperplasia with eosinophilia. Arch Dermatol 103:50–57
35. Mehregan DR, Hall MJ, Gibson LE (1992) Urticarial vasculitis. A histopathologic and clinical review of 72 cases. J Am Acad Dermatol 26:441–448
36. Mraz JP, Newcomer VD (1967) Erythema elevatum diutinum. Presentation of a case and evaluation of laboratory and immunological status. Arch Dermatol 96:235–246
37. Peltz S, Vestey JP, Ferguson A, Hunter JAA, Mclaren K (1993) Disseminated metastatic cutaneous Crohn's disease. Clin Exp Dermatol 18:55–59
38. Peterson WC Jr, Fusaro RM, Goltz RW (1964) Atypical pyogenic granuloma. A case of benign hemangioendotheliosis. Arch Dermatol 90:197–201
39. Pizzo SV, Murray JC, Gonias SL (1986) Atrophie blanche. A disorder associated with defective release of tissue plasminogen activator. Arch Pathol Lab Med 110:517–519
40. Reinauer S, Megahed M, Goerz G, Ruzicka T, Borchard F, Susanto F, Reinauer H (1995) Schönlein-Henoch purpura associated with gastric *Helicobacter pylori* infection. J Am Acad Dermatol 33:876–879
41. Requena L, Sangüeza OP (1997) Cutaneous vascular proliferations. Part II. Hyperplasias and benign neoplasms. J Am Acad Dermatol 37:887–920
42. Rosai J (1982) Angiolymphoid hyperplasia with eosinophilia of the skin. Its nosological position in the spectrum of histiocytoid hemangioma. Am J Dermatopathol 4:175–184
43. Rosai J, Gold J, Landy R (1979) The histiocytoid hemangiomas. A unifying concept embracing several previously described entities of skin, soft tissue, large vessels, bone, and heart. Hum Pathol 10:707–730
44. Roustan G, Sánchez Yus E, Salas C, Simón A (1999) Granuloma faciale with extrafacial lesions. Dermatology 198:79–82
45. Ryan TJ (1992) Cutaneous vasculitis. In: Champion RH, Burton JL, Ebling FJG (eds) Rook/Wilkinson/Ebling textbook of dermatology, 5th edn. Blackwell Scientific, Oxford, pp 1945–1951
46. Sheth AP, Olson JC, Esterly NB (1994) Cutaneous polyarteritis nodosa of childhood. J Am Acad Dermatol 31:561–566
47. Shum DT, Guenther L (1990) Metastatic Crohn's disease. Case report and review of the literature. Arch Dermatol 126:645–648
48. Smoller BR, McNutt NS, Contreras F (1990) The natural history of vasculitis. What the histology tells us about pathogenesis. Arch Dermatol 126:84–89
49. Soter NA, Mihm MC Jr, Gigli I, Dvorak HF, Austen FK (1976) Two distinct cellular patterns in cutaneous necrotizing angiitis. J Invest Dermatol 66:344–350
50. Strutton G, Weedon D, Robertson I (1995) Pustular vasculitis of the hands. J Am Acad Dermatol 32:192–198
51. Tasanen K, Raudasoja R, Kallioinen M, Ranki A (1997) Erythema elevatum diutinum in association with coeliac disease. Br J Dermatol 136:624–627
52. Weedon D (1997) Skin pathology. Churchill Livingstone, Edinburgh
53. Wells GC, Whimster IW (1969) Subcutaneous angiolymphoid hyperplasia with eosinophilia. Br J Dermatol 81:1–15
54. Winkelmann RK (1980) Granulomatous vasculitis. In: Wolff K, Winkelmann RK (eds) Vasculitis. Lloyd-Luke, London, pp 228–239
55. Yiannias JA, El-Azhary RA, Gibson LE (1992) Erythema elevatum diutinum. A clinical and histopathologic study of 13 patients. J Am Acad Dermatol 26:38–44

Chapter 8

Skin Lesions due to Abnormalities in Blood Components

8

Skin lesions may be triggered by transient or permanent abnormalities in the coagulation system or by the existence of antigen–antibody complexes, cryoglobulins, or hereditary deformed red blood cells in the circulation. Both arteries and veins are affected and display fibrinoid wall necrosis and/or thrombosis and extravasated erythrocytes. With the exception of lesions due to mixed cryoglobulinemia, there are very few perivascular inflammatory cells. The vascular damage gives rise to hemorrhagic, vesicular/bullous skin lesions, which may be followed by ulceration or infarctions. The lesions are dispersed or localized. To this group belong: disseminated intravascular coagulation, thrombotic-thrombocytopenic purpura, different kinds of hypercoagulability of minor severity, skin necrosis due to treatment with warfarin, cryoglobulinemia, and hereditary hemoglobulinopathies.

8.1 The Normal Coagulation/Fibrinolytic Balance in the Coagulation System

Under normal conditions anticoagulant forces prevail over procoagulant mechanisms. However, low-grade intravascular coagulation is a physiologic and continuous phenomenon required in the healing process of the many small injuries that occur on the endothelium due to the circulatory stress. Minute endothelial erosions are rapidly healed under the cover of a thin primary clot, and the healed lesions are as swiftly cleared by fibrinolytic activity.

External and internal damage to vessel walls triggers a series of enzymatic activities ending up with the formation of a clot. At the injured area, subendothelial collagen is exposed. Within minutes thrombocytes adhere to the collagen surface and at the same time become activated. The normally disc-like thrombocytes become spherical and release substances that attract more platelets. Tightly attached to each other, they cover the area. This phenomenon is called platelet aggregation and represents the primary hemostatic plug, which temporarily stops the bleeding, but does not contain enough fibrin to be reliable in the long run. At the endothelial injury, the tissue factor, a membrane protein present in the perivascular bed, is released. Together with activated coagulation factor VII, it starts the coagulation process and thrombin is formed. Thrombin initiates further platelet aggregation and converts soluble fibrinogen into fibrin. The latter is deposited in the primary plug as polymerized fibrin and gives rise to the strong permanent hemostatic plug. At this stage tissue plasminogen activator (t-PA), also produced by endothelial cells, is mobilized and converts plasminogen to plasmin, a proteolytic enzyme, which degrades fibrin. The fibrinolytic activity prevents further propagation of the thrombus. When an intravascular clot is formed both plasminogen and its activator bind to the clot. Plasminogen and activator closely contact each other and plasminogen is converted to plasmin. As long as plasmin is bound to fibrin it cannot be inactivated. As the fibrin clot dissolves, the plasmin is set free and is again inactivated.

8.2 Disseminated Intravascular Coagulation

Disseminated intravascular coagulation (DIC), in children called purpura fulminans, is a severe and life-threatening disorder. It starts with the release of thrombin in the circulation and gives rise to abnormal coagulation tests. The widespread intravascular coagulation consumes all factors involved in the coagulation (i.e., prothrombin, factors V and VIII, fibrinogen and thrombocytes) and this process forms the basis for hemorrhages, which are very difficult to treat. DIC most commonly occurs as a complication of obstetric conditions, major trauma, malignant neoplasia, and sepsis. Involvement of the skin gives rise to hemorrhages, large bullae and infarction.

8.2.1 Example

Case 1. Disseminated Intravascular Coagulation

An 82-year-old woman was admitted to hospital because of generalized purpura, ecchymoses, and hemorrhagic bullae. Coagulation studies indicated disseminated intravascular coagulation. She was given heparin and recovered temporarily, but died 3 weeks later. The underlying disease was never discovered.

A biopsy specimen from a bullous lesion included subcutaneous tissue. A thick layer of fibrin, erythrocytes and inflammatory cells replaced the epidermis and the upper half of the dermis. In the deep dermis and subcutaneous tissue there was conspicuous extravasation of red blood cells. Many venules, but also some arterioles and capillaries, were totally or partially occluded by fibrin thrombi. In the subcutis two large veins were involved. The vessel walls were preserved and surrounded by only a sparse number of inflammatory cells, mainly lymphocytes (Fig. 8.1).

8.3 Thrombotic-Thrombocytopenic Purpura/ Hemolytic-Uremic (TTP/HUS) Syndrome

This syndrome may be hereditary or acquired, chronic or acute. The acute acquired form is serious and life threatening. Thrombi obstruct arterioles, capillaries and venules over wide areas, and in many organs. The process starts with aggregation of platelets. Coagulation tests are normal. The unrestrained thrombus formation consumes thrombocytes and gives rise to thrombocytopenia, hemorrhages and infarctions. TTP has been described as a disease most often seen in adult women and is accompanied by fever, thrombocytopenia, microangiopathy, hemolytic anemia, transient neurologic deficits and renal failure; HUS is a disease most often seen in children and is accompanied by thrombocytopenia, microangiopathy, hemolytic anemia and renal failure, but without neurologic symptoms and fever. In children the TTP/HUS syndrome is mostly provoked by gastrointestinal infections, and in adults by various kinds of infections and drugs. Today the distinction between TTP and HUS is considered to be less sharp. For example, one or several accompanying symptoms may be missing in TTP and patients with HUS may have fever and neurologic dysfunction (Aster 1999). TTP only (i.e., without accompanying symptoms) may be caused by drugs, the most common of which is heparin, and may even occur in association with malignancy.

Drugs, such as heparin, quinine, quinidine, penicillins and thiazide diuretics, may induce thrombocytopenia by means of the type II cytotoxic hypersensitivity reaction (Sect. 4.3.2). The antigen, a metabolite of the drug, binds to the surface of the thrombocytes. In the presence of complement, antibodies directed against the surface antigen kill the thrombocytes and give rise to thrombocytopenia and, possibly, bleedings. Some patients with thrombocytopenia, due to treatment with heparin, simultaneously develop TTP. In these cases investigations have shown that IgG antibodies against a complex of heparin and platelet factor 4 have developed. The pathogenic IgG binds to Fc receptors on the platelets whereby platelets become activated and produce procoagulant microparticles followed by venous as well as arterial thrombosis and infarctions (Warkentin et al. 1994; Warkentin and Kenton 1996). Other drugs are also known to occasionally cause TTP; for example quinine, cyclosporine and mitomycin C (Cines et al. 2000).

8.3.1 Examples

Case 2. TTP Caused by Furosemide

A 79-year-old woman was hospitalized because of cardiac failure and treated with the diuretic furosemide. During the treatment she developed discoloration on the dorsal aspect of the feet and also a bulla in the same area on the right foot. Thrombocytes fell to 36×10^9/l (reference range 150–400×10^9/l). C3, C4, and cryoglobulins were negative. She recovered after withdrawal of the drug.

A biopsy specimen was taken from the dorsal aspect of the right foot and included most of the dermis. In the papillary and upper dermis, groups of small vessels were occluded by erythrocyte thrombi and surrounded by many erythrocytes, but no or very few inflammatory cells. In the middle part of the dermis, there were scattered larger venules filled with densely packed and disintegrating erythrocytes. Small thrombosed vessels were best observed in PAS-stained sections (Fig. 8.2).

Case 3. TTP in Association with Lymphoma

A 71-year-old man had for a full year noticed dark blue patches on the hands and feet, and on the fingers and toes even small ulcerations, which healed spontaneously. Over the previous month his skin condition had deteriorated. When he presented he had conspicuous and deep necrotic lesions on the hands and feet. It was found that the patient was suffering from a centroblastic-centrocytic lymphoma with massive involvement

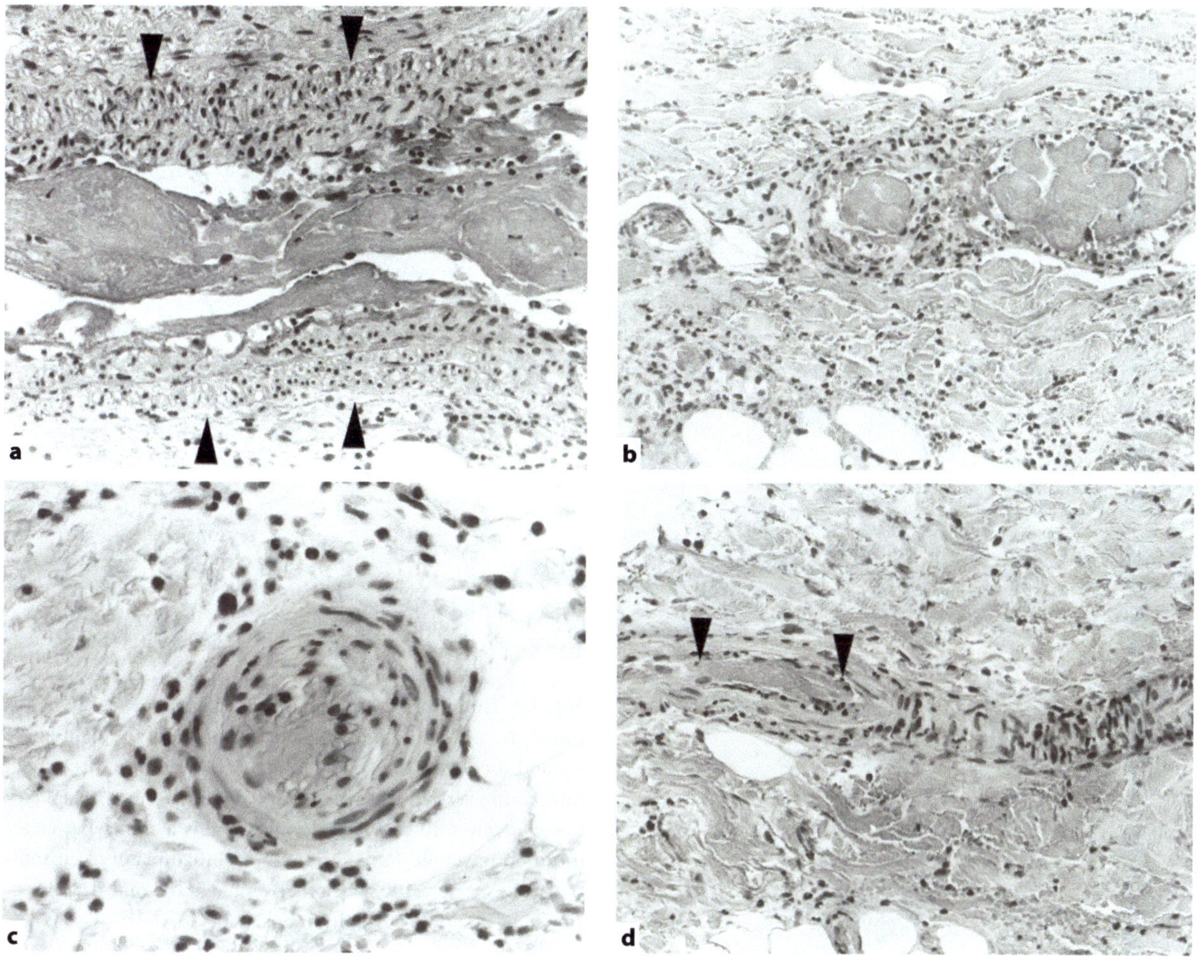

Fig. 8.1 Disseminated intravascular coagulation. **a** A large and longitudinally cut vein located in the subcutaneous tissue is obstructed by a fibrin thrombus (*arrowheads* vessel wall); ×200. **b** Thrombosed veins of different size at the dermal–subcutaneous interface; ×200. **c** An arteriole at the interface is obstructed by fibrin and erythrocytes; ×400. **d** Horizontally running thrombosed arteriole. Between the *arrowheads* the thrombus is exposed; ×200. H&E

of the bone marrow, lymph nodes, and spleen. He also had thrombocytopenia with the lowest value 40×10^9/l. There were no cryoglobulins and no circulating antigen–antibody complexes. The necrotic distal phalanx of the right little finger underwent spontaneous amputation. Other lesions healed after treatment, which included splenectomy. The weight of the spleen was close to 4.5 kg.

A biopsy specimen was taken from a non-ulcerated lesion on the left ring finger. The specimen comprised dermis and the uppermost part of the subcutaneous tissue. The epidermis was normal. In the dermis and upper subcutis, different kinds of vessels were obliterated by fibrin thrombi, or engorged with erythrocytes. In some of the vessels, fibrinoid wall necrosis was also observed. There were patchy sparse interstitial infiltrates of lymphocytes, neutrophils and eosinophils. Extravasation of red blood cells was conspicuous (Fig. 8.3).

8.3.2 Comment

Probably the pathway differs according to the cause of the TTP. Investigations have shown that in some patients with a chronic relapsing form of TTP/HUS, von Willebrand factor (vWF) seems to be involved (see Glossary). This factor is normally secreted from endothelial cells as ultralarge sticky molecules and is crucial for the adherence of platelets to collagen and other surfaces in the coagulation process. Normally large molecules are degraded by vWF-cleaving prote-

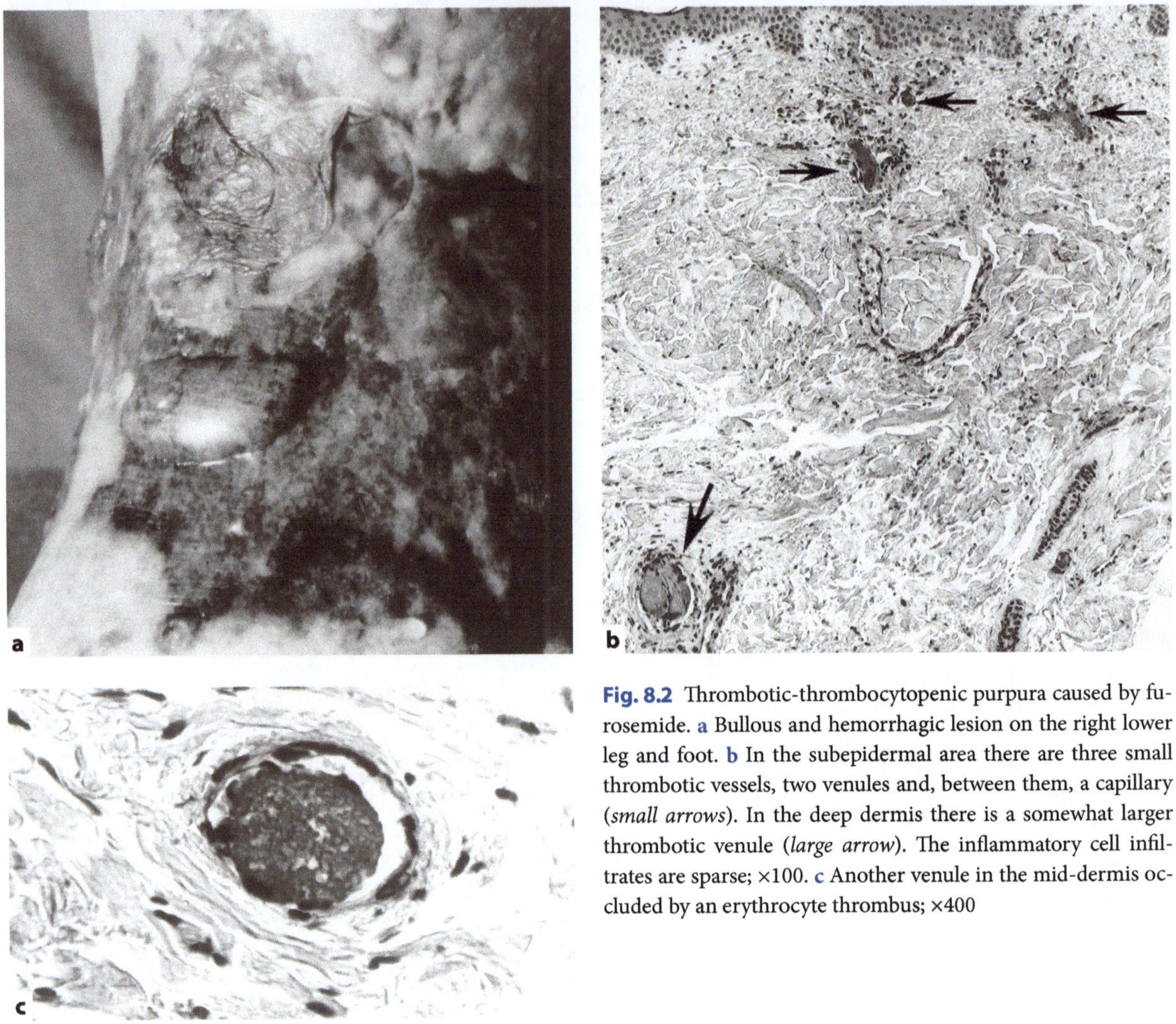

Fig. 8.2 Thrombotic-thrombocytopenic purpura caused by furosemide. **a** Bullous and hemorrhagic lesion on the right lower leg and foot. **b** In the subepidermal area there are three small thrombotic vessels, two venules and, between them, a capillary (*small arrows*). In the deep dermis there is a somewhat larger thrombotic venule (*large arrow*). The inflammatory cell infiltrates are sparse; ×100. **c** Another venule in the mid-dermis occluded by an erythrocyte thrombus; ×400

ase and are not found in the circulation. In patients with the chronic hereditary form of TTP/HUS syndrome extremely large polymeric forms of vWF may be found in the plasma and are therefore suspected of being involved in the disease. A study of patients with hereditary and acquired forms of chronic TTP/HUS showed that vWF-cleaving protease is lacking in the hereditary form, and that in patients with the acquired form the protease activity is blocked by IgG antibody (Cines et al. 2000). An acquired form of vWF-cleaving protease deficiency would be a plausible cause in Case 3.

8.4 Hypercoagulability of Minor Severity

With hypercoagulability is meant any alteration of the coagulation pathways that predisposes to thrombosis. The disorders may be primary or genetic and secondary or acquired. Inherited forms are due to mutations in the factor V gene or to lack of an anticoagulant (antithrombin III, protein C, or protein S). Acquired disorders are, among others, heparin-induced TTP (described above) and the antiphospholipid antibody syndrome (lupus anticoagulant syndrome) that may occur in patients suffering from autoimmune diseases. Sometimes concurrent factors cooperate (Sect. 8.4.2 and 8.5).

8.4.1 Examples

Case 4. Hypercoagulability

A 58-year-old woman at the age of 50 years had had a thrombus in the vena axillaris and was prescribed

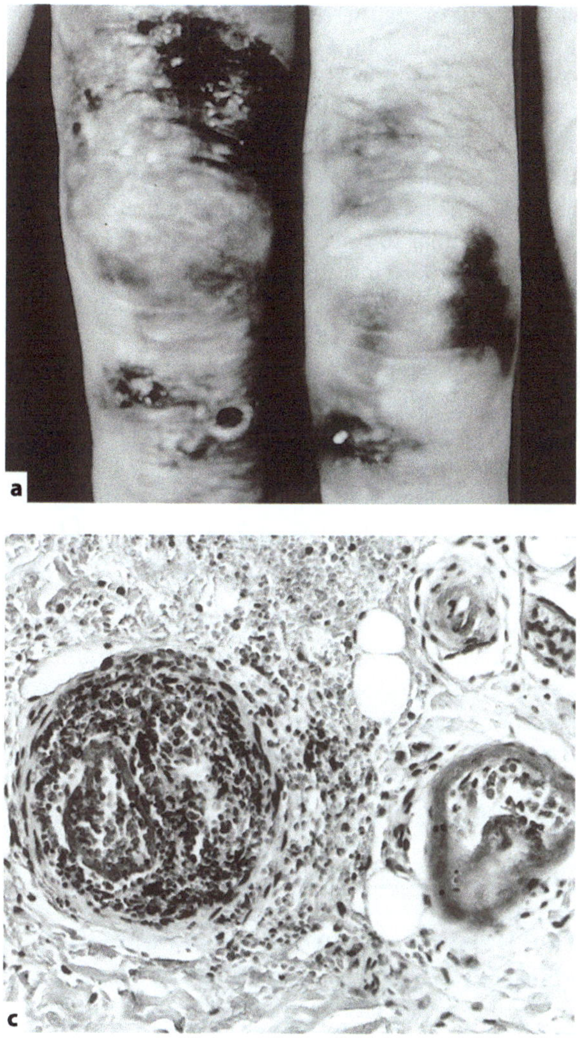

Fig. 8.3 Thrombotic-thrombocytopenic purpura associated with lymphoma. a Multiple hemorrhagic ulcerations on fingers. b In the papillary dermis there are two thrombosed capillaries (*arrows*) close two a dilated venule which contains a small aggregate of erythrocytes; ×400. c Two affected vessels in the subcutaneous tissue. The larger vessel is an arteriole stuffed with erythrocytes; the smaller has a totally necrotic wall. There is perivascular bleeding; ×200

continuous anticoagulant treatment with warfarin. At the age of 57 years, high blood pressure and seriously impaired renal function of uncertain origin were diagnosed. One kidney was completely silent, while the other one recovered one-third of normal capacity after surgical reconstruction of the obstructed renal artery. About 2 years after the operation she presented with bluish-red discoloration of both soles and complained of pain in the feet appearing after a short suspension of the warfarin treatment.

A biopsy specimen was taken from the edge of the foot and revealed scattered small thrombotic venules without necrosis or inflammatory cell infiltrates. Most of them were located in the deep dermis. The thrombi were easily recognized in PAS-stained sections, but difficult to perceive in sections stained with H&E (Fig. 8.4).

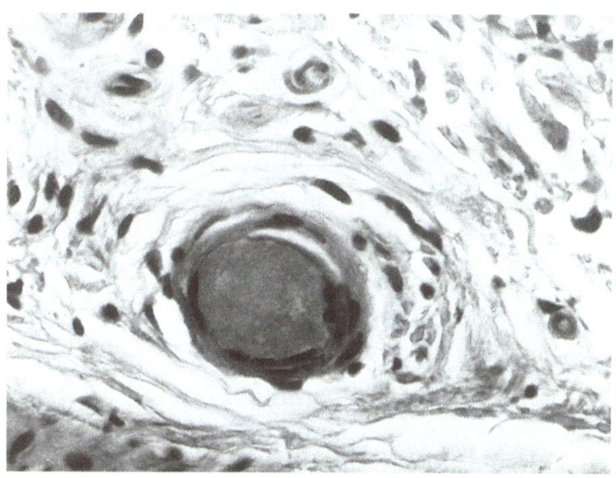

Fig. 8.4 Hypercoagulability. A small thrombotic vessel in the deep dermis with a sparse number of perivascular inflammatory cells; H&E, ×400

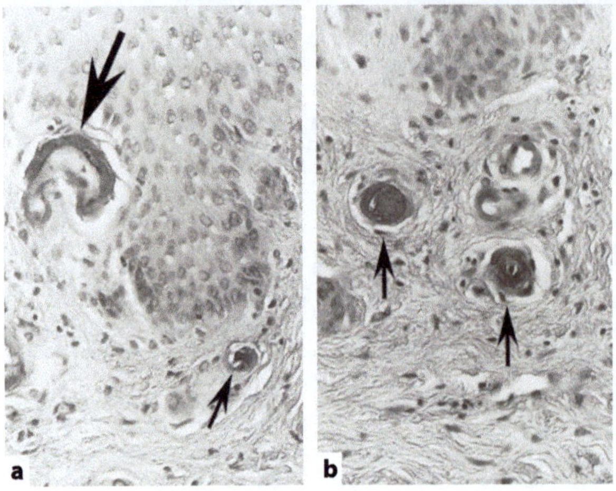

Fig. 8.5 Hypercoagulability. **a** A necrotic venule is seen at the top of a dermal papilla (*large arrow*). Below the rete ridge there is an occluded capillary (*small arrow*). **b** Two thrombotic venules in the subepidermal area (*arrows*). PAS, ×200

Case 5. Hypercoagulability

A 43-year-old woman suffered from severe asthma and was under continuous treatment with high doses of corticosteroids. For about a year and a half she had had recurrent erythematous and painful swellings on the lower legs and feet. There was also a small ulcer on the right sole.

Two biopsy specimens were taken from the sole at an interval of 1 month. They showed the same histopathologic pattern and involved both the dermis and subcutaneous tissue. In these locations there were thrombi and fibrinoid wall necrosis in small vessels (venules and capillaries) without any reaction or only a sparse amount of perivascular lymphocytes.

The result of routine coagulation analysis was normal. However, further investigation revealed a decreased value for tissue activator of plasminogen (t-PA) and an increased value for its inhibitor (t-PAI) (Fig. 8.5).

8.4.2
Comment

The results of laboratory investigations in Case 4 are not known. However, the occurrence of a vena axillaris thrombus at a relatively early age and the history of severe renal damage indicate that this patient probably suffered from a primary type of hypercoagulability, most likely protein C deficiency. Protein C is the key component in the anticoagulant system, which normally balances the coagulation system (Dahlbäck 2000). Without continuous anticoagulation therapy these patients run the risk of getting venous and/or arterial thrombi in different organs, for example the kidneys, giving rise to renal failure and/or hypertension. The lesions on the soles were interpreted as a consequence of the interrupted warfarin treatment.

Cases similar to Case 5 have been described. Thus Pizzo et al. (1986) investigated eight patients, thought to have *atrophie blanche*, with respect to their release of t-PA. They found that all patients had defective release of t-PA from blood vessels. Furthermore, in six patients diagnosed with *atrophie blanche* markedly elevated levels of serum fibrinopeptide A (a cleavage product of thrombin) were found, suggesting a thrombogenic state (McCalmont et al. 1992). During the 1990s elevation of the plasma concentration of t-PAI has been a common finding in patients with thrombotic disease and has therefore been the subject of much interest and investigation. However, so far the importance of elevated t-PAI values in thrombotic disease has not definitely been proved. Probably concurrent factors are involved (Wiman 1996). In Case 5 it is possible that a combination of a genetic variant of t-PAI and an extrinsic factor (high doses of corticosteroids) caused the thrombotic state.

8.5
Skin Necrosis Induced by Treatment with Warfarin

Skin necrosis induced by oral treatment with the anticoagulant warfarin is a serious complication. One or several lesions occur during the first 10 days after the treatment is started. Widespread thrombosis in the microvasculature gives rise to necrosis of the skin and underlying fat tissue, which may require surgery and even amputation. The lesions, which are well demarcated and erythematous, are preceded by paresthesia, or a sensation of pressure. Common sites are the breasts, buttocks and thighs. An initial large loading dose of warfarin given to patients with hereditary protein C deficiency may give rise to a transient hypercoagulable state, which is thought to trigger the phenomenon (Chan et al. 2000).

8.6
Cryoglobulinemia

Cryoglobulins are immunoglobulins which lack the carbohydrate groups present in normal immunoglobulins. This molecular difference probably explains the unique solubility characteristics of cryoglobulins:

Table 8.1 Cryoblobulins

Type of cryoglobulin	Components	Characteristics
Type I	Monoclonal IgM or IgG	May be associated with malignant diseases of the immune system and essential cryoglobulinemia
Type II, mixed	Polyclonal IgG and monoclonal IgM rheumatoid factor	Form circulating antigen–antibody complexes. May be associated with malignant diseases of the immune system, autoimmune diseases, hepatitis C virus infection, and essential cryoglobulinemia
Type III, mixed	Polyclonal IgG and polyclonal IgM rheumatoid factor	Form circulating antigen–antibody complexes. May be associated with autoimmune diseases, hepatitis C virus infection, and a variety of other infectious diseases

they are able to precipitate from plasma or serum on cooling and redissolve on warming. Small amounts of cryoglobulins are continuously produced together with ordinary immunoglobulins, but they are mostly rapidly taken care of in the liver by means of hepatocellular receptors for deglycosylated glycoproteins. However, trace amounts of cryoglobulins may appear in the serum of healthy individuals (Levo 1980).

There are three types of cryoglobulins. Type I consists of monoclonal cryoglobulins, type II consists of polyclonal IgG and monoclonal IgM rheumatoid factor (antiglobulin), and type III consists of polyclonal IgG and polyclonal IgM rheumatoid factor. Thus types II and III are mixed cryoglobulins and may form circulating antigen–antibody complexes (Pawlotsky et al. 1995). Types I and II occur in patients suffering from plasma cell neoplasia, malignant lymphoma, or leukemia, but also in patients without evidence of underlying disease; in such patients the condition is called essential cryoglobulinemia. Types II and III may be associated with autoimmune diseases. Finally, type III is found in a variety of infectious diseases (Table 8.1). In monoclonal cryoglobulinemia vascular lesions in the skin are due to intravascular precipitates, which can be local or widespread and give rise to ulcerations and necrosis of the same kind as those described above in Case 3 (where cryoglobulins were not found). In mixed cryoglobulinemia circulating antigen–antibody complexes may cause neutrophilic venular vasculitis (leukocytoclastic vasculitis). However, in type II, the requirements for both precipitation and neutrophilic venular vasculitis exist which may provoke a mixed histopathologic pattern as seen in Case 6, described below.

Investigations have shown that many cases of cryoglobulinemia types II and III, but not type I, are associated with chronic hepatitis C virus infection (Pawlotsky et al. 1995).

8.6.1 Example

Case 6. Cryoglobulinemia

A 41-year-old woman had suffered from recurrent tender lesions on the lower legs for 4 years. She presented with large, fresh, infiltrated, erythematous and purpuric nodules of up to 10 mm diameter on the lower legs. There were also older ulcerated lesions on the ankles. A knife biopsy specimen was taken from a fresh non-ulcerated nodule. Laboratory investigation had revealed transient cryoglobulinemia, cryofibrinogenemia, and kappa chains in the urine; however more detailed analysis of the cryoglobulins was never done

The specimen included the whole dermis and a generous piece of subcutaneous tissue. The most important changes were seen at the dermal/subcutaneous interface. Many different-sized venules, small veins, and scattered arterioles were affected. Some veins (venules) were partially or totally occluded by fibrin or erythrocyte thrombi without wall necrosis; in others the wall was totally necrotic or diffusely penetrated by red blood cells, lymphocytes or neutrophils. Involved arterioles were dilated and contained a thrombus made up of disintegrating erythrocytes and nuclear fragments. Interstitial inflammatory cell infiltrates consisted mainly of lymphocytes, but there were also patchy dense infiltrates of neutrophils, and a fair number of histiocytes and mast cells. Only scattered eosinophils were observed. There was massive extravasation of erythrocytes (Fig. 8.6).

8.7 Hereditary Hemoglobinopathies

Sickle cell anemia, congenital spherocytosis and thalassemia minor in adults may give rise to leg ulcers. The

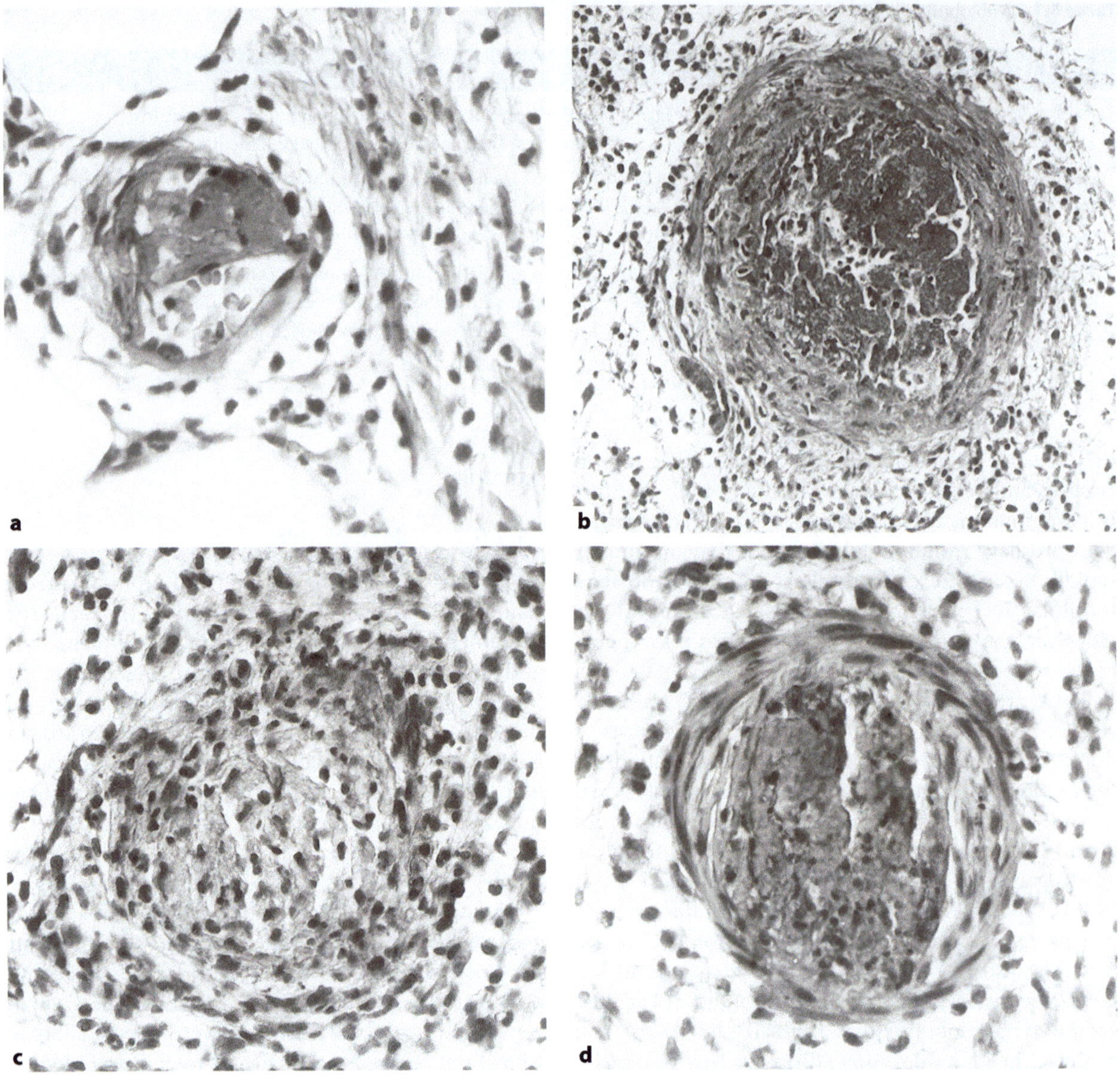

Fig. 8.6 Cryoglobulinemia. **a** A venule is partly obstructed by a fibrin thrombus; ×500. **b** A small vein is occluded by an erythrocyte thrombus and surrounded by a moderately dense infiltrate of lymphocytes; ×250. **c** Totally necrotic vessel filled with disintegrating red blood cells, neutrophils and nuclear fragments; ×500. **d** An arteriole is densely packed with disintegrating erythrocytes and nuclear fragments; ×500. H&E

abnormally shaped erythrocytes aggregate in small vessels and give rise to thrombi and wall necrosis.

8.7.1 Example

Case 7. Thalassemia Minor

The patient, a 31-year-old Greek woman, had no previous illnesses and did not use drugs. For 2 years she had noticed increasing pigmentation and small ulcerations on the lower legs and the dorsal aspect of the feet. She also complained of pain in the lower legs on exertion. When she presented there were some ten superficial and conspicuously walled-off ulcers from 2 to 10 mm in diameter, and white, atrophic and irregularly shaped scars on the dorsal and lateral aspects of the feet. Brownish discoloration and petechiae were also observed on the lower legs and feet. The clinical pattern was very similar to that described as atrophie

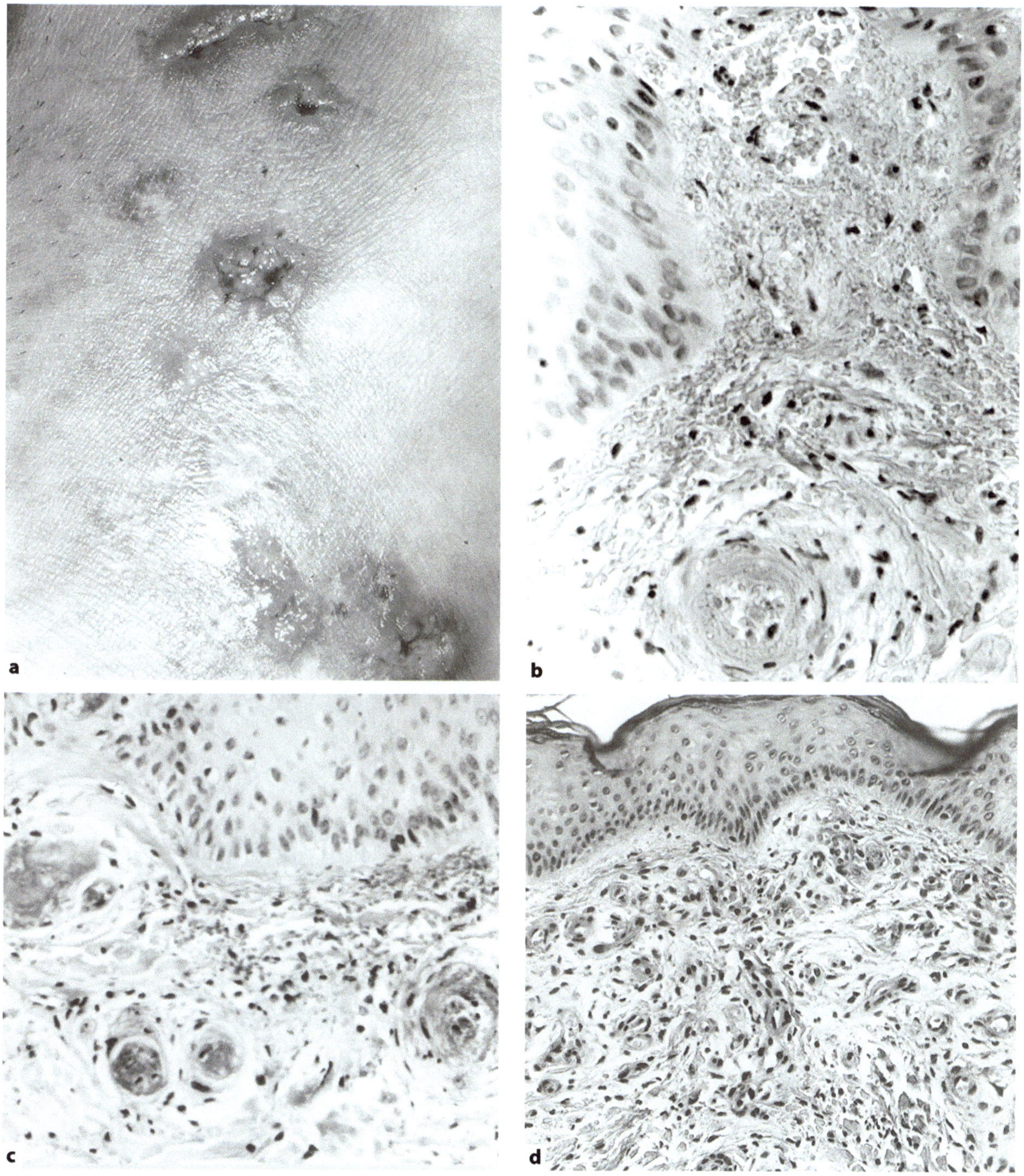

Fig. 8.7 Thalassemia minor. **a** Small walled-off ulcers and white scars on the dorsal aspect of the foot. **b** There is a fresh hemorrhage in a dermal papilla and below in the upper dermis a necrotic vessel filled with erythrocytes; ×400. **c** Several affected venules in the subepidermal area; ×250. **d** This section shows prominent capillary proliferation (angiogenesis); ×200 (a and c reproduced from Berge et al. 1970, with permission)

blanche. Laboratory investigations revealed that the patient was suffering from thalassemia minor (Berge et al. 1970).

A biopsy specimen was taken from a fresh purpuric lesion on the foot. The whole dermis was included, but not subcutaneous tissue. In the papillae and the subepidermal area and at the sweat gland level there were scattered groups of small vessels that contained fibrin or erythrocyte thrombi and/or showed partial or complete fibrinoid wall necrosis. The epidermis overlying involved vessels was flat and showed signs of imminent necrosis. However, in the subepidermal compartment there were also small areas with proliferating capillaries. Extravasation of red blood cells was conspicuous, but inflammatory cells were sparse and mainly lymphocytes (Fig. 8.7).

References

1. Aster J (1999) Red cells and bleeding disorders. In: Cotran RS, Kumar V, Collins T (eds) Robbins pathologic basis of disease. W.B. Saunders Company, Philadelphia, pp 636–643
2. Berge G, Brehmer-Andersson E, Rorsman H (1970) Thalassemia minor and painful ulcers of lower extremities. Acta Derm Venereol 50:125–128
3. Chan YC, Valenti D, Mansfield AO, Stansby G (2000) Warfarin induced skin necrosis. Br J Surg 87:266–272
4. Cines DB, Konkle BA, Furlan M (2000) Thrombotic thrombocytopenic purpura. A paradigm shift? Thromb Haemost 84:528–535
5. Dahlbäck B (2000) Blood coagulation. Lancet 355:1627–1632
6. Levo Y (1980) Nature of cryoglobulinaemia. Lancet 1(8163):285–287
7. McCalmont CS, McCalmont TH, Jorizzo JL, White WL, Leshin B, Rothberger H (1992) Livedo vasculitis: vasculitis or thrombotic vasculopathy? Clin Exp Dermatol 17:4–8
8. Pawlotsky J-M, Dhumeaux D, Bagot M (1995) Hepatitis C virus in dermatology. A review. Arch Dermatol 131:1185–1193
9. Pizzo SV, Murray JC, Gonias SL (1986) Atrophie blanche. A disorder associated with defective release of tissue plasminogen activator. Arch Pathol Lab Med 110:517–519
10. Warkentin TE, Kelton JG (1996) A 14-year study of heparin-induced thrombocytopenia. Am J Med 101:502–507
11. Warkentin TE, Hayward CPM, Boshkov LK, Santos AV, Sheppard J-AI, Bode AP, Kelton JG (1994) Sera from patients with heparin-induced thrombocytopenia generate platelet-derived microparticles with procoagulant activity: an explanation for the thrombotic complications of heparin-induced thrombocytopenia. Blood 84:3691–3699
12. Wiman B (1996) Plasminogen activator inhibitor 1 in thrombotic disease. Curr Opin Hematol 3:372–378

Chapter 9

Arteriosclerosis in the Skin

9

In the distal part of the lower legs arteriosclerosis in the deeper vessels may give rise to severe pain with or without nodules or ulceration. For obvious reasons, the most common variant of arteriosclerosis seen in punch biopsy specimens is arteriolosclerosis affecting arterioles and capillaries at the dermal subcutaneous interface. In specimens including deeper parts of subcutaneous tissue, even small affected arteries may be observed.

9.1 Arteriolosclerosis

There are two types of lesions: *hyaline* and *hyperplastic* arteriolosclerosis.

9.1.1 Hyaline Arteriolosclerosis

Hyaline arteriolosclerosis is thought to be due to a combination of leakage of plasma components through the endothelium and increased matrix produced by smooth muscle cells. The process starts beneath the endothelium and gradually extends to replace all the normal structures of the wall. When the process is active, the wall (pink in H&E-stained sections) is PAS-positive, but at the end-stage becomes PAS-negative. The vessel becomes thickened and tortuous, and its lumen narrow and even obliterated (Fig. 9.1a,b). Calcification is not seen. Hyaline arteriolosclerosis can be seen in all organs and tissues in elderly persons even without hypertension, but is accentuated by both benign and malignant hypertension.

9.1.2 Hyperplastic Arteriolosclerosis

Hyperplastic arteriolosclerosis is mostly related to severe hypertension. The wall is markedly thickened and the lumen is narrowed. The intima becomes hyaline, but may in the early phase show cell proliferation and infiltrates of lymphocytes. The media is composed of concentric rings of smooth muscle cells, some of which have a vacuolated or foamy cytoplasm due to accumulation of lipids. Rarely fibrinoid necrosis may appear. Deposition of calcium is not seen (Fig. 9.1c–e).

9.2 Arteriosclerosis

Arteriosclerosis may be seen in arteries in the deep subcutaneous tissue. In addition to the findings in hyperplastic arteriolosclerosis areas of calcification may be observed (Fig. 9.2a).

9.3 Examples

Case 1. Hyaline Arteriolosclerosis

A 58-year-old male suffered from malignant hypertension and had extremely painful leg ulcers and areas of brownish-red discoloration on the lower legs, slightly above the ankles.

A knife biopsy specimen was taken from a non-ulcerated area. A small brim of subcutaneous tissue was included. Along the dermal subcutaneous interface arterioles and capillaries with thickened walls and severely narrowed or obliterated lumina were observed. In H&E-stained sections the slightly concentrically laminated walls had a hyaline, pink appearance and contained some scattered, elongated or rounded nuclei. Hyaline material was in some areas strongly PAS-positive. There were no or very few perivascular lymphocytes. No normal arterioles could be identified. In the upper dermis extravasated erythrocytes and a sparse number of lymphocytes were seen (Fig. 9.1a,b).

Case 2. Hyperplastic Arteriolosclerosis[1]

A 56-year-old woman, who had been on treatment for hypertension for a long time, had recently acquired a painful ulcer on the lower leg.

1 Cases 2, 3 and 4: by courtesy of Dr. Mari-Anne Hedblad, Karolinska University Hospital, Stockholm, Sweden

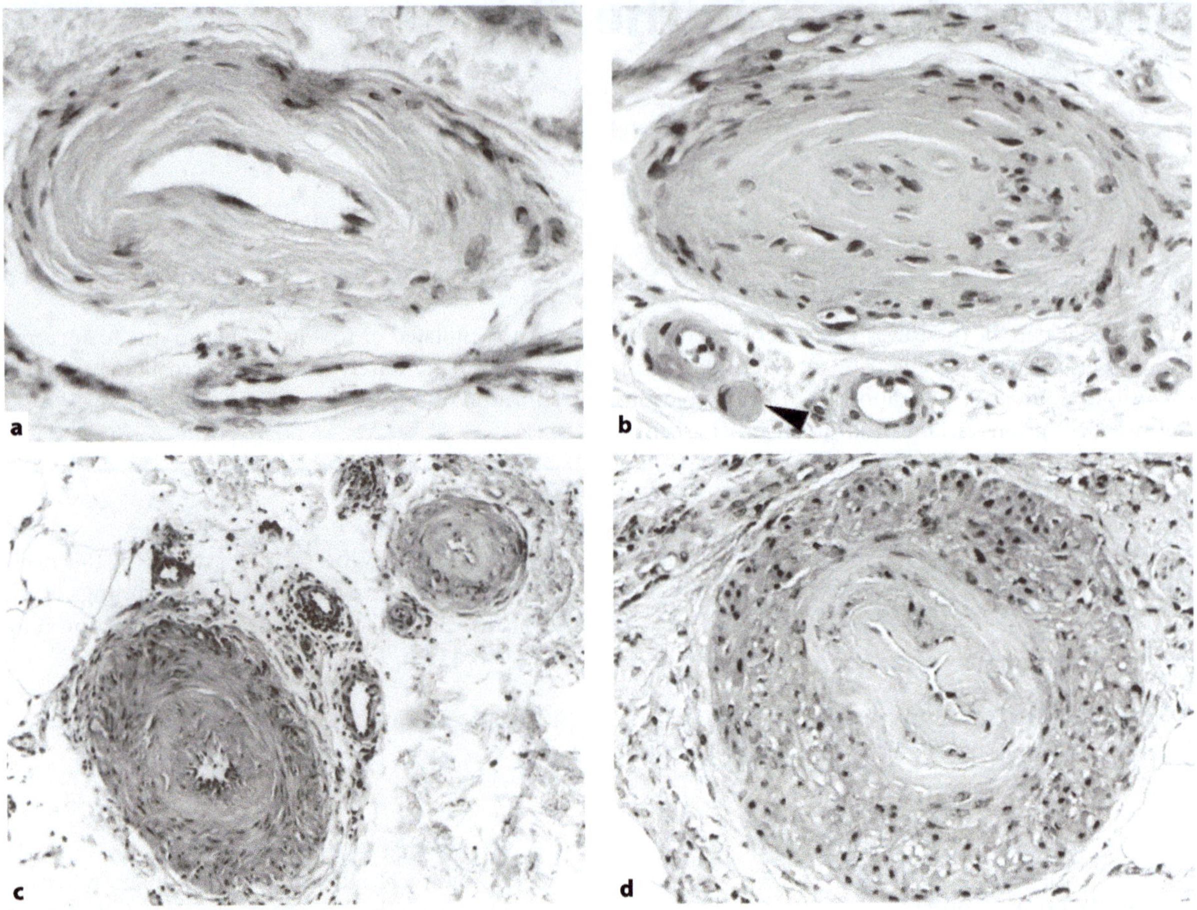

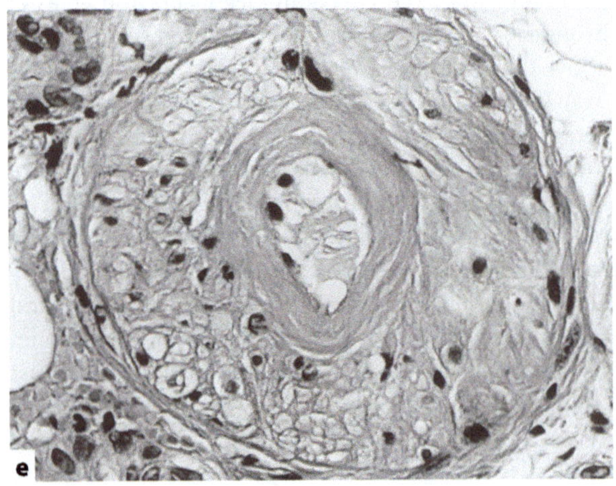

Fig. 9.1 Arteriolosclerosis. **a** A hyaline arteriole in the deep dermis has a thickened wall and narrowed lumen; ×300. **b** Another vessel is entirely occluded. The *arrowhead* indicates an obstructed capillary; ×300. **c** Hyperplastic arterioles in the upper subcutis with thickened muscular media, hyaline intima and narrow lumen; ×125. **d** A hyperplastic arteriole in subcutis. The intima is conspicuously thickened and hyaline. The media is diffusely infiltrated with lymphocytes and many muscle cells are vacuolated; ×250. **e** In this arteriole the changes in the media are more advanced. It is mainly hyaline, but contains an aggregate of vacuolated cells and scattered lymphocytes; ×400. H&E

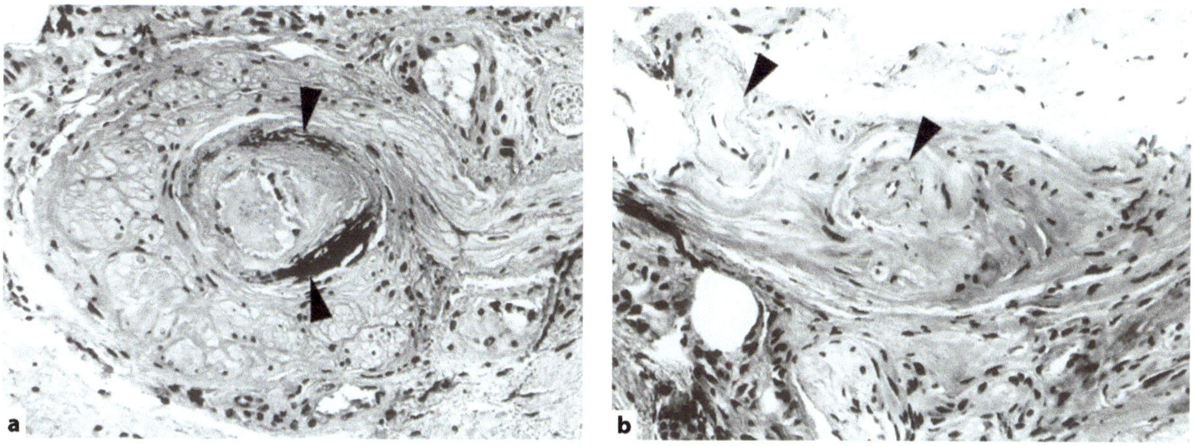

Fig. 9.2 Arteriosclerosis and arteriolosclerosis. **a** A small arteriosclerotic artery in the subcutaneous tissue. The intima is irregularly thickened and the lumen narrowed. The black deposits between the intima and media are calcium (*arrowheads*). The media is thickened and contains mainly vacuolated cells. **b** At the subcutaneous–dermal border this vessel ends up in a tortuous hyaline arteriole, cut at two levels (*arrowheads*). H&E, ×200

Three biopsy specimens taken over a short period of time showed principally the same histopathologic pattern. In the upper part of subcutis there were one or two arterioles with hypertrophic muscular media, thickened hyaline intima and narrowed lumen. Sparse lymphocytes were observed in the dermis. The epidermis was normal (Fig. 9.1c,d).

Case 3. Hyperplastic Arteriolosclerosis

A 72-year-old man with hypertension had for some months suffered from a very painful ulcer on the lower leg.

A biopsy specimen included a fair part of subcutaneous tissue, which contained a large arteriole. The vessel had a thick hyaline intima and a conspicuously thickened and hyaline media, in which an aggregate of lipophages and scattered lymphocytes were seen (Fig. 9.1e).

Case 4. Arteriosclerosis

A 76-year-old woman presented with a painful therapy-resistant ulcer on the lateral aspect of the lower leg. A knife biopsy specimen was taken from the margin of the ulcer.

The material included a large part of subcutaneous tissue, in the deepest part of which a small artery was observed. The lumen of the artery was partly obliterated by an irregular thickening of the hyaline intima. Between the intima and the media calcifications were observed. The media was conspicuously thickened and contained macrophages with rich, vacuolated/foamy cytoplasm. The vessel could be followed through the specimen and ended up as a hyaline arteriole at the dermal-subcutaneous interface (Fig. 9.2).

9.4 Differential Diagnosis

- Lesions due to a hypercoagulability state (Sect. 8.4) have to be distinguished from hyaline arteriolosclerosis in the active PAS-positive phase.
- Emboli from an atheromatous plaque are rarely seen in small arteries in subcutis. The embolus differs from changes developed at the place by containing elliptic clefts after dissolved cholesterol crystals and scattered giant cells of foreign body type.

10 Thromboangiitis Obliterans

Thromboangiitis obliterans, or Buerger disease, is an inflammatory, progressive disease which starts in the distal parts of the extremities and affects small and medium-sized arteries and veins. In 1879, Winiwarter described the first case and in 1908, Buerger published his first observations on a group of such patients (Joyce 1990). The mechanism is unknown. However, it is suspected to be an autoimmune reaction, obviously triggered by smoking (Joyce 1990).

10.1 Clinical Appearance

The patient suffering from Buerger disease is most often a man and a heavy smoker. It starts before the age of 35 years. Initial symptoms are ischemia and claudication of both legs and hands, which start distally and progress towards the head. The disease is chronic and the course rapid. After a few months to 1 or 2 years repeated partial or total infarctions of the extremities occur; it is thus a seriously disabling disease (Joyce 1990).

10.2 Histopathologic Appearance

Recurrent episodes of inflammation befall segments of small and medium-sized arteries and veins, mostly confined to vessels in the areas mentioned above. Fresh lesions start with a fibrin thrombus and characteristic dense focal infiltrates of neutrophils (microabscesses) in the thrombus. Also a few giant cells are commonly present. When the acute phase subsides, the thrombus becomes organized and lymphocytes and macrophages prevail over neutrophils. Finally the lesions heal with fibrosis and obstruction of the involved section. In contrast to arteriosclerosis, both arteries and veins are affected, there are no calcifications and in arteries the inner elastic membrane is preserved. It is said that the process begins in arteries and then spreads to veins and sometimes also to nerves (Crawford 1977). Typically, old lesions predominate and sometimes no fresh lesions are found in an amputation specimen. If lesions are widespread the condition may give rise to infarction and necessitate amputation.

10.3 Example

Case 1. Thromboangiitis Obliterans[1]

The patient, born in 1921, had undergone finger amputation at least five times between 1978 and 1981, and before that both lower legs had been amputated.

Pieces for histologic investigation were taken from amputated fingers or parts of fingers on seven occasions. In all specimens several different-sized arteries and veins with organized thrombi were observed. Acute inflammation was seen only in one specimen, where two veins were engaged. No connections between affected veins and arteries, or engagement of nerves were seen (Fig. 10.1).

References

1. Crawford T (1977) Thromboangiitis obliterans (Buerger's disease). In: Anderson WAD, Kissane JM (eds) Pathology. C.V. Mosby, St. Louis, pp 903–904
2. Joyce JW (1990) Buerger's disease (thromboangiitis obliterans). Rheum Dis Clin North Am 16:463–470

1 Courtesy of Dr. Bo Törnberg, Stockholm, Sweden

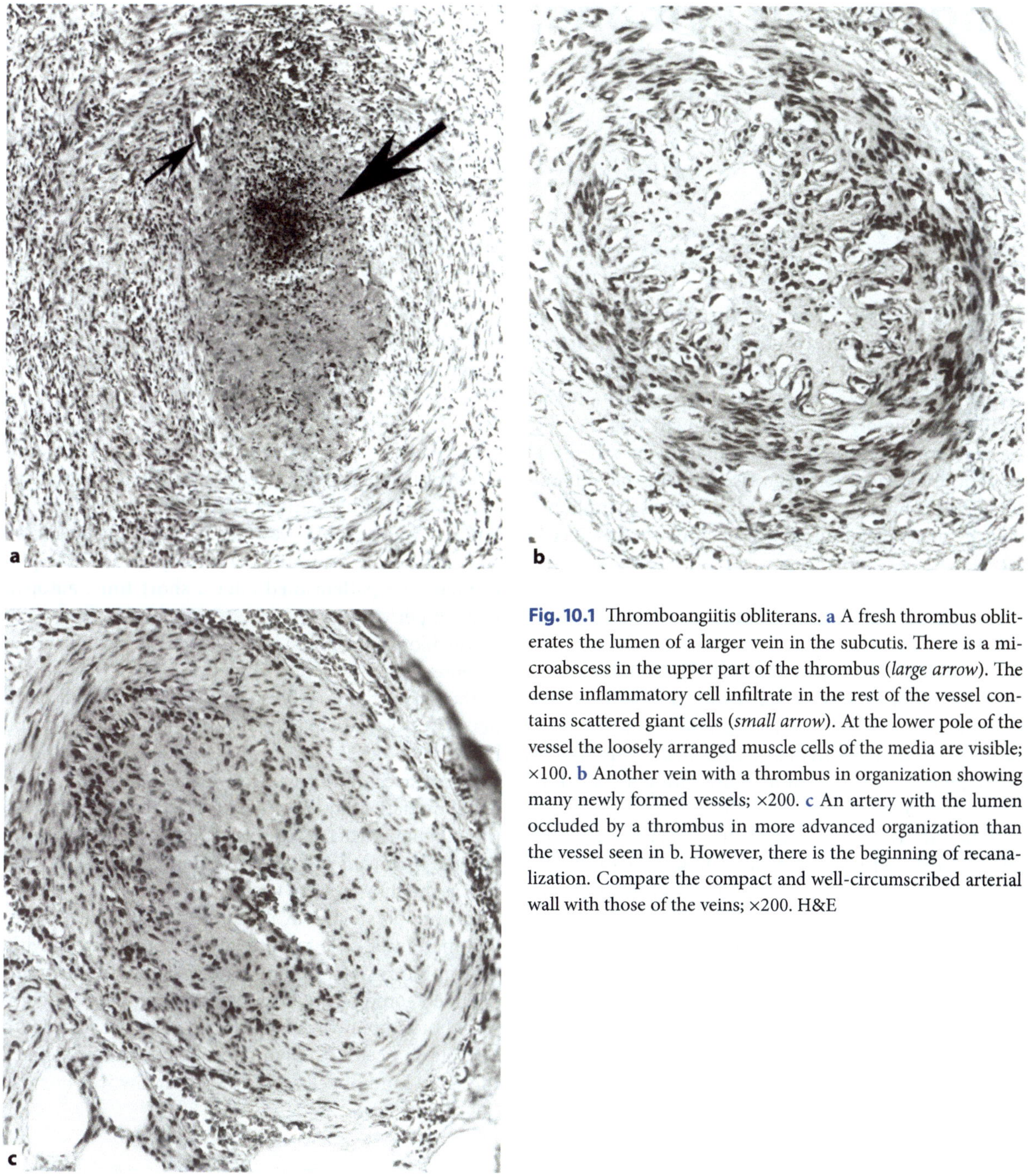

Fig. 10.1 Thromboangiitis obliterans. **a** A fresh thrombus obliterates the lumen of a larger vein in the subcutis. There is a microabscess in the upper part of the thrombus (*large arrow*). The dense inflammatory cell infiltrate in the rest of the vessel contains scattered giant cells (*small arrow*). At the lower pole of the vessel the loosely arranged muscle cells of the media are visible; ×100. **b** Another vein with a thrombus in organization showing many newly formed vessels; ×200. **c** An artery with the lumen occluded by a thrombus in more advanced organization than the vessel seen in b. However, there is the beginning of recanalization. Compare the compact and well-circumscribed arterial wall with those of the veins; ×200. H&E

11 Angiotropic Lymphoma

Intravascular tumor growth in the skin is rare, and is most commonly seen in lymphatic vessels with metastases from breast adenocarcinoma. In angiotropic lymphoma, a rare and very special form of lymphoma, venules are mainly affected. The growth was thought to develop from the endothelium and was called malignant angioendotheliomatosis until the early 1980s when the tumor cells were identified as lymphoma cells by means of immunohistochemistry (Ansell et al. 1982).

11.1 Clinical and Histopathologic Appearances

Most often the disease presents with skin lesions such as infiltrates, plaques or telangiectases, which may be accompanied by neurologic symptoms. Lymph nodes, bone marrow, spleen and liver are rarely involved, in contrast to other forms of lymphomas.

Often the diagnosis is first settled at autopsy, which may reveal widespread intravascular growth in the brain and other organs (Wrotnowski et al. 1985). In most reported cases the lymphoma has been of B cell origin, but also T cell lymphomas have been observed (Willemze et al. 1987; Calamia et al. 1999).

11.2 Examples

Case 1[1]

An 83-year-old woman had over a period of 6 months observed dark blue discoloration all over her body. Investigation revealed conspicuous telangiectases on the trunk and legs, and hard, deep, painful infiltrates on the thighs.

Biopsy specimens disclosed angiotropic B-cell lymphoma with, in principle, the same histopathologic pattern as described below in Case 2. The bone marrow was normal. The patient markedly improved after cytotoxic chemotherapy (Fig. 11.1a).

Case 2

A 76-year-old woman presented with a palm-sized infiltrated area with telangiectases on the upper medial part of the left thigh and enlarged lymph nodes in the groin. A knife biopsy was taken from the skin lesion and fine needle aspiration of a lymph node was performed. The patient died after a short time; autopsy was not performed.

The biopsy specimen included a large part of subcutaneous tissue. The epidermis was normal. In all levels of the dermis and in the subcutis as well, a high number of vessels were partly or totally occluded by notably atypical cells. Most of these vessels were veins of different size, but tumor cells were also seen in arteries and lymphatics, and as small perivascular infiltrates in the subcutaneous fat. Vessels, which were identified as arteries by means of vG-elastin stain, contained no or only a small number of tumor cells.

Immunohistochemical staining technique identified the tumor cells as immature B cells reacting with the antibody L26. Inflammatory cell infiltrates surrounded some of the occluded vessels and were composed of lymphocytes (which did not react with L26), and plasma cells. The lymph node aspiration yielded the same kind of cells. The bone marrow was normal. (Fig. 11.1b,c,d)

11.3 Differential Diagnosis

The differential diagnosis includes other kinds of intravascular tumor growth. For differential diagnosis immunohistochemical investigation is mandatory.

1 Courtesy of Dr. Eva Tegner, University Hospital, Lund, Sweden

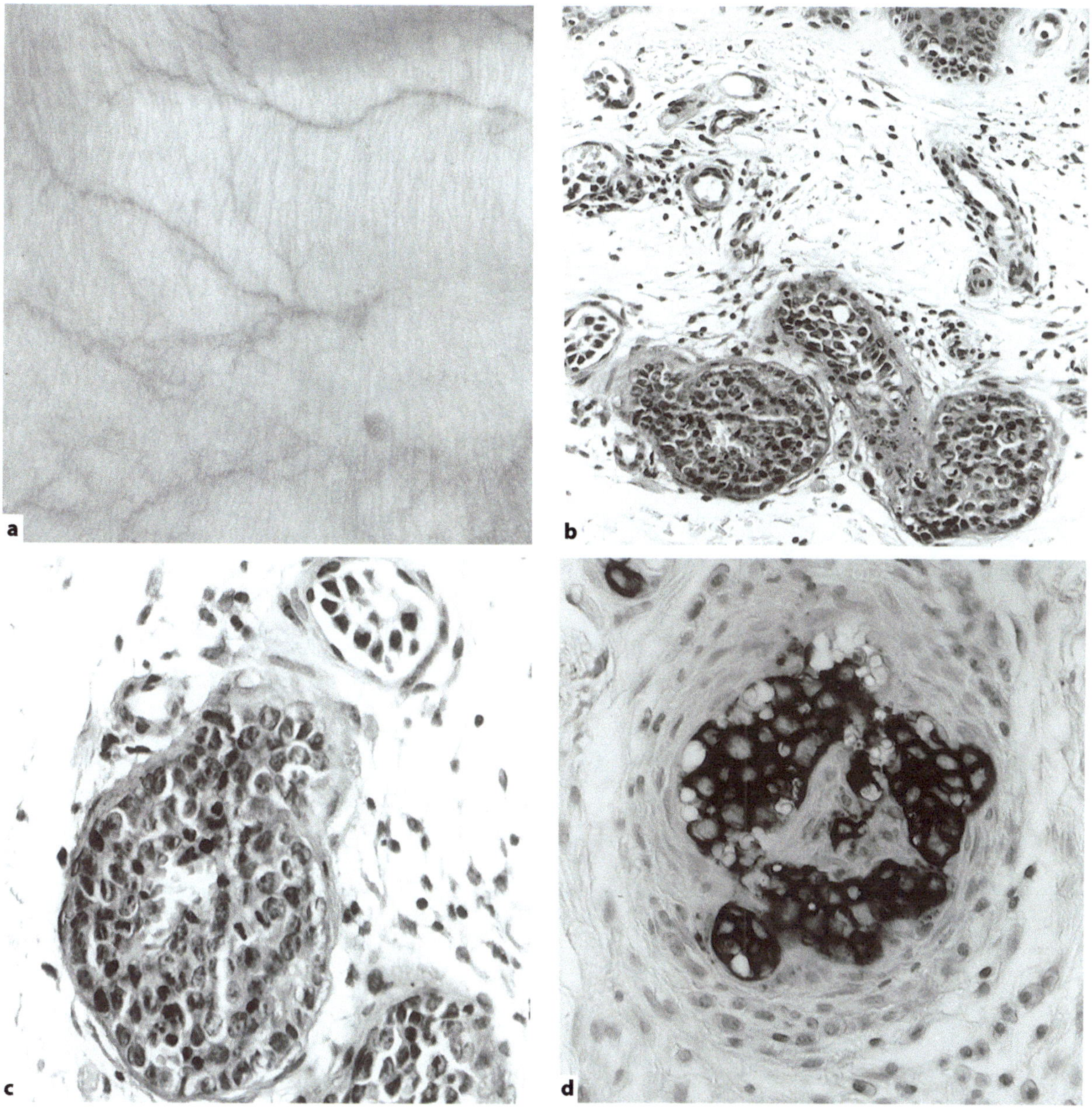

Fig. 11.1 Angiotropic B cell lymphoma. **a** Salient telangiectases on the abdomen. **b** Two distended venules in the mid-dermis are stuffed with tumor cells; H&E, ×200. **c** Close-up of the left vessel in b. In this venule tumor cells seem to fuse with the endothelium. However, in the small venule at the top it is clear that they are lying free in the lumen and that the endothelium is normal; H&E, ×400. **d** Immunohistochemical staining with the B-cell marker L26 is positive. The perivascular cell infiltrate consists of plasma cells and T cells, negative for B-cell markers; L26, ×400

References

1. Ansell J, Bhawan J, Cohen S, Sullivan J, Sherman D (1982) Histiocytic lymphoma and malignant angioendotheliomatosis. One disease or two? Cancer 50:1506–1512
2. Calamia KT, Miller A, Shuster EA, Perniciaro C, Menke DM (1999) Intravascular lymphomatosis. A report of ten patients with central nervous system involvement and a review of the disease process. Adv Exp Med Biol 455:249–265
3. Willemze R, Kruyswijk MRJ, De Bruin CD, Meijer CJLM, Van Berkel W (1987) Angiotropic (intravascular) large cell lymphoma of the skin previously classified as malignant angioendotheliomatosis. Br J Dermatol 116:393–399
4. Wrotnowski U, Mills SE, Cooper PH (1985) Malignant angioendotheliomatosis. An angiotropic lymphoma? Am J Clin Pathol 83:244–248

Chapter 12

Infections Caused by Common Pyogenic Bacteria

12

The most common pyogenic bacteria affecting skin, adnexa and subcutis are streptococci and staphylococci. They are not visible in H&E-stained sections, but may be demonstrated with Gram stain (see Glossary).

12.1 Streptococcal Infections

Beta-hemolytic streptococci give rise to an acute, diffusely spreading infection associated with malaise and fever. Located in the dermis, the infection is called erysipelas, located in the subcutis cellulitis. Cellulitis may be extended erysipelas or originate in the subcutis. The histopathologic pattern is that of an acute inflammation with edema, dilated vessels and dense infiltrates of neutrophils.

However, β-hemolytic streptococci may also give rise to non-bullous impetigo (see below).

12.2 Staphylococcal Infections

Staphylococcus aureus causes furuncles and carbuncles (i.e., follicular and perifollicular abscesses of variable extension) and impetigo. There are two types of impetigo, non-bullous and bullous.

12.2.1 Non-Bullous Impetigo

Non-bullous impetigo is the most common form. The cause is either infection by *Staphylococcus aureus* only, or by *Staphylococcus aureus* together with a β-hemolytic streptococcus, or by a β-hemolytic streptococcus only. Children of all ages are the most commonly affected. The bacteria gain entry through slightly damaged skin; predilection sites are the face and extremities. The lesions start as vesiculopustules, which rapidly transform into honey-colored crusts.

Histologically there are mainly unilocular pustules in the superficial part of the epidermis, which at first are covered by stratum corneum and later by crusts, composed of fibrin and neutrophils.

12.2.2 Bullous Impetigo

Bullous impetigo is caused by *Staphylococcus aureus*. It affects newborns and older infants, but is uncommon in adolescents and adults. The initial lesion is a clear vesicle that develops into a flaccid bulla, which bursts and gives rise to a honey-colored crust.

Histologic investigation shows a wide subcorneal vesicle. Thus the roof consists of the stratum corneum, to which a few cells from the stratum granulosum may be attached. The vesicle contains a small or moderate number of neutrophils and a few desquamated or acantholytic cells (see Glossary); it may even be empty or nearly empty, probably due to loss of the contents during processing. The floor includes the rest of the epidermis, which is edematous, but has a rather smooth surface. In the dermal papillae and upper dermis there are edema and inflammatory cell infiltrates.

12.3 Anonymous Bacterial Infections

Routine cultures for pathogenic bacteria are not always helpful, as demonstrated in Case 2, in which repeated cultures were negative.

12.4 Examples

Case 1. Bullous Impetigo

A 17-year-old boy without previous skin problems had had an eruption of blisters on the left buttock over a period of 3 weeks. He presented with small fresh vesicles, pustules, and crusts on a slightly erythematous area twice the size of a palm. There were also small

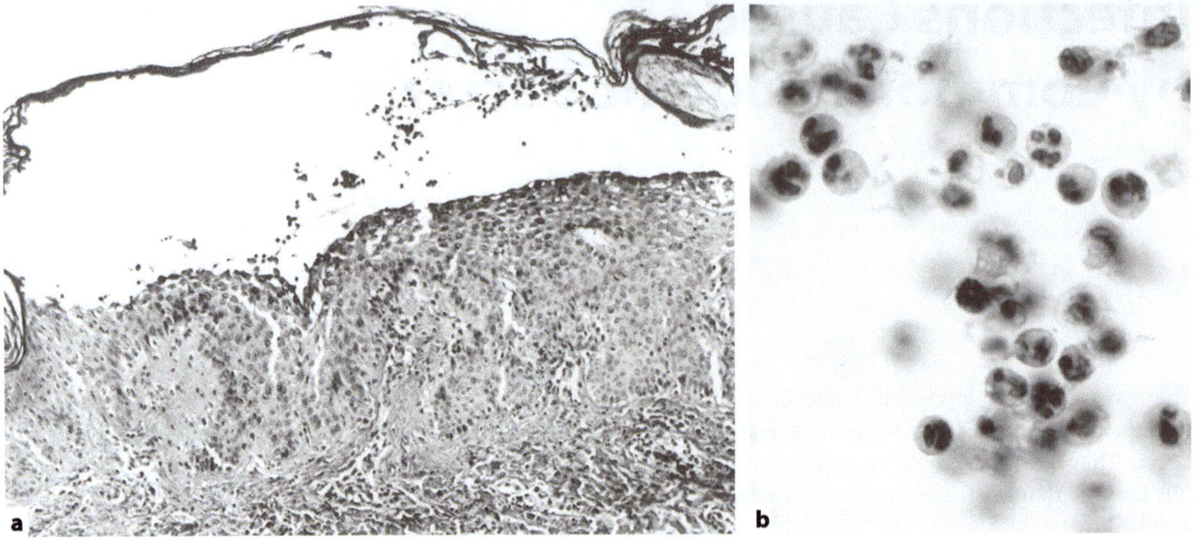

Fig. 12.1 Bullous impetigo. **a** The micrograph shows a part of a wide subcorneal bulla, which contains a sparse number of inflammatory cells. The underlying part of the epidermis is edematous, is slightly penetrated by inflammatory cells, and has several longitudinal clefts. **b** Close-up of the content of the bulla displays aggregates of neutrophils. Note the segmented nuclei, cut at different levels. H&E

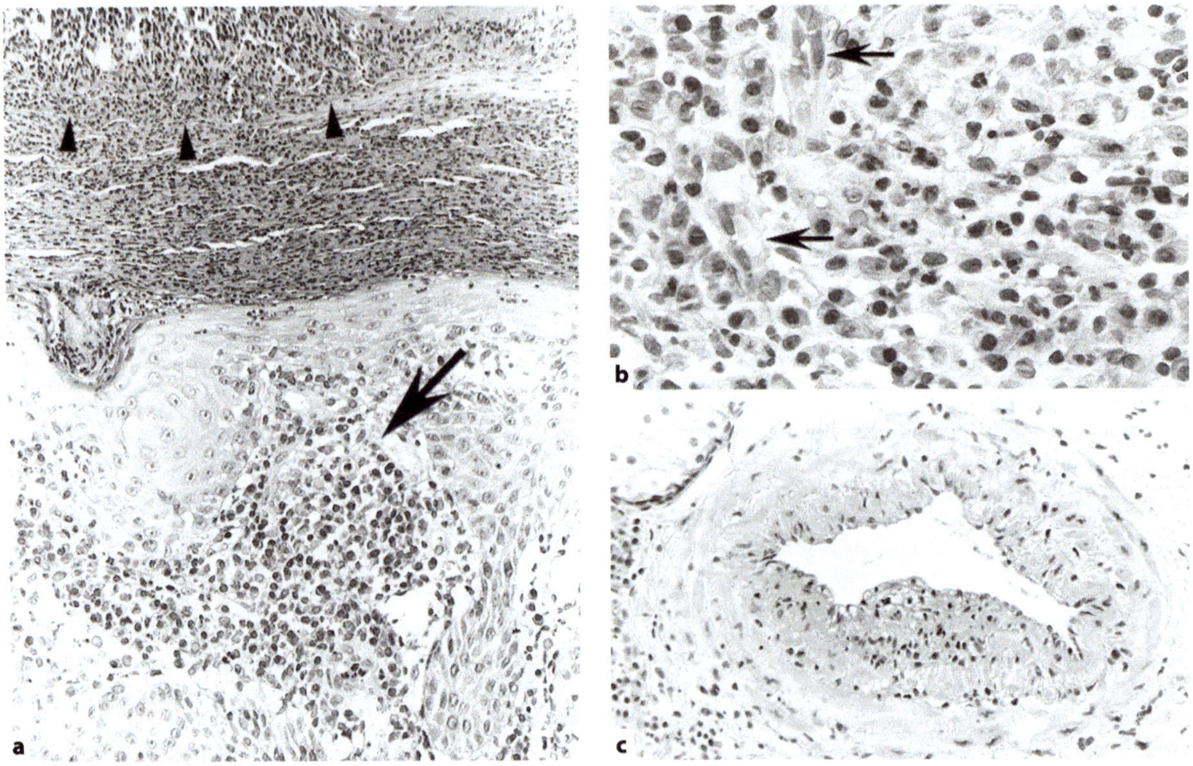

Fig. 12.2 Anonymous, chronic, purulent infection. **a** The horny layer is markedly thickened and infiltrated by neutrophils, which at the outermost part form a pustule (*arrowheads*). In the papillary dermis there is a dense mixed cell infiltrate (*arrow*). **b** Close-up of the dermal cell infiltrate shows a mixture of lymphocytes, plasma cells, histiocytes and neutrophils with a segmented nucleus. The arrows indicate two newly formed vessels. **c** A vein at the subcutaneous border, the intima of which is partly thickened and infiltrated by lymphocytes. H&E

lesions on the right thigh, and the right cheek and ear. Suggested diagnoses were pityriasis lichenoides et varioliformis acuta and atypical pyoderma.

Histologic investigation showed a wide subcorneal vesicle, which contained a small number of neutrophils and scattered desquamated keratinocytes. The floor of the vesicle consisted of an acanthotic and edematous epidermis with a rather smooth surface, and showed small vertical clefts. In the papillae and upper dermis there were moderately dense perivascular infiltrates of lymphocytes.

Culture yielded massive growth of *Staphylococcus aureus*. After antibiotic treatment the lesions healed (Fig. 12.1).

Case 2. Anonymous, Chronic, Purulent Infection

A 61-year-old man consulted for an erythematous and scaling lesion, 15 mm in diameter, located on the tip of the nose and present for a year. Investigations including cultures for bacteria and fungi and serologic tests for syphilis were negative. Two biopsy specimens were taken at an interval of 2 months. One year later (i.e., two years after the onset of the lesion) it remained unchanged and resistant to treatment.

The two biopsy specimens were reexamined. They had a similar pattern. The epidermis was thickened, spongiotic and sparsely infiltrated by neutrophils. The conspicuously thickened horny layer was permeated with neutrophils, which formed superficial pustules. In the dermis there was a confluent and very dense cell infiltrate, which mainly consisted of plasma cells and lymphocytes, but also contained many neutrophils and scattered eosinophils. Newly formed vessels were prominent and in one of the specimens a single thick-walled vein with a subendothelial infiltrate of lymphocytes was observed at the dermal–subcutaneous interface. Hair follicles were not involved. Fungal structures and bacteria were not found (Fig. 12.2).

Because of the dense mixed inflammatory cell infiltrate in the dermis combined with superficial pustules, some kind of bacterial infection was suspected in spite of repeated negative cultures. A broad-spectrum antibiotic was tried and the lesion healed.

12.4.1 Comment

The clinical appearance as well as histopathologic pattern and course in Case 2 have similarities to so-called blastomycosis-like pyoderma described by Su et al. (1979). The observed patients had had purulent, verrucous lesions on an extremity or in the head and neck area for a long time, which were resistant to treatment and histologically showed epithelial hyperplasia and purulent inflammation. Investigation excluded fungal and mycobacterial infections. However, culture was positive for at least one of the pathogenic bacteria *Staphylococcus aureus*, β-hemolytic streptococci, and *Pseudomonas aeruginosa*. Following treatment with systemic antibiotics and a topical wet antibacterial dressing the lesions rapidly healed.

12.5 Differential Diagnosis

Biopsies are rarely taken from lesions caused by pyogenic bacteria because of the well-known clinical patterns of these diseases, which are usually confirmed by successful treatment with antibiotics and/or by culture on material taken from the infected skin. Occasionally an atypical clinical appearance or failure in treatment leads to a biopsy.

- Folliculitis and perifolliculitis caused by fungal and mycobacterial infections may clinically be misinterpreted as furuncles or carbuncles and may also be missed histologically if not in the mind of the pathologist (Figs. 13.4c, 13.6c and 15.3a).
- Intraepidermal IgA pustulosis. As in bullous impetigo and other bacterial pustules, there may be subcorneal pustulosis and also some acantholytic cells. Culture from intact vesicles and pustules is decisive (Sect. 25.2).
- Pemphigus foliaceus shows a discreet superficial acantholysis without neutrophils or other inflammatory cells and very little inflammatory response in the upper dermis (Sect. 25.1.2).
- Staphylococcal scalded-skin syndrome (i.e., widespread bullae and exfoliation), seen in newborns and small children, is caused by exotoxins produced by staphylococci in an infectious focus located somewhere else in the body. Intact lesions are sterile.

Reference

1. Su WPD, Duncan SC, Perry HO (1979) Blastomycosis-like pyoderma. Arch Dermatol 115:170–173

13 Common Fungal Infections

With respect to the mode of presentation and propagation in tissue there are three categories of fungi:

1. *Yeast fungi* (unicellular fungi) exist only as spores and produce new spores by budding.
2. *Filamentous fungi* produce filaments (hyphae), but not yeast cells. Some kinds of filamentous fungi form septate hyphae (i.e., the hyphae consist of a chain of cells separated by septa); other kinds produce non-septate hyphae. Filamentous fungi may brake up into spores called arthrospores. A conglomeration of hyphae is called mycelium.
3. *Dimorphic fungi* are able to form both hyphae and yeast spores. They produce new yeast cells by budding from spores as well as from hyphae.

The most common kinds of fungal skin infections are dermatophytosis, *Malassezia furfur/pityrosporum* infections, candidiasis, and aspergillosis.

13.1 Dermatophytosis (Ringworm, Tinea)

Dermatophytes are species of pathogenic filamentous fungi, which belong to one of three genera: *Trichophyton, Microsporum* and *Epidermophyton* (see Table 30.1). They infect the stratum corneum of the skin and many of them also hair and/or nails. According to their natural setting they can be categorized as: anthropophilic fungi, which primarily infect humans and spread from one person to another; zoophilic fungi, which primarily infect animals and can be transmitted to humans; and geophilic fungi, which reside in the soil and occasionally infect animals and humans.

Trichophyton rubrum and *T. mentagrophytes* are common dermatophytes with a worldwide distribution. *Trichophyton rubrum,* which is anthropophilic, prevails in the western world, where it is the most common cause of chronic fungal infections. *Trichophyton mentagrophytes* exists as an anthropophilic and a zoophilic variant. Another common and ubiquitous zoophilic dermatophyte is *M. canis*. Handling an affected animal can result in infection.

13.1.1 Clinical Appearance

Different parts of the body may be affected. With respect to the location, the eruption may have a more or less characteristic appearance. This is the reason why the disease is named after the part of the body affected: tinea corporis (includes trunk and limbs), tinea faciei, tinea cruris, tinea manuum, tinea pedis, tinea capitis, tinea barbae, and tinea unguium.

For example, tinea circinata is the characteristic lesion usually seen in tinea corporis. It presents as a rounded, erythematous, slightly infiltrated, more or less scaling plaque, which extends gradually at the periphery and becomes circinate or annular due to central healing. The active border is clearly defined and slightly raised and may contain pustules.

However, not always do lesions express the pattern described as typical for the location or typical for a fungus lesion in general. They may be mainly papular, vesicular, pustular, follicular, or nodular. The intensity of the inflammatory reaction depends on several factors such as the type of fungus, the degree of follicular invasion, and the immune state of the patient. Thus, in contrast to the anthropophilic *T. mentagrophytes*, the zoophilic variant gives rise to vesicular and/or pustular lesions. Nodular lesions are caused by infection of deep-seated hair follicles.

Tinea capitis, infection of the scalp, may be inflammatory or non-inflammatory. Usually *M. audouinii* and *M. canis* give rise to only a slight inflammatory reaction. However, *M. canis* is sometimes the cause of kerion celsi, a painful tumefaction due to a purulent infection in the dermis and subcutaneous tissue that is always combined with cervical lymphadenitis. *Trichophyton schoenleinii* is the most common cause of a purulent infection of the scalp, called favus, characterized by thick yellow crusts consisting of hyphae and cellular debris (Hay et al. 1992; Elewski 1992).

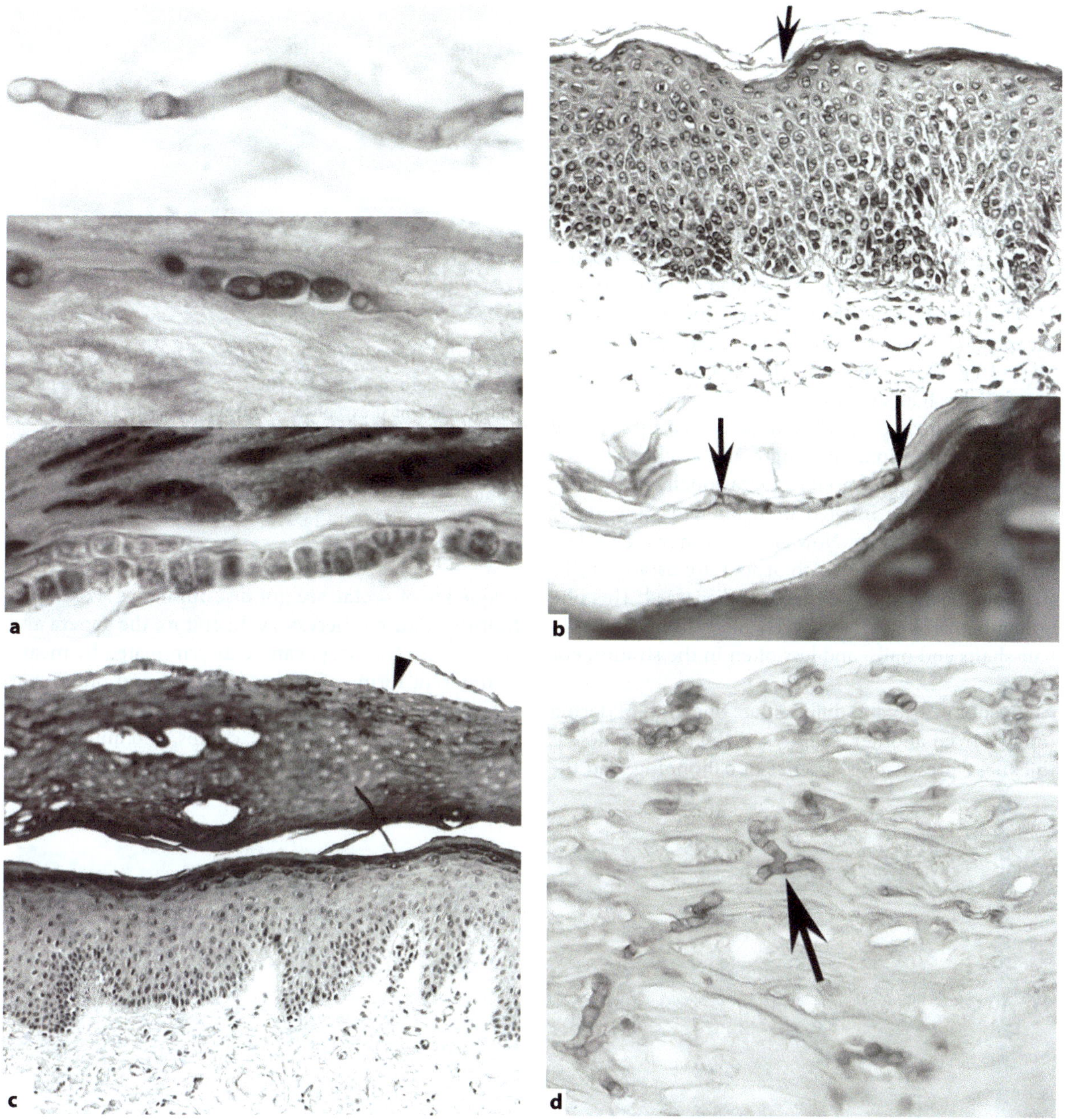

Fig. 13.1 Dermatophytosis. **a** *Top*: segmented hypha in the horny layer; PAS. *Middle*: a string of arthrospores in the horny layer; PAS. *Bottom*: a row of arthrospores located between the hair shaft and the internal root sheath of a hair follicle. H&E (detail from Fig. 13.5b). **b** *Top*: there is a single hypha in the horny layer (*arrow*). The epidermis is slightly spongiotic and in the papillary dermis there is a sparse infiltrate of lymphocytes. *Bottom*: close-up shows the hypha indicated above. The *arrows* indicate two septa. PAS. **c** In this case the horny layer is markedly thickened. The indicated superficial area of the horny layer (*arrowhead*) is permeated by thin, black structures, hyphae. **d** Close-up demonstrates a substantial number of tightly segmented hyphae, one of which is branching (*arrow*). PAS

13.1.2 Histopathologic Appearance

In sections stained with H&E and vG, hyphae and spores are transparent, and therefore, in most cases, are difficult or impossible to detect. For that reason it is necessary to use special fungal stains, such as PAS or silver stains (Gomori, Grocott). Hyphae and spores are stained red with PAS and black with silver stains. Both types of staining methods give equally good results, but the PAS reaction is faster and the procedure is less complicated than that for silver impregnation.

Dermatophytes are filamentous fungi which in tissue produce only septate hyphae and arthrospores (Fig. 13.1). These are found in the stratum corneum, hair follicles, hair shafts, and nails. Hyphae are distinct structures which, properly stained, are easily detected at low magnification. The length and thickness of the segments are highly variable. Occasionally one or several segments are inflated or ballooned. Sometimes hyphae are branching. Now and then they are broken up into arthrospores, which at first are arranged like strings of pearls and later become dispersed. This phenomenon can be seen relatively often in hair follicles, hair shafts and nails, and less often in the stratum corneum.

It is not possible to differentiate one kind of dermatophyte from another. Features of the hyphae such as thickness, presence or absence of ballooning, and the frequency of septae are not discriminative. For identification culture is necessary. In culture the genera and species (see Glossary) can be discriminated by means of different forms of spores (conidia) and other characteristic structures emerging from the hyphae such as spirals, nodules, racquets, combs, and antlers (Hay et al. 1992; Elewski 1992).

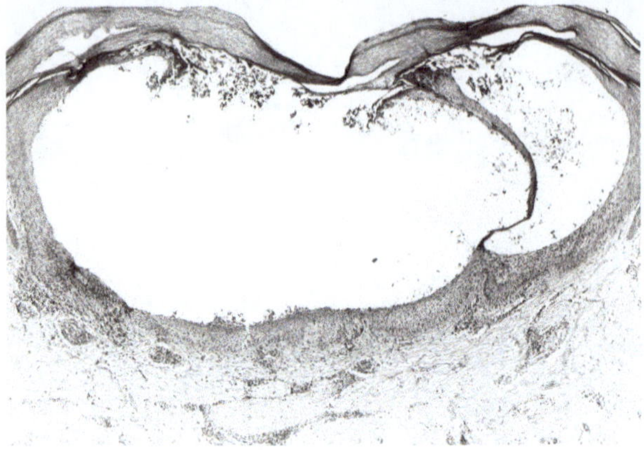

Fig. 13.2 Dermatophytosis. There is a bilocular intraepidermal vesicle which except for small aggregates of neutrophils is empty. The roof of the vesicle consists only of stratum corneum. In the subepidermal area there are perivascular infiltrates of inflammatory cells. One of the few hyphae observed in the horny layer is shown in Fig. 13.1a. PAS

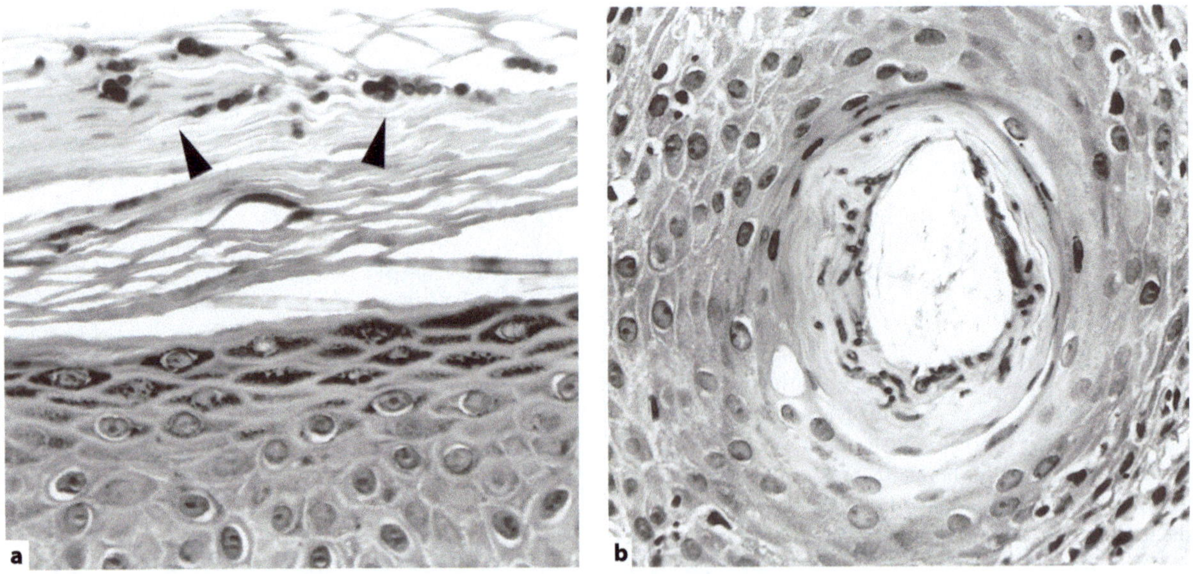

Fig. 13.3 Dermatophytosis. **a** There are arthrospores (*arrowheads*) in the superficial part of the horny layer. **b** A hair follicle in the upper dermis contains hyphae. These are lying in the keratin that surrounds the hair shaft. The hyphae are cut at different levels. Cross sections may be mistaken for spores which, however, are not present. The presence of keratin around the hair shaft indicates that the follicle is cut above the entrance of the sebaceous ducts. PAS

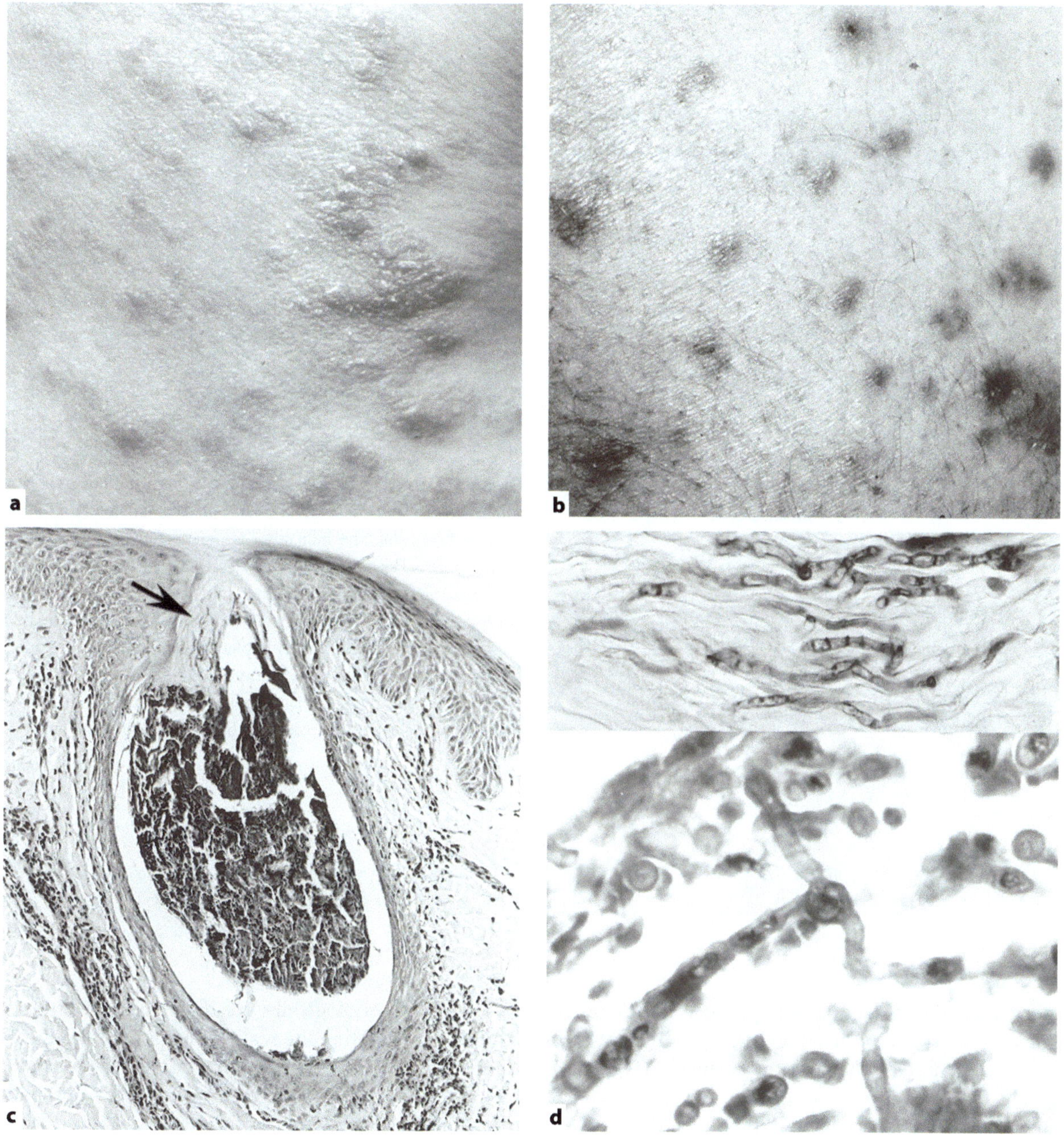

Fig. 13.4 Dermatophytosis. **a** Papular and slightly scaling eruption on the trunk. **b** Follicular papules on the buttock. **c** Biopsy specimen from the patient in **b**. A superficial hair follicle is dilated and filled with necrotic material. The orifice is blocked by a keratin plug which contains hyphae (*arrow*). **d** *Top*: close-up of the area indicated in **c** shows a conglomeration of hyphae which are tightly segmented and focally slightly ballooned. *Bottom*: close-up of the abscess demonstrates hyphae breaking up into spores and free-lying spores. PAS (**c** and **d** *bottom* are reproduced from Brehmer-Andersson 1970, with permission)

The intensity of the inflammatory tissue reaction differs substantially from one case to another and is in harmony with the clinical expression. There may be only small infiltrates of lymphocytes in the papillary dermis and slight or no spongiosis in the epidermis (Fig. 13.1b,c). However, usually there are moderate to dense cell infiltrates with dominance of neutrophils in both the dermis and the epidermis and sometimes vesiculopustules (Fig. 13.2).

In vellus hair-bearing skin, sometimes also called

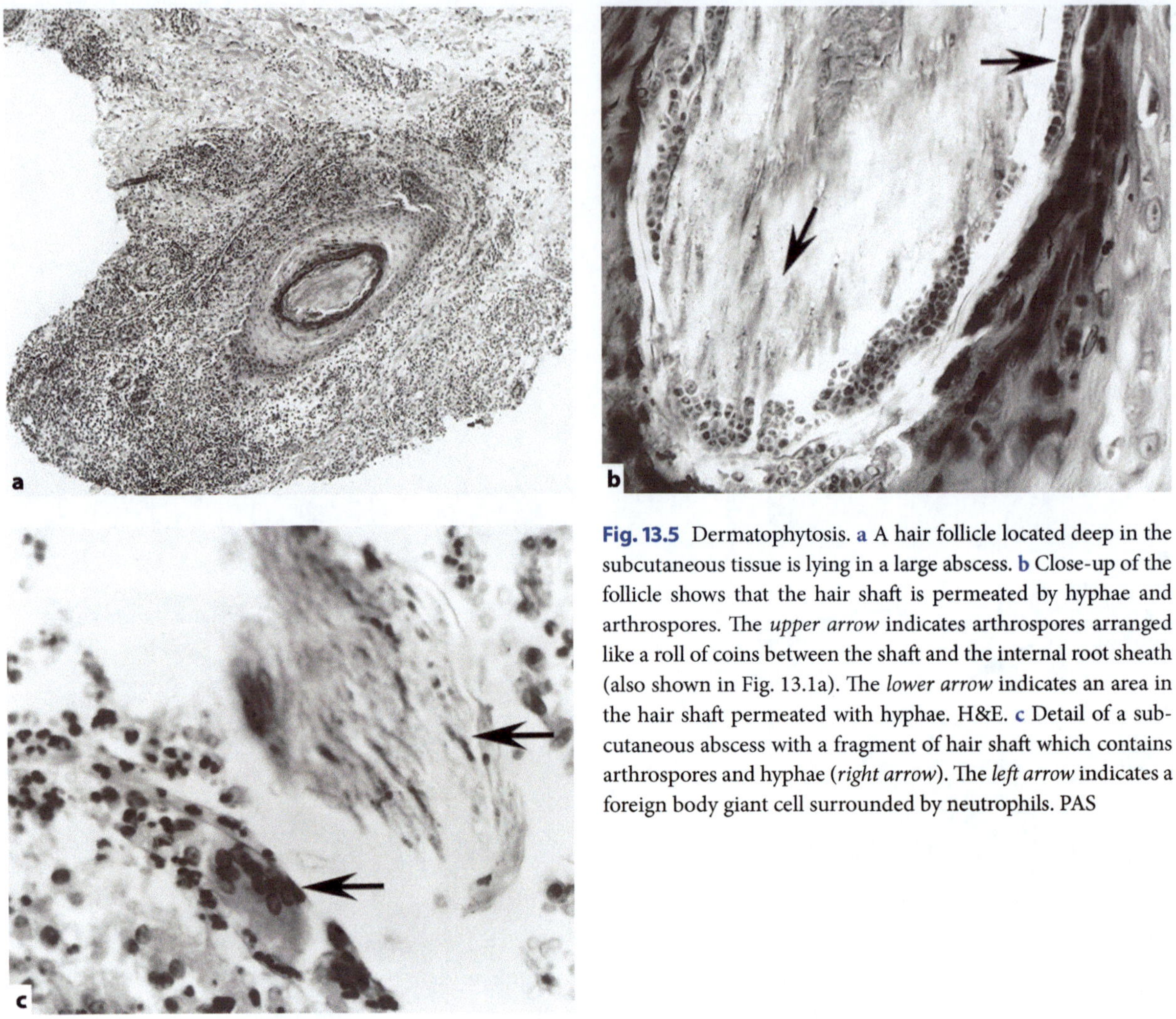

Fig. 13.5 Dermatophytosis. **a** A hair follicle located deep in the subcutaneous tissue is lying in a large abscess. **b** Close-up of the follicle shows that the hair shaft is permeated by hyphae and arthrospores. The *upper arrow* indicates arthrospores arranged like a roll of coins between the shaft and the internal root sheath (also shown in Fig. 13.1a). The *lower arrow* indicates an area in the hair shaft permeated with hyphae. H&E. **c** Detail of a subcutaneous abscess with a fragment of hair shaft which contains arthrospores and hyphae (*right arrow*). The *left arrow* indicates a foreign body giant cell surrounded by neutrophils. PAS

the glabrous skin (see Glossary), hair follicle infections are mostly superficial and thus an integral part of the infection in the stratum corneum (Fig. 13.3). Rarely the infection is confined only to superficial follicles (Fig. 13.4). Now and then deep folliculitis and perifolliculitis with abscess formation in the surrounding tissue are seen (Fig. 13.5a,b). In such cases fragments of hair shaft with fungal structures and/or spores lying free in an abscess may be the only clue to the diagnosis. Ruptured follicles may give rise to granulomas consisting of histiocytes, epithelioid cells and multinucleated giant cells (Fig. 13.5c).

13.1.3 Relevant Investigations

Kligman (1952, 1955) thoroughly studied tinea capitis caused by *M. audouinii* and *M. canis*, clinically as well as histopathologically. He infected children and adults by inoculating the scalp with spores from these fungi. He found two types of infection: scalp infection (i.e., infection of the stratum corneum only), and hair infection (i.e., infection of the follicle and hair shaft only). These two types of infection could exist together or each separately. The scalp infection corresponded to tinea corporis on the vellus hair-bearing skin and had the same course and gross appearance.

Kligman found that from the outermost part of the follicular orifice hyphae enter the infundibulum of the follicle and grow downwards on the outside of the hair shaft in a potential space between the horny layer of the external root sheath and the hair shaft. At about the level of the entrance of the sebaceous ducts, hyphae also penetrated the hair and continued to grow downwards in the hair, but stopped at the upper limit of the keratogenous zone (the matrix). Above the matrix, the fungus invaded the newly formed keratin at the same pace as the hair was growing. The fungus was then passively carried out with the hair. The fungi never invaded the hair matrix. Because of the shape of the matrix, the dividing line between infected and non-infected tissue acquired the form of an inverted V. This line is called the Adamson fringe. Arthrospores are thought to develop outside as well as inside the hair shaft and are therefore called ectothrix and endothrix spores, respectively. The opinion of Kligman was that *M. audouinii* and *M. canis* can produce only ectothrix spores, and thus he called them ectothrix fungi in contrast to endothrix fungi which give rise only to endothrix spores.

Later Graham (1972) studied biopsy specimens from many patients with tinea capitis that had occurred naturally and was caused by different types of *Microsporum* and *Trichophyton* fungi. He found that *M. audouinii, M. canis, M. gypseum, T. mentagrophytes, T. schoenleinii* and *T. rubrum* are able to form both ectothrix and endothrix spores, and therefore called them ecto-endothrix fungi. The only endothrix fungi observed by Graham were *T. violaceum, T. tonsurans* and *T. sulfureum*.

13.1.4 Examples

Case 1. Dermatophytosis

A 45-year-old male presented with widespread annular erythematous and slightly scaling lesions on the upper half of the trunk, hips and thigh. The only suggestion on the request form was multiple lesions of erythema migrans.

The histopathologic changes were slight spongiosis in scattered small areas of the epidermis and sparse infiltrates of lymphocytes in the upper dermis. The PAS staining revealed only a few hyphae: out of seven sections, one contained no hyphae and the others only one or two; they were not possible to detect in sections stained with H&E or vG. The patient recovered after antifungal treatment. However, he suffered multiple relapses, and a culture taken during one of these yielded *T. rubrum* (Fig. 13.1b).

Case 2. Dermatophytosis

A 24-year-old female presented with light brown maculae on the sole of the left foot. Clinical suggestions were fungal infection and lichen ruber.

In a thick stratum corneum PAS disclosed a substantial number of hyphae without any inflammatory reaction in the horny layer, epidermis or dermis. The hyphae were tightly segmented, and at the surface some of them had broken up into arthrospores. Even being aware of their presence, it was impossible to identify hyphae in sections stained with H&E.

In all probability this is a case of tinea nigra caused by *Phaeoanellomyces wernickii* (former name *Exophiala wernickii*); it is not a dermatophyte, but is usually grouped together with dermatophytes. Clinical characteristics are asymptomatic coin-sized, nonscaly, brown or gray patches on soles and palms; histopathologic characteristics are a thickened stratum corneum with branching septate hyphae and very little inflammatory reaction in the dermis (Elewski 1992) (Fig. 13.1c,d).

Case 3. Dermatophytosis

The patient had a vesicular and scaling eruption of the sole of one foot. Cultures were negative, and thus biopsy was performed.

Microscopic investigation showed a large and well-demarcated bilocular vesicle, empty except for small aggregates of neutrophils. PAS-stained sections displayed hyphae only in the keratinous roof of the vesicle. In the dermis there were perivascular infiltrates of inflammatory cells, mainly lymphocytes (Figs. 13.1a top, 13.2).

An important differential diagnosis in a case like this is pustulosis palmoplantaris (Fig. 23.5).

Case 4. Dermatophytosis

A 55-year-old male presented with vesicles on the palms of the hands. Fungal infection was not suspected.

The biopsy specimen showed vesiculopustules in the epidermis and dense cell infiltrates and hemorrhages in the dermis. PAS revealed a fair number of hyphae and arthrospores throughout the horny layer. It was then possible to identify some hyphae and arthrospores as slightly basophilic structures in H&E-stained sections. Culture yielded *T. mentagrophytes* (Fig. 13.1a middle).

Case 5. Dermatophytosis

A 56-year-old male suffered from diabetes mellitus. He presented with annular erythema beneath surgical stockings. Fungal infection was not suggested.

A biopsy specimen showed hyphae and arthrospores in the stratum corneum and moderate inflammatory infiltrates in the dermis. In a hair follicle located in the upper half of the dermis hyphae surrounded, but did not penetrate, the hair shaft. In this case the folliculitis was an integral part of tinea circinata infection. Culture yielded *T. rubrum* (Fig. 13.3).

Case 6. Dermatophytosis

Two days after childbirth a 32-year-old woman became aware of a widespread papular and slightly scaling eruption on the trunk, the right upper arm, and the left side of the neck. She was treated topically with corticosteroids without effect, and thus a biopsy specimen was taken from a fresh lesion. Fungus infection was not suggested.

Histologic investigation revealed two small hair follicles surrounded by dense inflammatory cell infiltrates in the upper dermis. In one of them PAS disclosed hyphae and arthrospores. The patient was referred to the dermatology outpatient clinic. The whole specimen was cut in series and every section was scrutinized. Nowhere were fungal structures found in the horny layer encompassing the follicle (Fig. 13.4a).

At the age of about 6 weeks the baby also showed lesions, highly suspected to be due to fungal infection, on the trunk and neck. Direct microscopy and repeated cultures on scrapings from both the mother and the untreated child were negative. The mother was given oral, and the child topical, antifungal treatment and both healed.

Case 7. Dermatophytosis

Every summer the last 16 years this 41-year-old man had suffered from spells of folliculitis on the buttocks, resistant to antibacterial treatment.

A biopsy revealed folliculitis with septate hyphae in the infundibulum and an intrafollicular abscess with hyphae and arthrospores. No hyphae were found in the stratum corneum outside the follicle. Later on a biopsy specimen taken for culture yielded *T. rubrum* (Fig. 13.4b–d).

Case 8. Dermatophytosis

A 38-year-old man, otherwise healthy, suffered from tinea cruris. He presented with a subcutaneous nodule located on the medial aspect of the left thigh. The skin above was unaffected, thus there was no connection with the tinea cruris lesion. The nodule was thought to be a pilomatricoma.

Histologic investigation revealed a large subcutaneous abscess without granulomatous reaction. In the middle of the abscess was a hair follicle with a disintegrating hair shaft. The shaft was permeated with hyphae, some of them breaking up into arthrospores. There was also a row of arthrospores located between the hair shaft and the internal root sheath. Both hyphae and spores were easily identified in sections stained with H&E. No fungal structures were found in epidermis or in other follicles. In new sections stained with PAS there was no hair follicle, only an abscess containing a few spores (Figs. 13.1a bottom, 13.5a,b).

Case 9. Dermatophytosis

A 70-year-old woman had multiple red infiltrates on the right lower leg, which clinically was thought to be vasculitis.

The biopsy specimen showed a huge abscess which involved both the dermis and subcutaneous tissue and also contained scattered small epithelioid cell granulomas and foreign body giant cells. The only sign of fungus infection was a disintegrating fragment of a hair shaft permeated with hyphae and spores lying in the subcutaneous abscess. Neutrophils, macrophages and multinucleated giant cells surrounded the fragment (Fig. 13.5c).

13.1.5 Comment

It has been asserted that the diagnosis of superficial fungal infections is rarely dependent on histologic investigation (Montgomery 1967; Hay 1992). However, if staining for fungi with PAS is routinely used for all biopsy specimens taken from non-tumorous skin lesions, histopathologic investigation is an easy and effective way to detect even clinically unexpected cases and to confirm suspected cases negative on direct microscopy (see Glossary) and/or culture. Clues such as the so-called sandwich sign with a cleft in the horny layer (Gottlieb and Ackerman 1986) and the presence of neutrophils in the horny layer in H&E-stained sections (Ackerman 1979) are not of value when there are only scattered hyphae and/or the inflammatory reaction is weak, or if the only inflammatory cells are lymphocytes.

The presence of hyphae always indicates infection. The detection of only one hypha is probably enough to settle the diagnosis. However, careful searching usually discloses a few more. The observation of spores only in the horny layer is not enough for diagnosis, though scattered spores in abscesses close to or affecting hair follicles, or located in the dermis–subcutis should arouse suspicion.

Negative results of culture and direct microscopy may be due to the presence of only scattered hyphae, as demonstrated in Case 1, or to the reality that the infection is strictly confined to hair follicles, as shown in Case 7 and Case 8. If the histopathologic investigation shows that only follicles are involved, a biopsy specimen instead of scraped material should be taken for a new culture. An early or a late stage of the lesion may explain a sparse number of hyphae in the stratum corneum. This is in accordance with the investigations of Kligman (1952, 1955), which proved that when a scalp infection, analogous to tinea corporis on the vellus hair-bearing skin, reaches its maximum size, the hyphae in the stratum corneum disappear. Dermatophyte infections do not appear secondary to other dermatoses, but can occasionally coexist with other skin diseases.

13.2 *Malassezia furfur/Pityrosporum* infections

The yeasts *P. orbiculare* and *P. ovale* are present in small amounts as saprophytes in the stratum corneum of normal skin, especially in areas containing sebaceous glands, but can also be found in large aggregates in the scales of, for example, actinic keratoses and discoid lupus erythematosus. They are today thought to be variants of the same yeast which, depending on predisposing factors, can change into the pathogen fungus *M. furfur* (Faergemann 1992). *Malassezia furfur* is dimorphic and lipophilic (i.e., to grow in culture the medium needs supplementation with fatty acids). It is the cause of pityriasis (tinea) versicolor. The yeasts may give rise to *Pityrosporum* folliculitis, and under special conditions to systemic manifestations.

13.2.1 Pityriasis (Tinea) Versicolor

Pityriasis versicolor is a worldwide chronic skin disease, which is most common in areas with high temperatures and high relative humidity. Predisposing factors are seborrhea and hyperhidrosis and treatment with corticosteroids. The disease is mainly present in adults with a peak in the third decade. It is equally common in men and women.

13.2.1.1 Clinical appearance

Malassezia furfur infection gives rise to well-demarcated, finely scaling, light to reddish-brown, oval patches which often coalesce into large areas. In untanned patients the affected areas are darker than the surrounding skin; in tanned patients they are paler, and thus can be misinterpreted as vitiligo. Typical locations are seborrheic areas such as the upper part of the trunk, but even other parts of the body including the face and scalp may be affected. The hair, nails and mucous membranes are never affected.

13.2.1.2 Histopathologic Appearance

In pityriasis versicolor the stratum corneum is usually thickened. *Malassezia furfur* structures (i.e., hyphae and spores) are found at all levels of the horny layer and often also in the loose keratin of the outermost part of the follicular orifices without signs of folliculitis. Such a finding should *not* be interpreted as *Malassezia* folliculitis. Both hyphae and spores are easily recognized in sections stained with H&E, though they are accentuated by PAS staining (Fig. 13.6). Hyphae are segmented, slender, even, and in histologic sections mainly long structures. A characteristic phenomenon is two hyphae arranged one after the other with abruptly "cut" ends separated by a small even gap. Rarely single such gaps can be seen also in *Candida* infections. The yeasts are mostly spherical (*P. orbiculare*), sometimes oval (*P. ovale*). They have double-contoured walls, and often lie in groups. Some of them are budding. Spores can be missing. In such cases identification is based on the easily detected long and short hyphae and typical gaps in routinely stained sections. In the dermis there is usually only a slight inflammatory reaction with small perivascular infiltrates of lymphocytes.

13.2.2 *Pityrosporum* folliculitis

Pityrosporum folliculitis, which is a disease separate from pityriasis versicolor, was first described in some detail by Potter et al. (1973). It is, as mentioned above, caused by the yeasts *P. orbiculare* and *P. ovale*.

13.2.2.1 Clinical Appearance

Discrete, erythematous, and/or pustular follicular lesions up to 4 mm in diameter are scattered on the back, chest, and upper arms. The papules may be severely itchy. Predisposing factors are, as in pityriasis versicolor, a warm and humid climate, occlusion, and treatment with corticosteroids.

13.2.2.2 Histopathologic Appearance and Pathogenesis

Due to obstruction of the orifice by a keratin plug, the follicle in *Pityrosporum* folliculitis is markedly dilated. The dermal part of the follicle shows more or less widespread necrosis. Both in the plug and in the follicle there are dense aggregates of spores, some of which are budding (Fig. 13.6c,d). Hyphae are not seen.

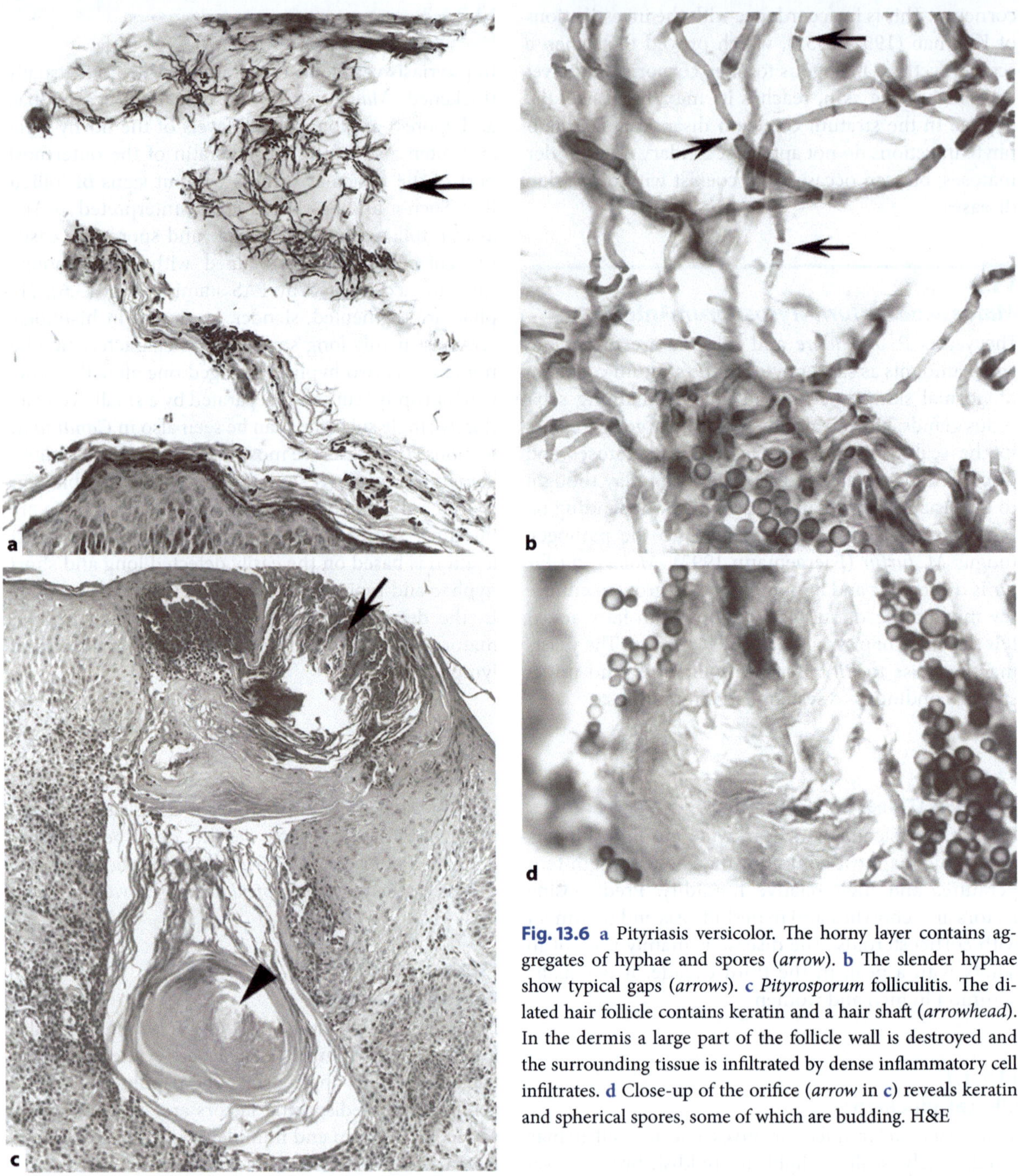

Fig. 13.6 a Pityriasis versicolor. The horny layer contains aggregates of hyphae and spores (*arrow*). b The slender hyphae show typical gaps (*arrows*). c *Pityrosporum* folliculitis. The dilated hair follicle contains keratin and a hair shaft (*arrowhead*). In the dermis a large part of the follicle wall is destroyed and the surrounding tissue is infiltrated by dense inflammatory cell infiltrates. d Close-up of the orifice (*arrow* in c) reveals keratin and spherical spores, some of which are budding. H&E

The degree of inflammatory tissue reaction is variable. However, in spite of extensive necrosis, the inflammatory cell infiltrate is often sparse. If the follicle is ruptured, there can be perifollicular abscesses and a granulomatous reaction with foreign body giant cells.

Predisposing factors and follicular occlusion may stimulate the propagation of yeasts. Free fatty acids and other products generated from the yeasts then provoke an inflammatory reaction (Faergemann 1992).

13.2.3 Systemic Manifestation

Systemic spreading of *Pityrosporum* yeasts has been described in neonates and older children who had received prolonged intravenous lipid infusion (Redline et al. 1985).

13.3 Candidiasis

Candida species are dimorphic fungi, some of which give rise to candidiasis. The most common is *C. albicans*. Other less-common species are *C. glabrata* and *C. parapsilosis*. As commensal yeast organisms, *Candida* spores may be present without symptoms in the mouth and the gastrointestinal tract of most individuals, and in the vagina of some women, but usually not on the skin. As a pathogenic dimorphic fungus producing both hyphae and spores, it may affect mucous membranes, skin, and nails. It is opportunistic (i.e., it is more common in individuals with a predisposing factor such as immunosuppression or diabetes mellitus than in healthy persons). Candidiasis may also be secondary to other skin and mucous membrane disorders such as diaper dermatitis (of which it may also be the primary cause), inverse psoriasis, oral lichen planus, and mucous membrane malignancies including squamous cell carcinoma (Ray 1992).

13.3.1 Clinical Appearance

The appearance varies with respect to the area affected.

13.3.1.1 Skin Lesions

In the skin, *Candida* infection usually affects intertriginous regions. The lesions, which form erythematous, oozing, or pustular areas, may be pruritic or give rise to a burning sensation. Pustules outside the main lesion are considered typical.

13.3.1.2 Oral Lesions

Oral candidiasis presents in different forms:

- *Pseudomembranous candidiasis* or *thrush* appears as one or several well-demarcated patches covered with white membranes, which are easily detached and leave an erythematous denuded surface. The condition is seen in newborn children, in HIV-infected and other immunocompromised individuals, severely ill patients, and in patients treated with corticosteroids.
- *Erythematous candidiasis* presents as ill-defined erythematous areas that may be painful. It is associated with treatment with broad-spectrum antibiotics and corticosteroids, and with HIV infection.
- *Hyperplastic candidiasis* consists of firm white plaques, difficult to remove, on the tongue or bucca. The condition is particularly seen in smokers and may be secondary to a precancerous lesion or carcinoma.
- *Candida-associated denture stomatitis* is related to dental plates or braces.
- *Angular cheilitis* (i.e., fissures and soreness at the angles of the mouth) may be due to *Candida* infection emanating from the oral cavity; it is often associated with denture stomatitis

13.3.1.3 Mucocutaneous Infection

Mucocutaneous infection may give rise to *Candida* vulvovaginitis or *Candida* balanitis.

13.3.1.4 Chronic Mucocutaneous Candidiasis

Chronic mucocutaneous candidiasis occurs in a heterogeneous group of syndromes due to different kinds of defects of the cell-mediated immune system, and sometimes also includes endocrinopathy. The infection usually starts in early childhood and affects skin, nails and mucous membranes.

13.3.1.5 Systemic Manifestation

Systemic manifestations due to hematogenous dissemination are rare, but are seen in immunocompromised patients, especially if they are suffering also from neutropenia.

13.3.2 Histopathologic Appearance

As a dimorphic fungus *Candida albicans* produces both yeast spores and hyphae (Fig. 13.7). The fungal structures are found in a thickened and parakeratotic horny layer. Spores are oval or round (when transversely cut), and are on average bigger than *Pityrosporum* spores. Some spores are budding. Spores seem to aggregate in the outermost part of the stratum corneum, which is easily detached during the taking and processing of the samples. This could be the reason why spores are often missing in sections.

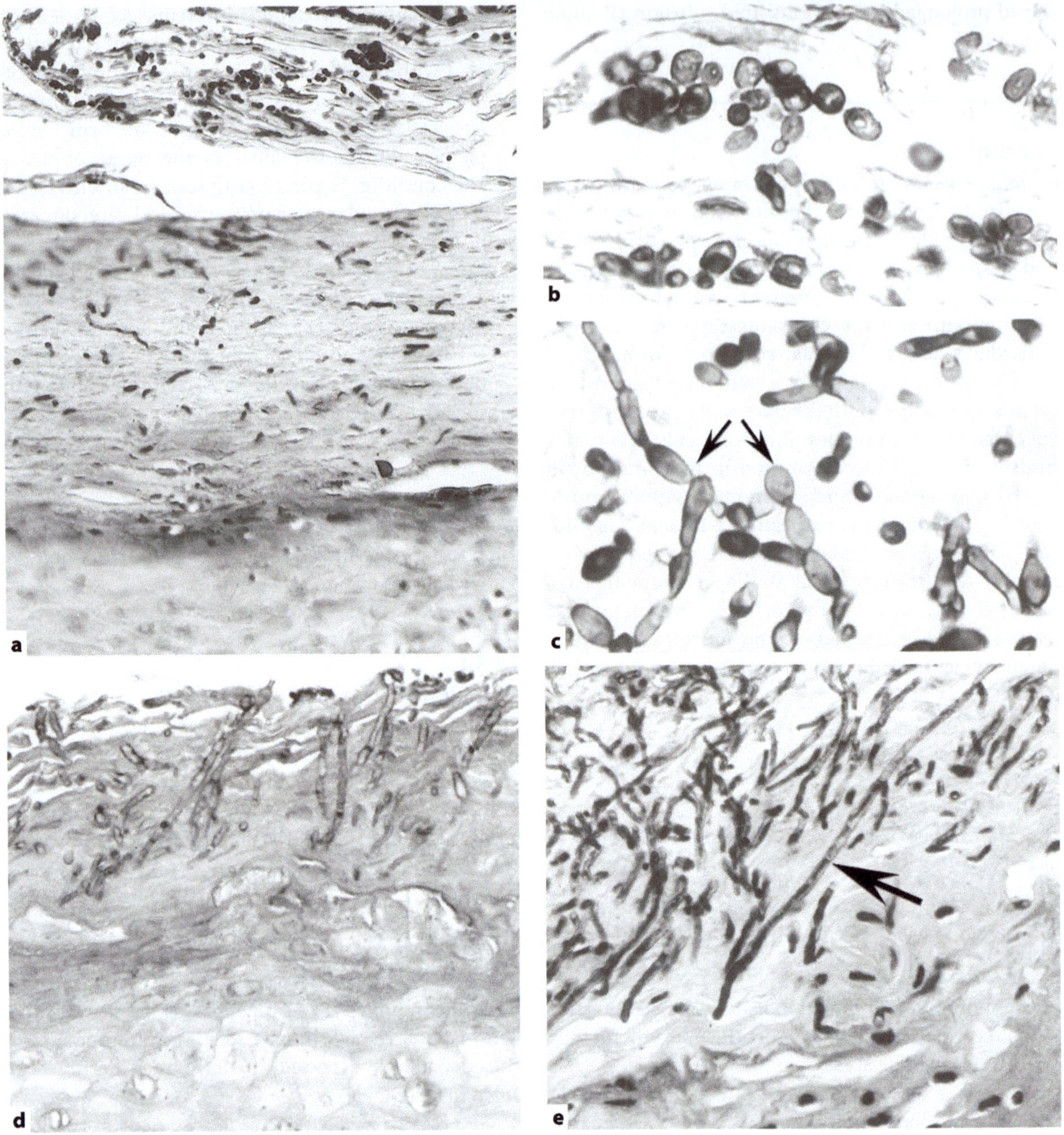

Fig. 13.7 Candidiasis. **a** The horny layer is strikingly thickened and permeated with hyphae running in all directions. In the outermost and partly detached fraction there is aggregation of spores. **b** Close-up of this part shows oval spores. In the center there is a budding spore. **c** The micrograph demonstrates so-called pseudohyphae in necrotic material from a ureter (*arrows*). **d** Hyphae pervade the horny layer and some are "diving" towards the epithelium. They are septate and in the right upper corner one is slightly ballooned. **e** In this case the hyphae are long, slender and branching. The *arrow* indicates a septum in a long hypha giving off three branches. Below the *arrow* some hyphae seem to be penetrating into the epithelium. PAS

Hyphae are septate, mostly unevenly thick, in areas ballooned, and may be branched. They are found throughout the thickness of the horny layer and are disorderly running in all directions; however, now and then they look as if they are "diving" towards the epithelium and seem to penetrate into its outermost vital cell layer. Now and then so-called pseudohyphae are seen. By pseudohypha is meant a series of yeast spores which have remained attached to each other. It is often said to be a common and characteristic phenomenon in *Candida* infections. However, in the experience of the author, pseudohyphae are rare in skin and mucous membrane lesions, and are usually short. Figure 13.7c shows pseudohyphae in necrotic material removed from the ureter in a patient suffering from *Candida* sepsis.

In immunocompetent persons the inflammatory reaction is often strong. The epithelium is thickened, there is marked hyper- and parakeratosis, neutrophils and pustules in the epithelium, and in the subepithelial tissue dense inflammatory cell infiltrates. In immunocompromised patients there are hyper- and parakeratosis but no or very few inflammatory cells.

In a skin lesion it is not possible to differentiate between *Candida* and dermatophytes if there are only hyphae and no yeasts or arthrospores. However, a "diving" pattern and a tendency to penetrate into vital epithelium indicate *Candida*. Also *Candida* hyphae are mostly easier to identify in sections stained with H&E than are dermatophyte hyphae. The presence of only yeasts is never enough to establish the diagnosis of candidiasis.

13.3.3 Examples

Case 10. Candidiasis

An 80-year-old male patient presented with a rather large and infiltrated lesion on the mucosa of the lower lip. The lesion was covered with crusts and small superficial ulcers had been noticed over about 18 months. Culture yielded *Candida albicans*, but because of unsuccessful treatment and the risk of underlying squamous cell carcinoma the whole lesion was excised.

Histologic investigation showed *Candida* hyphae and spores in large numbers, conspicuous epithelial hyperplasia, a dense inflammatory cell infiltrate, and moderate cell atypia (Fig. 13.7a,b).

Cases 11 and 12

The patients were two young men who were suffering from advanced HIV infection and clinically had lesions on the tongue border suspected to be so-called hairy leukoplakia.

Histologic investigation showed the same pattern in both patients. The horny layer was markedly thickened and permeated by *Candida* hyphae. There were strikingly few inflammatory cells in the epithelium as well as in the submucosa (Fig. 13.7d,e).

13.4 Aspergillosis

The most important species of *Aspergillus* are *A. fumigatus*, *A. niger*, and *A. flavus*. They are opportunistic and are seen in immunocompromised patients with chronic neutropenia. However *A. niger* is also able to infect immunocompetent humans.

13.4.1 Clinical Appearance

In primary infection of the skin, the lesions usually appear in a location exposed to trauma. They may occur in several forms such as erythematous and crusted plaques, hemorrhagic vesicles, bullae, or necrotic nodules (Khardori et al. 1989). Systemic manifestations mostly start in the lungs where the fungus grows into vessels leading to widespread dissemination (Binford and Dooley 1979).

13.4.2 Histopathologic Appearance

Aspergillus produces septate hyphae that branch regularly and dichotomously with acute angles. They are possible to identify in sections stained with H&E, but are easier to find when PAS stained. For the discrimination of species, culture is necessary (Binford and Dooley 1979).

In the lungs and paranasal sinuses, besides hyphae and spores, the lesions may contain conidiophores (fruiting bodies) which are structures seen in culture but usually not in tissue. Presumably the exudate in alveoli and sinuses serves as a culture medium.

13.4.3 Examples

Case 13. *Aspergillus*

The patient was suffering from AIDS and had small white patches on the tongue border.

A biopsy specimen showed multiple scattered hyperkeratotic foci. These contained a superficial conglomeration of spores from which dichotomously branching hyphae grew down towards the epithelium. No culture was done, but the characteristic growth pattern with dichotomously dividing hyphae permits a presumptive diagnosis of *Aspergillus* (Figs. 13.8a,b).

Case 14. *Aspergillus*

The patient was an otherwise healthy 26-year-old male. For 2 years he had had a right-sided blocked nose, nasal catarrh and pain over the right maxilla. During a Caldwell-Luc operation (see Glossary) a thickened and markedly changed mucous membrane with a large core of necrotic yellow–black tissue was found.

Histologic investigation revealed brownish hyphae, spores and conidiophores easily identified in H&E-stained sections. Culture yielded *Aspergillus niger* (Fig. 13.8c).

References

1. Ackerman AB (1979) Subtle clues to diagnosis by conventional microscopy. Neutrophils within the cornified layer as clues to infection by superficial fungi. Am J Dermatopathol 1:69–75
2. Binford CH, Dooley JR (1979) Deep mycoses. In: Binford CH, Connor DH (eds) Pathology of tropical and extraordinary diseases. Castle House Publications, London, pp 562–597
3. Brehmer-Andersson E (1970) Value of biopsies of superficial mycoses (in German). Hautarzt 21:160–165
4. Elewski BE (1992) Superficial mycoses, dermatophytoses, and selected dermatomycoses. In: Elewski BE (ed) Cutaneous fungal infections. Igaku-Shoin, New York, pp 12–59
5. Faergemann J (1992) Pityrosporum infections. In: Elewski BE (ed) Cutaneous fungal infections. Igaku-Shoin, New York, pp 69–83
6. Gottlieb GJ, Ackerman AB (1986) The "sandwich sign" of dermatophytosis. Am J Dermatopathol 8:347–350
7. Graham JH (1972) Superficial fungus infections In: Graham JH, Johnson WC, Helwig EB (eds) Dermal pathology. Harper & Row, New York, pp 137–253
8. Hay RJ (1992) Introduction to medical mycology. In: Elewski BE (ed) Cutaneous fungal infections. Igaku-Shoin, New-York, pp 1–11
9. Hay RJ, Roberts SOB, Mackenzie DWR (1992) Mycology. In: Champion RH, Burton JL, Ebling FJG (eds) Rook/Wilkinson/Ebling textbook of dermatology. Blackwell Scientific Publications, Oxford, pp 1127–1160
10. Khardori N, Hayat S, Rolston K, Bodey GP (1989) Cutaneous *Rhizopus* and *Aspergillus* infections in five patients with cancer. Arch Dermatol 125:952–956
11. Kligman AM (1952) The pathogenesis of tinea capitis due to *Microsporum audouini* and *Microsporum canis*. I. Gross observations following the inoculations of humans. J Invest Dermatol 18:231–246
12. Kligman AM (1955) Tinea capitis due to *M. audouini* and *M. canis*. II. Dynamics of the host-parasite relationship. Arch Dermatol 71:313–337
13. Montgomery H (1967) Dermatopathology. Harper & Row, New York

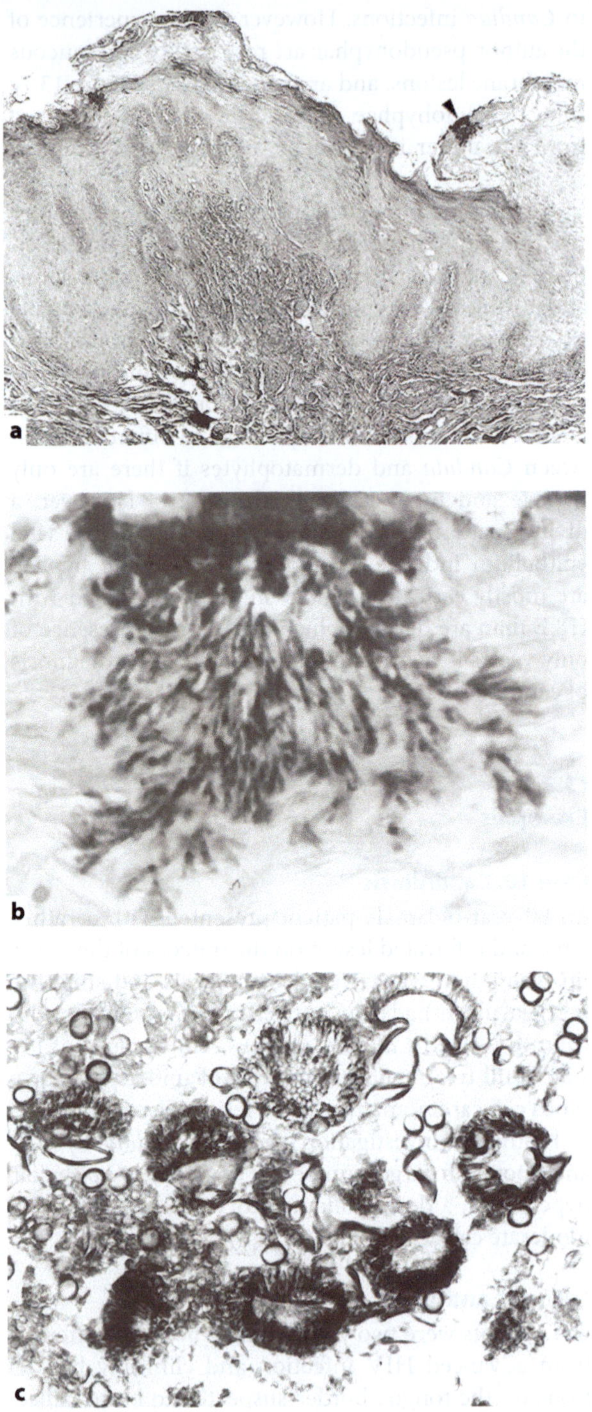

Fig. 13.8 Aspergillosis. **a** Lesion on the tongue border. There are areas with hyperkeratosis and in one of them a black spot (*arrowhead*). **b** Close-up of the black spot reveals a superficial conglomeration of spores from which a "broom" of dichotomously dividing hyphae are growing towards the epithelium; PAS. **c** *Aspergillus niger* in a paranasal sinus. Conidiophores and spores are lying in necrotic material; H&E

14. Potter BS, Burgoon CF, Johnson WC (1973) Pityrosporum folliculitis. Report of seven cases and review of the *Pityrosporum* organism relative to cutaneous disease. Arch Dermatol 107:388–391
15. Ray TL (1992) Cutaneous and disseminated skin manifestations of candidiasis. In: Elewski BE (ed) Cutaneous fungal infections. Igaku-Shoin, New York, pp 84–105
16. Redline RW, Redline SS, Boxerbaum B, Barett Dahms B (1985) Systemic *Malassezia furfur* infections in patients receiving intralipid therapy. Hum Pathol 16:815–822

14 Demodicidosis

Demodicidosis means infestation of the skin by *Demodex* mites. These are commonly found in skin biopsies, especially when taken from sebaceous areas. The predilection site is the face. Usually there is no inflammatory reaction. Aylesworth and Vance (1982) investigated a high number of consecutive skin biopsies and found that 10% of all specimens and 12% of all follicles contained mites. Infestation increases with age. Males are more often affected than females. Children are rarely affected.

14.1 Characteristics of Demodex Mites

In humans there are two species: *D. folliculorum* and *D. brevis*. They occupy different anatomical sites. *Demodex folliculorum*, the longer of the two, is found in hair follicles above the level of the entrance of the sebaceous ducts and *D. brevis* in the sebaceous glands and ducts. They both have life cycles including ova, larvae, protonymphs, nymphs and adults. *Demodex folliculorum* has large and arrowhead-like eggs. The eggs of *D. brevis* are oval. Both species can be seen in the same host. A large number of *D. folliculorum* may be present in one follicle. *Demodex brevis* mites are less frequent. Usually there is only one mite; occasionally there may be two. The mites feed on epithelial and glandular cells (Desch and Nutting 1972).

14.2 Pathogenesis and Clinical Appearance

The pathogenicity of *Demodex* mites is an unsettled question. Association with rosacea has been discussed. Bonnar et al. (1993) investigated the population density of *Demodex* mites in patients with rosacea and that of normal individuals. They used cyanoacrylate glue to remove the superficial layer of the stratum corneum and the follicular contents in a measured area. The retrieved material was then analyzed by light mi-

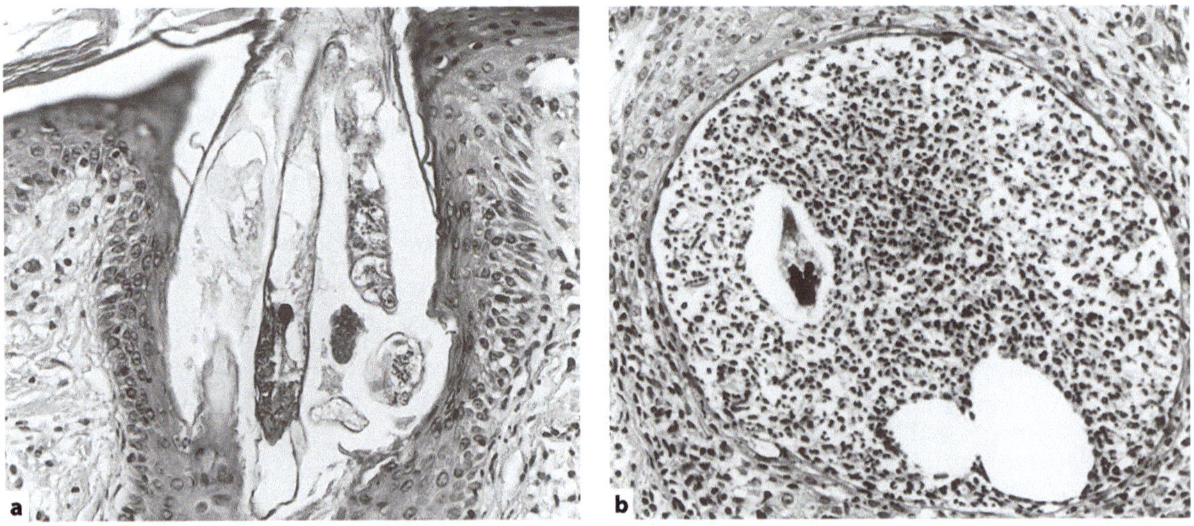

Fig. 14.1 *Demodex folliculorum*. **a** Parts of several mites are blocking the infundibulum of a hair follicle without inflammatory response. **b** A superficial follicular abscess (pustule) contains a *D. folliculorum* egg. H&E

croscopy and the mites were counted. They found a statistically significant increase in mites in different kinds of rosacea, but no significant difference in the number of mites after treatment of the rosacea. The authors concluded that, even if not the main cause of rosacea, *Demodex* may play a part in the pathogenesis by provoking an allergic reaction, by blocking the follicular orifice, or by acting as vectors for microorganisms. Pustular folliculitis and papulonodules, caused by overgrowth of *Demodex* mites (rosacea-like demodicidosis), have also been described in both immunocompetent and non-immunocompetent patients. A very high number of mites have been found in material scraped from the skin lesions of these patients (Purcell et al. 1986; Dominey et al. 1989; Ivy et al. 1995).

14.3 Example

Case 1. Pustular Folliculitis and Infestation with *D. Folliculorum*

A 29-year-old man presented with a somewhat unusual facial eruption consisting of minute and closely set follicular pustules. The suggested clinical diagnosis was comedo acne.

A biopsy showed a follicular abscess containing a *Demodex* structure, an ovum, which in *D. folliculorum* has the shape of an arrowhead. The follicular epithelium was edematous and sparsely infiltrated by neutrophils, but not disrupted. In the perifollicular tissue there were infiltrates of lymphocytes and neutrophils. A second mite was found in another follicle without any inflammatory reaction (Fig. 14.1).

Unfortunately, the patient was lost to follow-up, so further investigation could not be done. Whether the mite is the cause of the pustule or only an accidental finding remains an open question.

References

1. Aylesworth R, Vance JC (1982) *Demodex folliculorum* and *Demodex brevis* in cutaneous biopsies. J Am Acad Dermatol 7:583–589
2. Bonnar E, Eustace P, Powell FC (1993) The *Demodex* mite population in rosacea. J Am Acad Dermatol 28:443–448
3. Desch C, Nutting WB (1972) *Demodex folliculorum* (Simon) and *D. brevis* (Akbulatova) of man: redescription and reevaluation. J Parasitol 58:169–177
4. Dominey A, Rosen T, Tschen J (1989) Papulonodular demodicidosis associated with acquired immunodeficiency syndrome. J Am Acad Dermatol 20:197–201
5. Ivy SP, Mackall CL, Gore L, Gress RE, Hartley AH (1995) Demodicidosis in childhood acute lymphoblastic leukemia: an opportunistic infection occurring with immunosuppression. J Pediatr 127:751–754
6. Purcell SM, Hayes TJ, Dixon SL (1986) Pustular folliculitis associated with *Demodex folliculorum*. J Am Acad Dermatol 15:1159–1162

15 Infections Caused by *Mycobacterium Tuberculosis, M. Bovis,* and Atypical Mycobacteria

Tuberculosis is a worldwide infection caused by *M. tuberculosis* and *M. bovis*, which primarily affects the respiratory and intestinal tracts and is one of the main causes of death in poor parts of the world. *Mycobacterium bovis* has, because of pasteurization of milk, practically been eradicated in developed countries. Also for a long time the rates of *M. tuberculosis* infections and deaths have been low in Europe and the US because of improved hygiene, more spacious living and effective antibiotics. However, since the mid-1980s, due to a high rate of HIV infection and multidrug-resistant mycobacteria, tuberculosis has once again become an increasing problem in the western world.

Mycobacteria are non-motile, non-sporulating comma-like rods, most of which are slow growing. They are intracellular parasites and in infected persons multiply in the cytoplasm of macrophages, where they also may remain latent for a long period of time. It is not possible to identify mycobacteria in routinely stained sections. However, they are acid-fast and thereby can be visualized and differentiated from other pathogenic rods by the Ziehl-Neelsen stain (i.e., stained with carbolfuchsin the organisms retain their red color after exposure to acid alcohol). Most mycobacteria have a low virulence and only a small fraction of exposed individuals become infected and ill.

15.1 *Mycobacterium Tuberculosis* and *M. Bovis* Infections in the Skin

Mycobacterium tuberculosis and *M. bovis* are closely related and the description below is relevant to both of them. The kind of skin lesion, the histopathologic pattern, and the number of bacteria present depend on the immunologic state of the individual and the degree of tuberculin sensitivity (Sect. 5.3.1.1). The diagnosis is verified by the presence of acid-fast bacteria in histologic sections and/or a positive culture. If the number of bacteria is low they may be very difficult to find in sections. The best site to look for them is in necrotic tissue close to preserved tissue. All kinds of skin tuberculosis may be met, but the prevalence is low. In a Spanish cohort investigation, which included 10,304 patients seen from 1980 through 1993, tuberculosis was found in 651 patients (0.14%), of whom 16 (2.4%) had cutaneous tuberculosis (Farina et al. 1995).

15.1.1 Primary Inoculation (Primary Complex, Tuberculous Chancre)

This kind of lesion is due to inoculation of mycobacteria through a slightly injured skin or mucous membrane in a non-sensitized person. It occurs in poor countries with a high incidence of tuberculosis and mostly affects children. In the western world inoculation is rare, but may happen for example to medical and veterinary personnel. A small suppurating ulceration appears, which slowly increases in size and does not heal; also the regional lymph nodes become infected and enlarged.

Histopathologic investigation of a biopsy specimen taken in the early stage shows acute inflammation with infiltrates of neutrophils. The number of acid-fast bacilli is high. After 3 to 6 weeks the inflammatory response becomes granulomatous and bacteria are difficult to find (Lever and Schaumburg-Lever 1990).

15.1.2 Tuberculosis Verrucosa Cutis

Tuberculosis verrucosa cutis appears as a result of exogenous inoculation of the mycobacteria through injured skin or mucous membranes in a person who has already experienced a primary infection, and thus is sensitized for tuberculin and also has acquired a certain degree of immunity against mycobacteria. Like primary inoculation, tuberculosis verrucosa is rare in western countries. Lesions are mostly located on the hands and start as small papules or papulopustules. They slowly increase in size and in the beginning may be mistaken for common warts.

Histologic investigation shows epidermal hyperplasia and hyperkeratosis. In the upper dermis there are signs of acute inflammation with abscesses; in the mid-dermis usually epithelioid cell granulomas are observed. Tubercle bacilli may be found (Lever and Schaumburg-Lever 1990).

15.1.3 Lupus Vulgaris

Lupus vulgaris appears in patients with a moderate degree of immunity against the mycobacteria and a high degree of tuberculin sensitivity. The source of the skin infection is an often occult tuberculous focus elsewhere in the body. It is a remarkably chronic and progressive manifestation that may cause ulcerations of the skin and underlying tissue, and/or atrophic scarring. It occurs at all ages, and is more common in females than in males. Like other forms of skin tuberculosis, the incidence in developed countries is low, and today, if not imported, in Scandinavia is seen only in elderly persons without other obvious signs of tuberculosis.

15.1.3.1 Clinical Appearance

Usually there is only one lesion. Most common locations are the head and neck, and here the preferential sites are the earlobes with surrounding areas of the cheek and neck, and the nose. The initial lesion is a small flat plaque that consists of reddish-brown papules with soft consistency, and on diascopy (i.e., seen through a glass slide pressed to the surface of the lesion) shows the color of apple-jelly. The plaque slowly grows in size. During progression, the appearance of the lesion may change according to the degree of inflammatory infiltration of the underlying tissues, ulceration, and scarring.

15.1.3.2 Histopathologic Appearance

The histopathologic pattern commonly referred to in lupus vulgaris includes densely packed epithelioid cell granulomas, which surrounded by dense infiltrates of lymphocytes form typical tubercles. The granulomas are preferentially confined to the upper dermis and contain a variable number of giant cells mostly of Langhans type. There are only small areas of necrosis or none at all. However, discrepancies from this classical pattern occur. Large necroses are sometimes present and in older lesions the lymphocytic infiltrate is sometimes scant. Furthermore, complications such as ulceration, secondary infection, and scarring may camouflage the typical pattern. It is very difficult to find mycobacteria in sections, and even culture is sometimes negative. In the latter case a positive result of the given therapy proves the diagnosis.

15.1.3.3 Examples

Case 1. Lupus Vulgaris

A 55-year-old woman had suffered for more than 27 years from slowly increasing lesions in the face. She presented with two bluish-red papular lesions measuring about 20×30 mm, one on the left eyelid and the other below the right ear. The diagnosis was verified by culture. Staining for mycobacteria was negative.

Histologic investigation revealed closely set epithelioid cell granulomas in the dermis and upper subcutis. The granulomas contained many giant cells of both foreign body type and Langhans type. Necrosis was not observed. Granulomas were surrounded by dense cell infiltrates composed mainly of lymphocytes. The epidermis was flat, but otherwise normal (Fig. 15.1a,b).

Case 2. Lupus Vulgaris

A 76-year-old woman was referred to the hospital because of a fractured femoral bone. It was then observed that she had a large scaling plaque with partly confluent brownish-red papules and central scarification on the right cheek. She did not know the duration of the lesion. Culture revealed the presence of *M. tuberculosis*.

The epidermis was edematous, thin and covered by a crust. In the dermis there were conspicuous edema and large areas of fibrinoid necrosis bordered by epithelioid cell granulomas and dense infiltrates of lymphocytes. Only a single giant cell of foreign-body type was observed (Fig. 15.1c,d).

15.1.4 Other Types of Skin Lesions due to Spreading from Internal Organs

Scrofuloderma implies a direct extension of tuberculous infection to the skin from underlying tissues such as lymph nodes or bone.

Orificial tuberculosis is due to inoculation of bacteria at the mucosal–cutaneous interface from internal organs.

Tuberculosis cutis miliaris disseminata and *meta-*

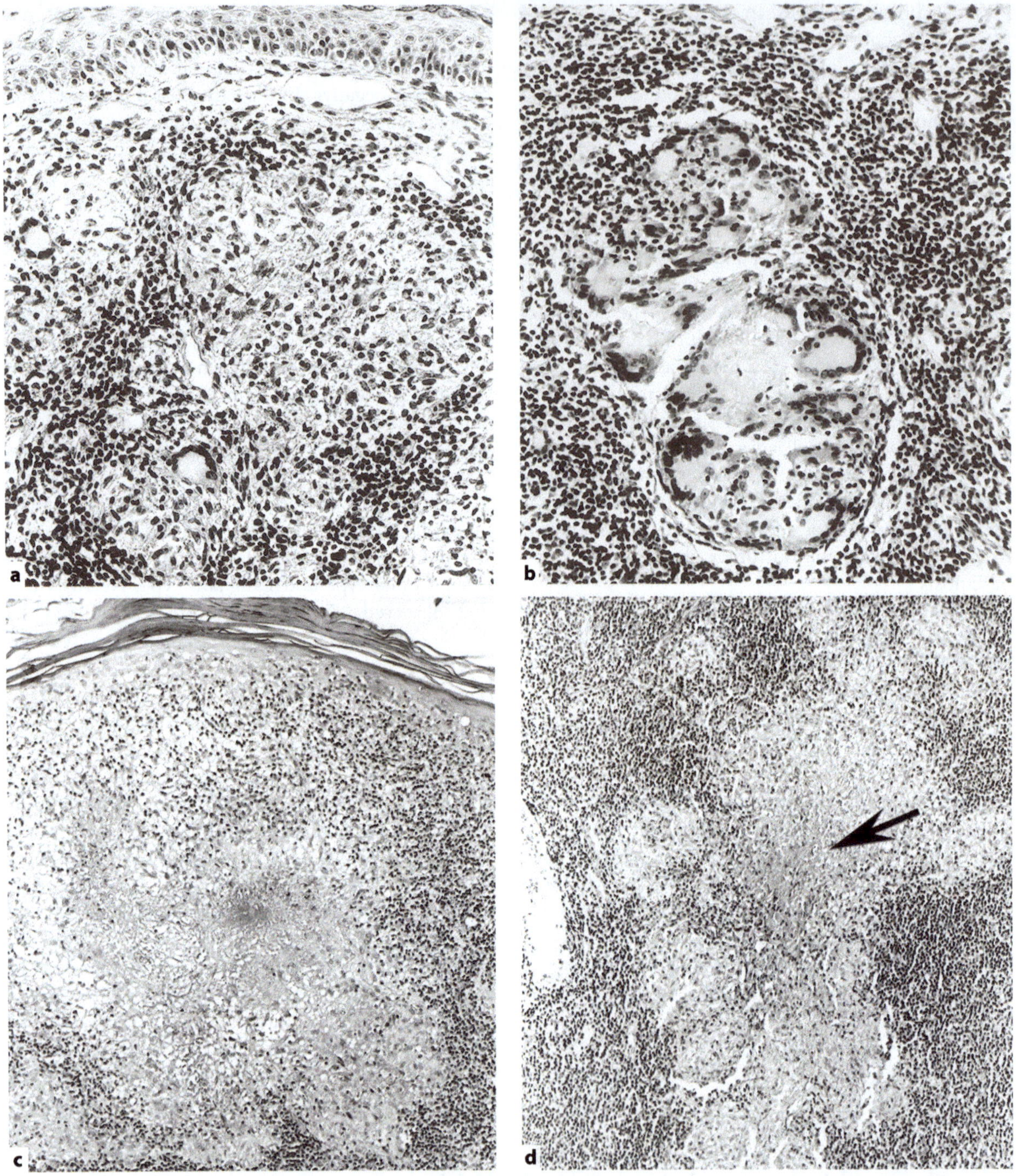

Fig. 15.1 Lupus vulgaris. **a** The epidermis is flat, but otherwise normal. In the dermis there are epithelioid cell granulomas surrounded by dense infiltrates of lymphocytes. They contain scattered giant cells of Langhans type, but no necrosis; H&E. **b** In another area there is a conglomeration of giant cells. **c** In this case there is a large, irregular fibrinoid necrosis, the lower part of which is bordered by epithelioid cell granulomas. The surrounding tissue is conspicuously edematous. Also the epidermis is edematous and infiltrated with lymphocytes. The horny layer is thickened and parakeratofic; PAS. **d** Accumulation of different-sized granulomas with a small central fibrinoid necrosis; arrow vG

static tuberculous abscesses are caused by hematogenous spread in undernourished and immunodeficient individuals.

15.2 Infections in the Skin Caused by Atypical Mycobacteria

During recent decades infections caused by atypical mycobacteria (i.e., mycobacteria other than *M. tuberculosis*, *M. bovis* and *M. leprae*) have been an increasing problem. Atypical mycobacteria comprise a number of pathogens, which on culture give rise to colonies of acid-fast bacilli. They may infect humans, but not guinea pigs, as do *M. tuberculosis* and *M. bovis*. Runyon (1959) presented a classification based on bacteriologic criteria and included four groups. Members of groups I–III are slow growing, but can be differentiated from each other in culture according to the color the colonies take on after exposure to light. The members of group IV are rapidly growing.

Infections with atypical mycobacteria are in several aspects different from infection with *M. tuberculosis* (Woods and Washington 1987). Usually person-to-person transmission does not occur. Isolates of *M. tuberculosis* from a person always indicate tuberculosis, while isolates of atypical mycobacteria, from for example the respiratory tract, are not always equated with disease. They may be present without giving rise to disease; often a predisposing condition such as a concurrent disease or damaged tissue is required for tissue invasion. Also, it is important to know that a few nonpathogenic atypical mycobacteria may be found accidentally in inflammatory skin lesions of other causes. Some relevant atypical mycobacteria infections are discussed below.

15.2.1 Infection with *M. Avium–Intracellulare* Complex

The bacteria, which belong to the *M. avium–intracellulare* complex are slow growing, exist in the environment, for example in soil and water, and infect animals (poultry, rabbits). The complex was recognized as a pathogen for humans in 1943, and is today the most common cause of atypical mycobacterial infection in humans. It is primarily a lung disease and usually occurs in patients with a preexisting pulmonary disease such as bronchiectasis, chronic bronchitis, emphysema, healed tuberculosis, or pneumoconiosis. *Mycobacterium avium–intracellulare* is also an important cause of infection in immunocompromised patients and, when present in HIV-infected individuals, is an AIDS-defining condition. Skin lesions in patients with disseminated disease have been reported (Horsburgh et al. 1985; Friedman et al. 1988; Maurice et al. 1988). The histopathologic pattern is variable (Woods and Washington 1987).

15.2.2 Infection with *M. Malmoense*

Mycobacterium malmoense, a slow growing atypical mycobacterium, was first described and isolated from four patients with lung disease in the Swedish city of Malmö in 1977 (Henriques et al. 1994). The infection is most common in northern Europe and Great Britain. In adults it is mainly a pulmonary disease. In children it appears as lymphadenitis (Jenkins and Tsukamura 1979; Henriques et al. 1994). As in infections with *M. avium–intracellulare* complex, there is often an underlying disease. Skin lesions seem to be rare, but in some patients tenosynovitis localized to a wrist or a hand, as in the case described below, has been observed (Syed and O'Flanagan 1998). In Sweden *M. malmoense* is second only to the *M. avium–intracellulare* complex as the cause of atypical mycobacterial infection (Henriques et al. 1994). The incidence is increasing and a number of cases have also been reported from central and southern Europe, USA and Canada (Enzensberger et al. 1999). *Mycobacterium malmoense* has been isolated from soil and water and probably is ubiquitous (Portaels et al. 1995).

15.2.3 Infection with *M. Marinum*

Mycobacterium marinum is a slow growing atypical mycobacterium that may give rise to cutaneous lesions in otherwise healthy persons. It was described by Aronson (1926) as the cause of an infectious disease in fish living in salt-water and later by Nordén and Linell (1951) as a human pathogen. The disease is contracted in swimming pools and by contact with infected aquariums and fish. Linell and Nordén (1954) presented a study on two epidemics caused by *M. marinum* infection. These occurred in two small Swedish cities and affected schoolchildren and adults who regularly and frequently visited the public swimming pool. The two epidemics involved more than 100 persons. The authors found an atypical mycobacterium in the skin lesions and named it *M. balnei*, which was later proved to be identical to *M. marinum* (Woods and Washington 1987).

15.2.3.1
Clinical Appearance

The organisms enter the skin through a slightly damaged epidermis. Two to three weeks after transmission a red papule appears at the site of inoculation, which in the series of Linell and Nordén in most cases was an elbow. The lesion slowly increases in size, becomes scaly, infiltrated, and sometimes centrally ulcerated. Usually after several months the lesion heals leaving a scar. However, in some cases the infection may go on for years, healing in the center but spreading peripherally.

15.2.3.2
Histopathologic Appearance

Biopsy specimens taken at different ages of the lesion have shown that the inflammatory cell infiltrate during the first months is nonspecific and sometimes purulent. After 2 to 4 months, giant cells and epithelioid cell granulomas appear (Månsso et al. 1970). In some cases granular or fibrinoid necroses in epithelioid cell granulomas have been observed (Linell and Nordén 1954). *Mycobacterium marinum* is as acid-fast as the *M. tuberculosis*, but is very seldom found in histologic sections (Linell and Nordén 1954).

15.2.4
Infection with *M. Fortuitum–Chelonae* Complex

The *M. fortuitum–chelonae* complex belongs to the rapidly growing group IV of atypical mycobacteria. Most of the lesions are located in the skin and are caused by a penetrating injury, or by surgery. Also individuals who are not immunocompromised may be affected (Woods and Washington 1987).

15.2.5
Examples

Case 3. *Mycobacterium Malmoense* Infection

A 62-year old woman suffered from systemic lupus erythematosus (SLE) and hypothyroidism. Over a period of 2 years she had noticed a slowly progressing swelling and erythema of the proximal part of the right little finger. It was thought to be a synovitis and a manifestation of SLE.

Excision biopsies from the tendon sheath of the base of the finger showed fibrous tissue with multiple closely set, large and often stellate, glossy, eosinophilic (fibrinoid) necrotic areas, enclosed by a wide border of macrophages and epithelioid cells and scattered giant cells together with other inflammatory cells, mainly lymphocytes. Surrounding these large granulomas, in a pattern very similar to that present in rheumatic nodules, there were smaller well-developed epithelioid cells granulomas with scattered giant cells, but no

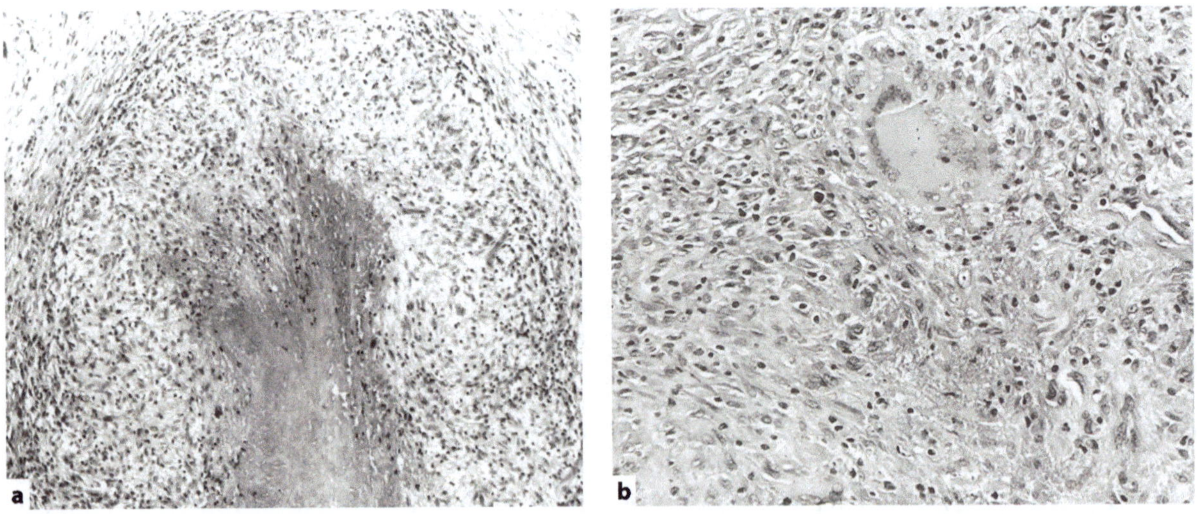

Fig. 15.2 *Mycobacterium malmoense*. **a** The micrograph shows a part of a large, stellate, fibrinoid necrosis surrounded by a broad rim of epithelioid cells. **b** Close-up of the granulomatous area discloses that in addition to epithelioid cells there is a slight admixture of lymphocytes and scattered giant cells. H&E

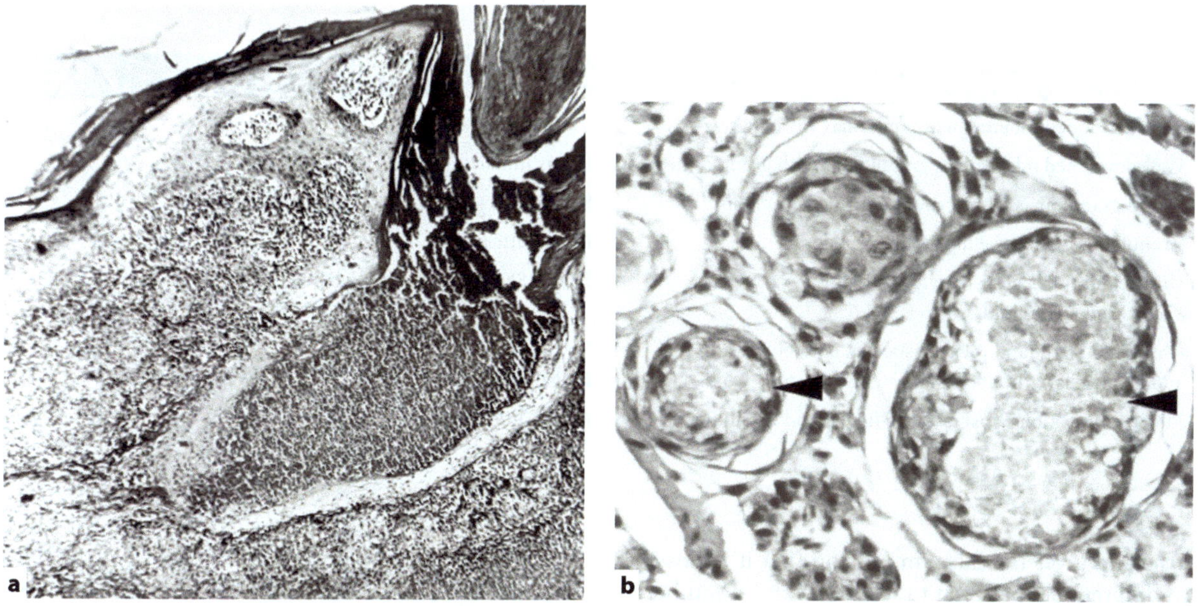

Fig. 15.3 *Mycobacterium marinum*. **a** A markedly distended and plugged hair follicle is filled with neutrophils and in the upper dermis walled off by small epithelioid cell granulomas. **b** Epithelioid cell granulomas in the liver of an aquarium fish. The indicated granulomas show granular necrosis. *(arrowheads)* H&E (reproduced from Månsso et al. 1970, with permission)

necrosis. Due to the impressive granulomas with fibrinoid necrosis, the diagnosis of rheumatoid nodule was suggested.

However, the biopsy wound did not heal and culture of discharged material was positive for *M. malmoense*. When the slides were reexamined a few acid-fast bacilli were found in necrotic areas. Also the small well-developed epithelioid cell granulomas outside the large necrotic granulomas were more in accordance with a tuberculous lesion than with a rheumatoid nodule (Fig. 15.2).

Case 4. *Mycobacterium Marinum* Infection

This 55-year old man presented with a 4×2.5 cm large bluish-red scaling lesion with marginal pustules on the dorsal aspect of the right lower arm. The lesion had developed during the previous 3 weeks. Fungal infection was suspected, but culture was negative and antifungal treatment had no effect. The lesion increased slowly at the periphery and healed in the center. Bacterial cultures were done and grew *M. marinum*.

During the course of the disease repeated biopsies were performed. Three months after occurrence of the lesion, investigation showed epithelial hyperplasia and nonspecific inflammatory cell infiltrates. Four months after occurrence of the lesion, small epithelioid cell granulomas were observed in the upper dermis. Finally, when the lesion was about six months old, the presence of well-developed granulomas without necrosis were obvious. Acid-fast bacilli were not observed. In addition to granulomas there were intrafollicular abscesses composed of neutrophils. The source of the infection was traced to the patient's aquarium. *M. marinum* was cultured from several components of the aquarium. A sick fish had liver granulomas with necrosis, in which acid-fast bacteria were found (Månsso et al. 1970) (Fig. 15.3a,b).

15.3 Comment

An important subject in the discussion on the histopathology of epithelioid cell granulomas is the kind of necrosis that may occur. Most often the areas of necrosis in epithelioid cell granulomas due to tuberculosis have a noneosinophilic, amorphous and slightly granular appearance in H&E-stained sections. In most textbooks and articles this kind of necrosis is called caseation necrosis. This concept is used as contrasted with the eosinophilic glossy, often angular, necrosis designated fibrinoid necrosis seen in rheumatic nodules and sometimes in sarcoidosis and leprosy. As already mentioned the concept caseation necrosis refers to the gross appearance of necrotic tissue in advanced lung tuberculosis (Sect. 5.3.1.1). Therefore the term caseation necrosis forms an association with tubercu-

Table 15.1 Mycobacterial infections differential diagnoses

Histologic pattern	Differential diagnosis
Well-developed tuberculoid granulomas without necrosis	Sarcoidosis (Sect. 5.3.1.2)
Well-developed tuberculoid granulomas with granular necrosis	Lupus miliaris disseminatus faciei
Naked granulomas with scattered fibrinoid necrosis	Sarcoidosis (Sect. 5.3.1.2), leprosy (Sect. 16.3.3)
Granulomas with large fibrinoid necrosis	Rheumatic nodule
Diffuse infiltrates of histiocytes with only a few or no epithelioid cells	Lepra (Sect. 16.3.3), syphilis (Sect. 17.2.2,), ACA (Sect. 18.4.2)
Chronic inflammation with dispersed epithelioid cells and giant cells without tendency to aggregate	Syphilis (Sect. 17.2.2), ACA (Sect. 18.4.2), fungal infections (Sect. 13.1.3)
Purulent infections, abscesses (follicular and nonfollicular)	Fungal infections (Sect. 13.1.3)

losis and gives the false impression that it is possible to differentiate between tuberculous and nontuberculous granulomas based on the histologic appearance of the necrosis. That this is a chimera is demonstrated in Case 2 (infection with *M. tuberculosis*) and Case 3 (infection with *M. malmoense*). In both cases granulomas containing large areas of fibrinoid necrosis were observed (Figs. 15.1c and 15.2a).

Also nontuberculous granular necrosis surrounded with epithelioid cell granulomas may appear in the skin as in lesions of lupus miliaris disseminatus faciei (today considered a variant of rosacea). It is therefore preferable to talk about granular necrosis instead of caseation necrosis and granulomas without necrosis instead of noncaseating granulomas.

15.4 Differential Diagnosis

Santa Cruz and Strayer (1982) investigated biopsy specimens from well-documented nonlepromatous mycobacterial lesions in the skin and subcutis from 31 patients, which included infections with *M. tuberculosis* as well as with different kinds of atypical mycobacteria. They found a wide range histopathologic patterns. These are matched with possible differential diagnoses in Table 15.1.

References

1. Aronson JD (1926) Spontaneous tuberculosis in saltwater fish. J Infect Dis 39:315–320
2. Enzensberger R, Hunfeld K-P, Krause M, Rüsch-Gerdes S, Brade V, Böddinghaus B (1999) Mycobacterium malmoense infections in immunocompetent patients. Eur J Clin Microbiol Infect Dis 18:579–581
3. Farina MC, Gegundez MI, Pique E, Esteban J, Martin L, Requena L, Barat A, Fernandez Guerrero M (1995) Cutaneous tuberculosis: a clinical, histopathologic, and bacteriologic study. J Am Acad Dermatol 33:433–440
4. Friedman BF, Edwards D, Kirkpatrick CH (1988) Mycobacterium avium-intracellulare: cutaneous presentations of disseminated disease. Am J Med 85:257–263
5. Henriques B, Hoffner SE, Petrini B, Juhlin I, Wåhlén P, Källenius G (1994) Infection with Mycobacterium malmoense in Sweden: report of 221 cases. Clin Infect Dis 18:596–600
6. Horsburgh CR Jr, Mason UG, Farhi DC, Iseman MD (1985) Disseminated infection with mycobacterium avium-intracellulare. A report of 13 cases and review of the literature. Medicine 64:36–48
7. Jenkins PA, Tsukamura M (1979) Infections with Mycobacterium malmoense in England and Wales. Tubercle 60:71–76
8. Lever WF, Schaumburg-Lever G (1990) Histopathology of the skin. J.B. Lippincott Company, Philadelphia
9. Linell F, Nordén Å (1954) Mycobacterium balnei, a new acid-fast bacillus occurring in swimming pools and capable of producing skin lesions in humans. Acta Tuberc Scand Suppl 33:1–84
10. Månsso T, Brehmer-Andersson E, Wittbeck B, Grubb R (1970) Aquarium-borne infection with Mycobacterium marinum. Acta Derm Venereol 50:119–124
11. Maurice PDL, Bunker C, Giles F, Goldstone A, Holton J (1988) Mycobacterium avium-intracellulare infection associated with hairy-cell leukemia. Arch Dermatol 124:1545–1549
12. Nordén Å, Linell F (1951) A new type of pathogenic Mycobacterium. Nature 168:826
13. Portaels F, Larsson L, Jenkins PA (1995) Isolation of Mycobacterium malmoense from the environment in Zaire. Tubercle Lung Dis 76:160–162
14. Runyon EH (1959) Anonymous mycobacteria in pulmonary disease. Med Clin North Am 43:273–290

15. Santa Cruz DJ, Strayer DS (1982) The histologic spectrum of the cutaneous mycobacterioses. Hum Pathol 13:485–495
16. Syed AA, O'Flanagan J (1998) Mycobacterium malmoense infection: an unusual cause of wrist swelling. J Hand Surg 23B:811–812
17. Woods GL, Washington JA (1987) Mycobacteria other than Mycobacterium tuberculosis: review of microbiologic and clinical aspects. Rev Infect Dis 9:275–294

16 Leprosy

Leprosy, caused by *Mycobacterium leprae* is one of the longest known and most chronic diseases that affects humankind. Today the disease is highly prevalent in central Africa, South-East Asia and South America, endemic in some parts of the US and endemic at a low level in southern Europe (i.e., Portugal, Spain, Italy, Greece, Turkey and southern Russia) (Thangaraj and Yawalkar 1987). In northern Europe observed cases are imported.

16.1 Pathogenesis

Secretions from the upper respiratory tract of infected persons with generalized leprosy contain a high number of bacteria which are able to survive for several days outside the body. Consequently, inhalation of infected droplets is thought to be the main means of transmission. In the alveoli the bacteria are taken up by macrophages and are then thought to disseminate in the body through the circulation. However, most individuals exposed to the bacteria develop a subclinical infection and never become ill. Only about 5% show symptoms.

Leprosy bacilli cannot be cultured on artificial media. In vivo they grow and multiply mainly in Schwann cells of the neurilemma and in macrophages in the skin. Consequently, the principal targets are peripheral nerves and skin. Even if not clinically detectable, peripheral nerves are always affected. The nerves may be involved at any level from the periphery to the dorsal root ganglia. Spinal cord and brain are not affected (Thangaraj and Yawalkar 1987).

16.2 Primary Neuritic Leprosy

In primary neuritic leprosy one or several peripheral nerve trunks are infected. The ulnar nerve is the most commonly affected. There is no cutaneous involvement and no history of previous skin lesions. Symptoms are paresis, hypotonia and atrophy of involved muscles. Histologic investigation of the nerve trunk shows the pattern of tuberculoid or borderline leprosy (Thangaraj and Yawalkar 1987).

16.3 Cutaneous Leprosy

In the skin, the disease is expressed as indeterminate leprosy, tuberculoid leprosy, borderline leprosy, or lepromatous leprosy. The leprosy bacteria are straight or slightly curved, Gram-positive rods. The number of bacteria present in the tissue varies with the type of expression of the disease. In sections they lie singly, in clumps, or in compact masses known as globi. A globus is surrounded by a membrane and may contain more than 50 bacteria. Like *M. tuberculosis*, *M. leprae* stains red with Ziehl-Neelsen stain, but is less acid-fast than *M. tuberculosis*. This means that if leprosy is suspected a modified stain with a shorter exposure to the acid–alcohol mixture has to be used.

16.3.1 Indeterminate Leprosy

This is the initial lesion characterized by one or several asymmetric, ill-defined, slightly hypopigmented, or erythematous macules. Sensation is usually normal.

Histologically there are small infiltrates of lymphocytes around vessels, peripheral nerves, sweat glands and hair follicles, but usually no granulomas. A thorough search may reveal a few bacilli, most likely in peripheral nerves. The lesion heals spontaneously if the level of cell-mediated immunity of the host to the bacilli is high enough. However, depending on the level of immunity, indeterminate leprosy may give rise to any of the other forms of leprosy.

16.3.2 Tuberculoid Leprosy

Usually there is only one well-demarcated, infiltrated rounded to oval skin lesion (up to 10 cm in diameter), which has a reddish or brownish color, or is hypopigmented. An irregular and raised border, scaling, and satellite lesions outside the border are signals of high activity of the disease and a decreasing cell-mediated immunity level of the patient (Thangaraj and Yawalkar 1987). In some patients an enlarged and hard cutaneous nerve may be seen or felt in or close to the affected area. Sensation is markedly impaired or lost. If the lesion is located on a hairy area, hairs are lacking or scanty.

Histologic investigation shows well-developed epithelioid cell granulomas, which are encircled by a dense or moderately dense infiltrate of lymphocytes and contain giant cells of Langhans type. The granulomas are spread in the dermis, but characteristically some of them are located close to the epidermis and even appear to gnaw on its base. Nerves are infiltrated and often destroyed. Bacilli are usually not present.

16.3.3 Borderline Leprosy

This form is subdivided into borderline-tuberculoid leprosy, mid-borderline leprosy, and borderline-lepromatous leprosy. There may be widespread erythematous or copper-colored infiltrated plaques and nodules. Also annular lesions due to central clearing are typical of borderline leprosy. The closer the patient is to the lepromatous pole, the more numerous and less well-defined the lesions are. However, hypoesthesia and impairments of hair growth are more marked in the borderline-tuberculoid than in the borderline-lepromatous form.

A clear subepidermal zone is the most important histopathologic difference between tubercular and borderline leprosy. In the borderline-tuberculoid variant, epithelioid cell granulomas contain only a few giant cells, mainly of foreign body type, and lymphocytes are sparse. Dermal appendages and nerves are infiltrated by granulomas, and partly destroyed nerves may be seen. In the mid-borderline form the epithelioid cell granulomas are more diffuse, lymphocytes few and diffusely spread; giant cells are lacking. Nerves are less involved. In the borderline-lepromatous form the inflammatory cell infiltrate is mainly composed of macrophages with abundant granular or foamy cytoplasm and a variable number of epithelioid cells. Lymphocytes may be present in patchy, large aggregates close to some granulomas. The perineurium of small nerves is often infiltrated by inflammatory cells and shows an onion-skin pattern (Ridley 1985). The number of acid-fast bacilli successively increases from borderline-tuberculoid leprosy to lepromatous leprosy.

16.3.4 Lepromatous Leprosy

Most cases develop from borderline leprosy; however a lepromatous nodule, usually situated in the face, may be the first sign of the disease. Usually the lesions are many and widespread. Macules appear in the early phase and are later followed by infiltrated and nodular lesions. The nodules are situated in the dermis.

Histologic investigation of skin lesions shows, below a flat epidermis and a cell-free subepidermal zone, large granulomas composed entirely of macrophages with abundant, clear or hazy cytoplasm containing very large numbers of *M. leprae*. Lymphocytes are sparse or absent. Nerves may have an onion-skin appearance without cell infiltrates (Ridley 1985).

Lepromatous leprosy is a generalized disease. A very high number of proliferating bacteria are found in both normal-appearing skin and lesional skin, in the mucous membranes of the upper respiratory tract, and also in inner organs, breast milk, semen and feces. The patients are specifically anergic to *M. leprae* (i.e., there is no general immune deficiency); this is mirrored by a negative lepromin test and a sparse number of lymphocytes in the lesions.

16.3.5 Example

Case 1. Lepromatous Leprosy[1]

The patient, a woman, was born in 1937 and in the mid-1960s immigrated to Sweden from Greece; she worked as a cleaner. For several years she had suffered from diffuse pain in the left arm and leg. In 1981, paresis of the left foot developed and she noticed an anesthetic area on the left lower leg and foot. She also complained of backache and numbness of the left arm. Lumbagosciatica was diagnosed, and at the end of 1985 she was granted a sickness pension.

In 1985, she consulted for urticaria-like efflorescences on the face and extremities; a drug reaction was suspected. A biopsy specimen revealed dilated dermal venules and moderate perivascular infiltrates of lymphocytes and scattered eosinophils. She presented 18 months later with up to palm-sized brownish-red and non-itching maculae on the arms, legs and lower back. Histologic investigation showed several small epithelioid cell granulomas with an admixture of lym-

1 Courtesy of Dr. Roland Nilsson, Capio Diagnostic, Stockholm, Sweden

phocytes in the dermis; giant cells were not observed. Sarcoidosis was suggested, but could not be proved. After a further 18 months nummular infiltrates and nodules up to 10 mm in size had developed on the extremities.

A biopsy specimen from a nodule showed a flat epidermis and a distinct, narrow and cell-free subepidermal area. Below this area the markedly thickened dermis was totally obliterated by closely set, dense aggregates of macrophages containing a very high number of acid-fast bacilli. There were a sparse number of diffusely spread lymphocytes, but no giant cells. Staining for acid-fast bacilli disclosed a high number of organisms also in biopsy specimens taken 3 years and 1.5 years earlier (Fig. 16.1).

At the time of diagnosis, in 1988, slit-skin smears (see Glossary) taken from three different skin lesions and an ear lobe revealed a high number of bacteria. After 18 months treatment for lepromatous leprosy the bacterial index according to Ridley (see Glossary) in ear-lobe smears was +4. The number of bacteria in ear-lobe smears then slowly diminished, and in 1994 and 1995 bacilli were not observed.

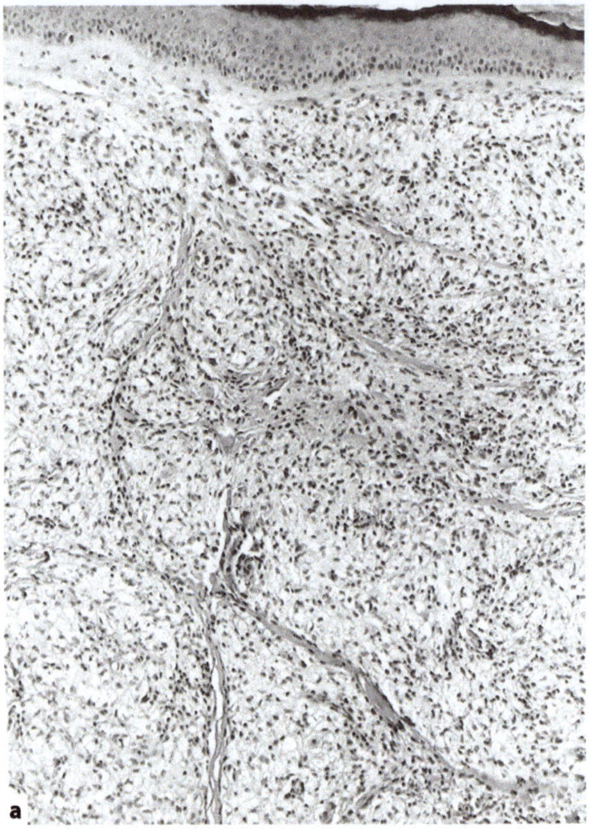

a

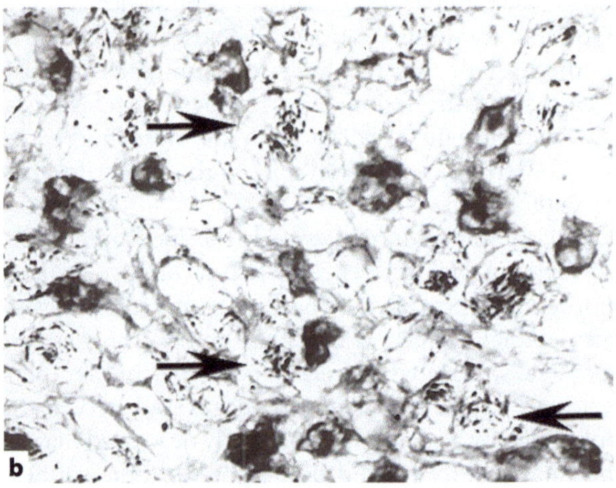

b

Fig. 16.1 Lepromatous leprosy. **a** Below a narrow and cell-free subepidermal area, the dermis is totally obliterated by different-sized granulomas, separated from each other by strings of connective tissue. The granulomas are composed of macrophages with abundant hazy or clear cytoplasm. There is a sparse admixture of lymphocytes; H&E, ×100. **b** Close-up shows that some macrophages contain clusters of bacteria (*arrows*); ×1000, Modified Ziehl-Neelsen stain

16.3.5.1
Comment

The related case with a history of disease over at least two decades demonstrates well the chronicity of leprosy and also highlights the difficulty in diagnosing leprosy in a leprosy-free country. The biopsy specimen from the urticaria-like lesion indicates that the patient was suffering from advanced leprosy as early as 3 years before the diagnosis was settled. The fact that the disease started as a primary neuritic leprosy added to the complexity.

16.3.6
Reactions in Leprosy

During the usually chronic course of the disease, acute and severe inflammatory exacerbations may appear in every type of leprosy except in the early indeterminate stage (Thangaraj and Yawalkar 1987). Reactions may be provoked by, for example, intercurrent infections, mental and physical stress, pregnancy, surgical interventions and inadequate treatment, but also by effective chemotherapy and reduction in the bacillary load. They are called reactions in leprosy, and are of two types.

16.3.6.1 Type I

Type I is regarded as a delayed-hypersensitivity reaction type IV (Sect. 4.3.4) and is most common in borderline-lepromatous leprosy. Exacerbations appear in preexisting skin and nerve lesions and are caused by a shift of the disease either to the tubercular pole (reversal or upgrading reaction) or to the lepromatous pole (downgrading reaction). Upgrading reactions may follow treatment and downgrading reactions are seen in patients with inadequate treatment. The most important histopathologic feature seems to be edema, which may be fibrinous (Ridley 1985)

16.3.6.2 Type II (Erythema Nodosum Leprosorum)

Type II reaction is a hypersensitivity reaction type III (Sect. 4.3.3). It is most common in lepromatous leprosy and has clinical and histopathologic characteristic patterns. Crops of new lesions, which come and go, appear in the skin and subcutaneous tissue. Histologic investigation shows vasculitis and infiltrates of neutrophils (Ridley 1985).

16.3.7 The Paucibacillary and Multibacillary Groups

According to the number of bacteria in the tissue, leprosy may be divided into two groups. The paucibacillary group includes indeterminate leprosy, primary neuritic leprosy, borderline-tuberculoid leprosy, and tuberculoid leprosy. No or only a few bacilli are found. Slit-skin smears are negative. The immunity state of the patient is good, which is mirrored by a positive lepromin skin test (see Glossary). The disease is stable. The multibacillary group includes mid-borderline leprosy, borderline-lepromatous leprosy, and lepromatous leprosy. Bacilli are usually found in slit-skin smears in increasing numbers from borderline tuberculoid-leprosy to lepromatous-leprosy. With the exception of the borderline-tuberculoid form, the lepromin test is negative. The immunity is poor and the disease is unstable.

16.3.8 Classification According to Ridley

The classification (including its special abbreviations) developed by Ridley and his group in 1974 is still in use (Lever and Schaumburg-Lever 1990):
Indeterminate leprosy (I)

- Tuberculoid leprosy (polar tuberculoid leprosy) (TT)
- True borderline form (BB)
- Borderline lepromatous form (BL)
- Lepromatous leprosy (LL) divided into:
  - Subpolar leprosy (LLs)
  - Polar leprosy (LLp)

16.3.9 Differential Diagnosis

- Sarcoidosis (Sect. 5.3.1.2), tuberculosis (Table 15.1), early lesions of secondary syphilis (Sect. 17.2.2) and other infections showing epithelioid cell granulomas are differential diagnoses of tuberculoid leprosy.
- Xanthoma and lepromatous leprosy may be mixed up.

References

1. Lever WF, Schaumburg-Lever G (1990) Histopathology of the skin. J.B. Lippincott Company, Philadelphia
2. Ridley DS (1985) Skin biopsy in leprosy: histological interpretation and clinical application. Ciba-Geigy, Basle
3. Thangaraj RH, Yawalkar SJ (1987) Leprosy for medical practitioners and paramedical workers. Ciba-Geigy, Basle

17 Syphilis

Syphilis is caused by the spirochete *Treponema pallidum*, a helical bacterium, which measures 6–15 μm in length and 0.10–0.18 μm in width. It divides through transverse fission, which may explain the large variation in length. *Treponema pallidum* is pathogenic only to humans and cannot be cultured. In fixed tissue the bacterium is waved. It cannot be seen in routinely stained sections, but may be visualized by means of different silver stains (Warthin-Starry, Steiner, Bosma-Steiner).

Untreated the disease passes through four stages: primary syphilis, secondary syphilis, latent syphilis, and late or tertiary syphilis. The concept "early syphilis" includes the two first stages. In adults, syphilis is usually contracted by sexual contact with a person suffering from either primary or secondary syphilis. The disease is contagious only during these two stages.

Humoral and cell-mediated immune responses are both necessary for the development of resistance to reinfection, and immunity to reinfection develops only in untreated individuals (Sanchez 1999). The primary syphilitic lesion elicits both the humoral and cell-mediated immune defense systems, which together kill most of the spirochetes, and the chancre heals. However, some spirochetes escape, proliferate, and finally give rise to secondary syphilis that is an expression of spirochetemia. During the period between the primary and secondary stages the cell-mediated response is suppressed while the antibody levels increase in response to the rising number of spirochetes. Late syphilis in the skin takes the form of infectious immune granulomas (Sect. 5.3.1). They are due to a cell-mediated hypersensitivity reaction provoked by a small number of spirochetes still present in the tissue.

17.1 Primary Syphilis

The spirochetes pass through mucous membranes or slightly damaged skin, and on the site of inoculation give rise to the primary lesion, the so-called chancre. The time between inoculation and appearance of the chancre varies between 10 and 90 days, but is on average 3 weeks.

17.1.1 Clinical Appearance

The chancre is a painless rounded, firm, button-like and well-circumscribed ulceration with a raised border. The oozing surface is crowded with spirochetes and thus is highly contagious. The predilection sites in men are the glans penis and prepuce, and in women, the vulva and uterine cervix. There can be more than one lesion. Extragenital chancres may appear on the lips, in the oral cavity, pharynx, rectum, and on the nipple. The regional lymph nodes become enlarged. The chancre may pass unnoticed, especially in females where it may be concealed due to the location. If not treated, it disappears after 3–12 weeks with an inconspicuous scar or without scarring.

17.1.2 Histopathologic Appearance

In the middle of the lesion there is ulceration, the floor of which consists of the upper dermis. The surface is covered with fibrinous exudate and inflammatory cells, mainly neutrophils. The surrounding epidermis is thickened and acanthotic. Below and around the ulceration the dermis is edematous and richly vascularized. Dilated venules have protruding endothelial cells and there are dense infiltrates of lymphocytes, plasma cells and histiocytes. Histiocytes sometimes aggregate and form granulomas. Larger veins in the subcutaneous tissue may be thrombotic and infiltrated by inflammatory cells (thrombophlebitis). A silver stain demonstrates the presence of spirochetes (Engelkens et al. 1991).

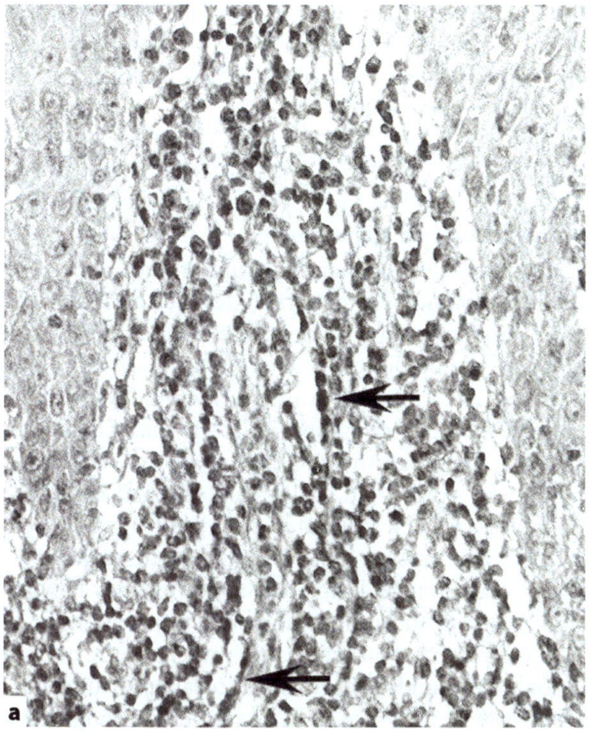

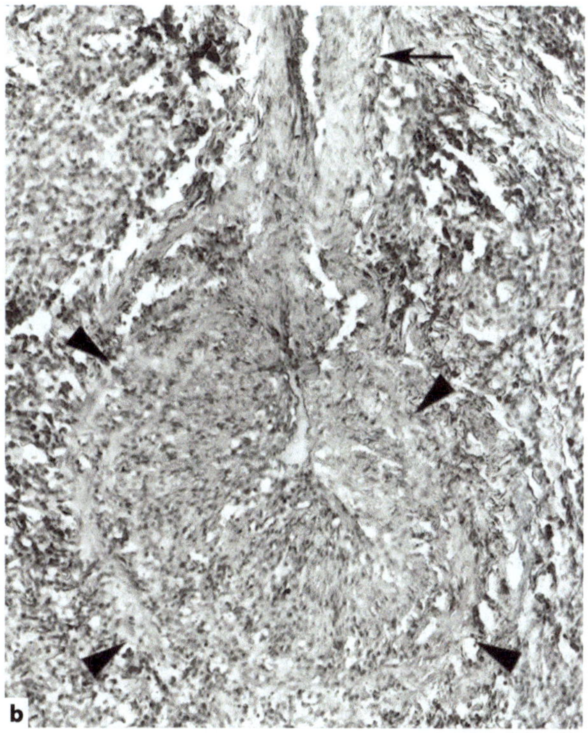

Fig. 17.1 Primary syphilis (chancre). **a** The papillary dermis contains a conspicuously dense cell infiltrate, consisting of lymphocytes and plasma cells. There are two dilated venules with protruding endothelial cells (*arrows*). **b** In the subcutis a longitudinally cut larger vein (*arrow*) joins a transversally cut vein. The latter is obliterated by a thrombus in organization (*arrowheads*). The surrounding tissue is permeated with inflammatory cells. H&E

17.1.3 Examples

Case 1. Primary Syphilis (Verified by Serologic Tests)

A 48-year-old man consulted because of phimosis. There was an ulcer on the dorsal part of the prepuce, a part of which was excised. The specimen measured 5×2 cm. On a fibrous base there was a shallow ulcer about 1 cm in diameter.

Histologic investigation revealed an ulcer covered with a crust of fibrin and neutrophils. The surrounding epidermis was acanthotic and parakeratotic. The dermis consisted of richly vascularized granulation tissue, which contained venules with protruding endothelial cells and very dense confluent inflammatory cell infiltrates, composed mainly of lymphocytes and plasma cells. Histiocytes were not conspicuous and epithelioid cell granulomas were not observed. At the dermal–subcutaneous border several veins were obliterated either by dense infiltrates of lymphocytes or by a thrombus in organization (thrombophlebitis). Extravasation of erythrocytes was a conspicuous phenomenon (Fig. 17.1).

Case 2. Primary Syphilis (Verified by Serologic Tests)

A 38-year-old man, presented with phimosis due to a striking edema. Investigation showed an ulcerated lesion that involved the glans penis and the dorsal part of the prepuce. A biopsy specimen was taken from the prepuce.

The histopathologic pattern was very much like that described above in Case 1, and also included thrombophlebitis. In addition there were aggregates of histiocytes.

17.2 Secondary Syphilis

In this stage the skin as well as mucous membranes are affected. The interval between the first and second stage is highly variable. The latter may appear before the primary lesion has completely vanished, or weeks or months after the healing of the chancre.

17.2.1 Clinical Appearance

There are two kinds of eruption, which appear one after the other. The first is called the *macular syphilid* and the second the *papular syphilid*. The papular syphilid may follow the macular syphilid or for a period of time exist together with it thus appearing as a maculopapular eruption.

17.2.1.1 Macular Syphilid

A macular syphilid occurs only in about 10% of infected individuals. It is evanescent and consists of light reddish-brown, nonscaling, round or oval macules symmetrically spread mainly over the trunk and upper extremities.

17.2.1.2 Papular Syphilid

The papules are disseminated all over the body including the face, soles, palms, mucous membranes, and the border between skin and mucous membranes. The early papules are shiny and copper-red, but change with the age of the lesion. An eruption may become slightly scaling and simulate more common skin diseases such as pityriasis rosea, psoriasis, and lichen planus. However, the eruption is associated with general lymph node enlargement, which differentiates secondary syphilis from those more common skin diseases. Sometimes there are symptoms such as general malaise, fever, headache and arthralgias.

In the genital area, papules coalesce to hypertrophic lesions called *condylomata lata*. Scalp hair follicles may be affected giving rise to the irregular and patchy so-called *moth-eaten alopecia*. Sometimes the eyebrows and beard are also involved. During recent years a variant of secondary syphilis called *lues maligna* with widespread noduloulcerative or vesiculonecrotic lesions and general symptoms has been described in HIV-infected patients (Don et al. 1995).

In immunocompetent patients, the papules and condylomata disappear after 4–12 weeks without treatment, but new eruptions may occur one or several times after symptom-free intervals. In many patients the secondary stage can also pass unnoticed. If untreated, the disease enters the latent stage, *latent syphilis*, the only marker of which is persistent positive serologic tests for syphilis. This stage may last for many years or forever.

17.2.2 Histopathologic Appearance

The first evanescent macular eruption has an nonspecific histopathologic pattern (Alessi et al. 1983). In early papular lesions patchy cell infiltrates are located close to the epidermis and around vessels and hair follicles. The infiltrates consist of lymphocytes and a variable number of plasma cells. In many cases diffusely scattered epithelioid cells and/or small loosely composed epithelioid cell granulomas also appear. Subepidermal cell infiltrates are mixed up with neutrophils and nuclear dust and invade the epidermis. In the center of the lesion the epidermis may be very thin (close to ulceration) and sometimes attains a lichenoid pattern. Spirochetes are present in the dermis (submucosa) and epidermis (mucosal epithelium); in condylomata lata they may be numerous (Engelkens et al. 1991) (Fig. 17.4). In older papular lesions epithelioid cell granulomas with giant cells of Langhans or foreign-body type may appear throughout the dermis below a normal epidermis. Venules are often slightly to moderately dilated and filled with red blood cells. They show more or less protruding endothelial cells. Changes in the subcutaneous tissue are inconspicuous.

17.2.3 Examples

Case 3. Secondary Syphilis (Serologically Verified)

A 36-year-old homosexual man presented with a generalized skin eruption observed for 6 weeks. The lesions were nummular or circinate and had a slightly raised border and a pale or atrophic center. Suggested diagnoses were: granuloma annulare, systemic lupus erythematosus, and sarcoidosis. A biopsy specimen was taken from the border of a lesion.

Histologic investigation revealed a large subepidermal inflammatory cell infiltrate and in the deeper dermis smaller infiltrates around vessels and hair follicles. The cell infiltrates were composed of lymphocytes, plasma cells, and diffusely dispersed epithelioid cells. Here and there epithelioid cells formed small and loosely composed granulomas. Over the subepidermal cell infiltrate the epidermis was markedly thin

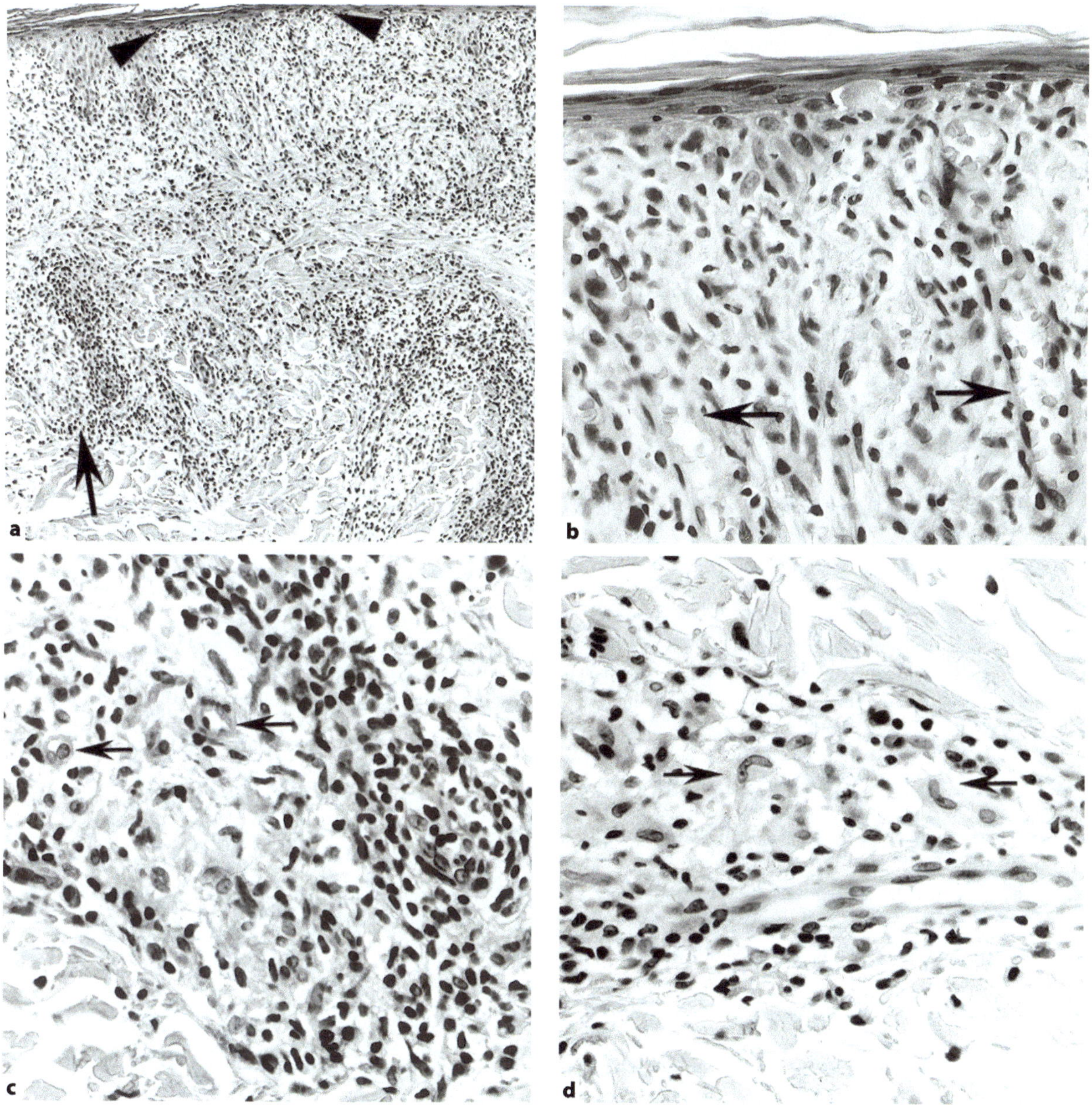

Fig. 17.2 Secondary syphilis (papular syphilid). a In the dermis there are patchy, dense inflammatory cell infiltrates, which contain lighter areas (*arrow*). One of the infiltrates is located close to a markedly thinned epidermis (*arrowheads*). b Close-up of the area indicated with arrowheads in a reveals that the infiltrate is gnawing into the epidermis, which shows the pattern of atrophic lichen planus; there is a sawtooth rete ridge and an apoptotic body. The mixed cell infiltrate is penetrated by dilated venules (*arrows*). c Close-up of the area indicated with an arrow in a. The cell infiltrate is composed of a group of loosely arranged epithelioid cells surrounded by lymphocytes and scattered plasma cells. The arrows indicate two capillaries. d Close to a dilated venule there is a small epithelioid cell granuloma with two banana-like epithelioid cells (*arrows*). Halfway between them there is a mitotic figure in early metaphase. H&E

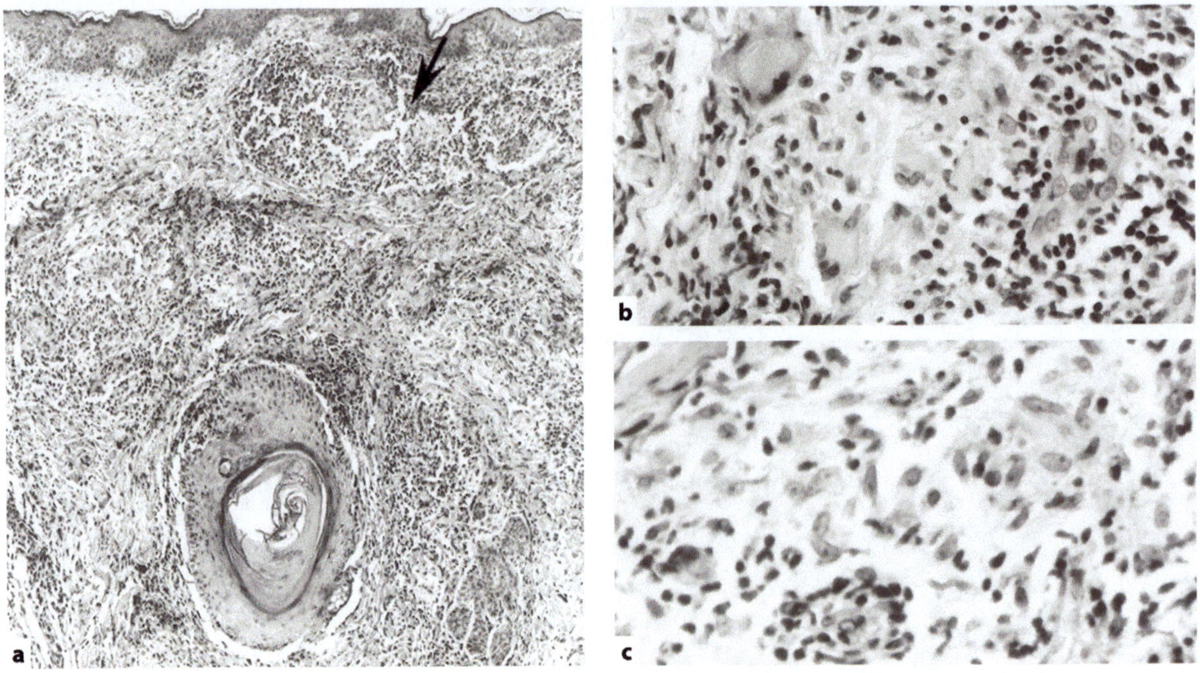

Fig. 17.3 Secondary syphilis (papular syphilid). **a** A hair follicle is surrounded by a dense inflammatory cell infiltrate which also contains small epithelioid cell granulomas. The *arrow* indicates two of them separated by a cleft. **b** Close-up shows a granuloma with two giant cells of Langhans type. **c** In another area there is a loosely composed epithelioid cell granuloma. H&E

and showed a lichenoid pattern. Venules were dilated and often filled with red blood cells. Vasculitis was not observed (Fig. 17.2).

Case 4. Secondary Syphilis (Serologically Verified)

A 46-year-old man had had casual sexual contacts. About 2 months later he experienced a transient lesion, probably an ulcer, on the prepuce. A month thereafter he got a widespread skin eruption, which vanished after a short period of treatment with oral penicillin prescribed for another reason. After a further 3 months the skin lesions recurred. Nearly a year after the occasion of the transmission he consulted for this latest eruption, which had started on the chest and then had successively spread to arms, legs and face. A great number of scaling papules were observed in these areas and also on the soles. He denied itching and pain.

A punch biopsy showed at all levels in the dermis, but with accentuation around a hair follicle, well-established epithelioid cell granulomas with giant cells of Langhans type or foreign-body type. Dense infiltrates of lymphocytes and aggregates of plasma cells surrounded the granulomas. Scattered venules were slightly dilated. There were no signs of vasculitis. The epidermis was normal (Fig. 17.3).

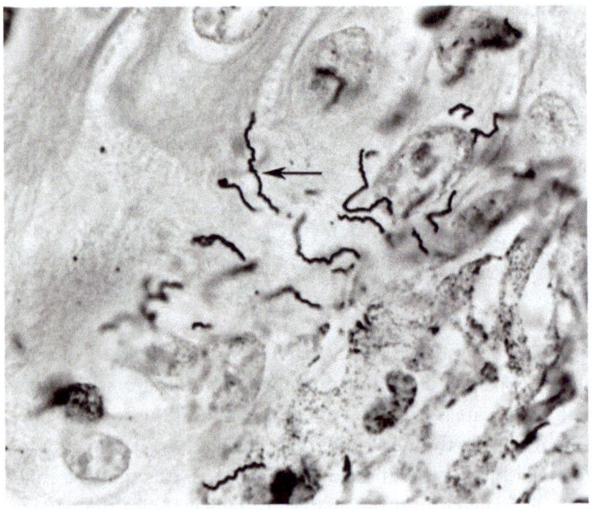

Fig. 17.4 Early syphilis. A cluster of *T. pallidum* in the papillary dermis close to the epidermal–dermal interface. The upper half of the indicated spirochete is lying in the epithelium (*arrow*). Note the desmosomes between the two basal cells. Bosma-Steiner stain, ×1250. The specimen was a gift from Dr. Johannes de Koning, Leeuwarden, The Netherlands

17.2.4 Differential Diagnosis

- *Sarcoidosis*. Papular syphilid with well-developed epithelioid cell granulomas but few or no plasma cells may be misinterpreted as sarcoidosis (Sect. 5.3.1.2).
- *Leprosy* with epithelioid cell granulomas (Sect. 16).
- *ACA* with epithelioid cell granulomas and/or diffusely scattered epithelioid cells (Sect. 18.4.2).
- *Tuberculosis* (Table 15.1).

17.3 Late Benign Syphilis (Tertiary Syphilis) in the Skin

After a variable and often long period (up to 20 years) manifestations of late syphilis may appear in the skin as well as in many other organs. Manifestations appearing in organs outside the cardiovascular and nervous systems are called late benign syphilis. Because of their gummy consistency they are called *gummas*.

17.3.1 Clinical Appearance

In the skin gummas may be up to 10 cm in diameter and appear as reddish tumors or plaques. They ulcerate and give rise to punched-out ulcers, which gradually heal with the formation of scars. In addition there may be smaller lesions, nodules, which appear in groups. Nodules coalesce and by growing at the periphery and healing in the center form annular or circinate figures. Like gummas they may give rise to punched-out ulcers and scars.

17.3.2 Histopathologic Appearance

As already mentioned, late lesions in the skin are immune granulomas. They consist of slowly growing granulomatous/necrotizing bulks, which are gradually replaced by fibrotic scar tissue. In the tegmen (the covering of the body) the gummatous process usually starts in the deep subcutis, but sometimes is due to extension from a gumma involving an underlying muscle or bone. When the lesion is expanding even the skin becomes involved. Nodules are from the beginning located in the skin. They are less destructive than gummas.

Gummas consist of areas of fibrous tissue densely penetrated with inflammatory cells of different types alternating with epithelioid cell granulomas and abscess formation. The presence of thrombophlebitis is emphasized in the older literature (Montgomery 1967). With the exception of thrombophlebitis similar changes are described in nodular tertiary lesions (Wu et al. 2000).

17.3.3 Example

Case 5. Tertiary Syphilis (Serologically Verified)[1]

A 63-year-old woman had suffered for 6 years from widespread ulcerated lesions on the buttocks. She also had scars from healed ulcers on the left hip and left shoulder. A large and deep excision biopsy including subcutaneous tissue was taken.

Histologic investigation revealed on one side of the specimen a large part of an abscess located in the subcutis. The abscess was composed of areas with densely packed neutrophils and nuclear dust and areas with loosely organized epithelioid cell granulomas and giant cells of Langhans type. Towards the central part of the specimen inflammatory cells, mainly lymphocytes and plasma cells imbedded in fibrous tissue walled off the abscess. Below the abscess several veins of different size were thrombotic or densely permeated and filled with inflammatory cells. Arteries were not involved. The dermis contained large, patchy and mainly perivascular cell infiltrates composed of lymphocytes, plasma cells and scattered epithelioid cells. The otherwise acanthotic epidermis was in one area ulcerated and covered by a crust of fibrin and neutrophils (Fig. 17.5).

17.4 Comment

Primary lesions of syphilis are usually diagnosed by means of dark-field microscopy and/or short interval checkups of serologic tests for syphilis. According to the experience of the author they are seldom excised or subjected to biopsies. A biopsy specimen is sometimes taken quite accidentally or for scientific investigations (Engelkens et al. 1991). Today tertiary syphilitic lesions are very rare, at least in Scandinavia. Case 5 was presented at a seminar in dermatopathology in Oslo, Norway, in 1964, organized and held by Dr. Kai Dammert. The main reason for discussing these rare lesions is the notable thrombophlebitis observed both in the

1 Courtesy of Dr. Kai Dammert, University of Oulu, Oulu, Finland

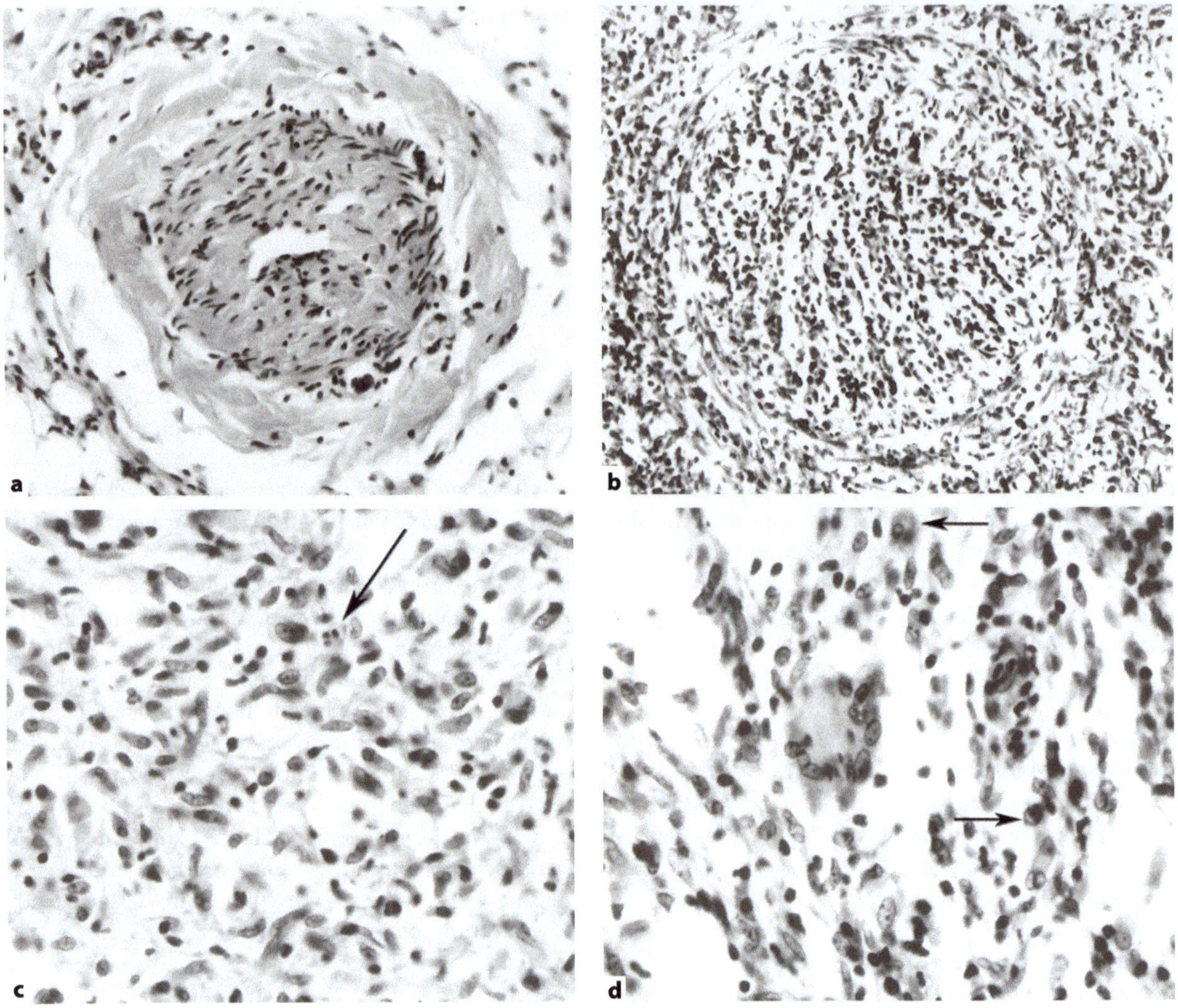

Fig. 17.5 Tertiary syphilis (gumma). **a** A large vein in the subcutaneous tissue is obliterated by an organized thrombus with central recanalization. **b** Another vein in the subcutis is stuffed with lymphocytes and surrounded by a very dense inflammatory cell infiltrate composed of different types of cells. **c** Edematous and disintegrating epithelioid cell granuloma with admixture of lymphocytes and scattered neutrophils (*arrow*). **d** Another area of the granuloma shows scattered giant cell and some plasma cells (*arrows*). H&E

biopsy specimens from the two patients with primary lesions and in the excised gumma. The involvement of both small and large vessels in syphilitic skin lesions is emphasized in the older literature (Holzmann and Hassenpflug 1962; Montgomery 1967).

Following investigations which included light microscopic studies of 29 primary syphilitic lesions, Engelkens et al. (1991) did not mention the presence of thrombophlebitis in the subcutis. However, the biopsies (not further characterized) could have been too superficial to be entirely representative. In the old literature endarteritis obliterans (i.e., thickening and fibrosis of the intima of small arteries followed by narrowing of their lumen) was reported to be significant for the diagnosis of both primary and secondary syphilitic lesions. This interpretation, which still remains in some modern textbooks, probably referred to the presence of high endothelial venules in the dermis, interpreted as obliterated capillaries before activated venules were focused on. Also activation of the venular endothelium in secondary syphilis has been demonstrated in immunohistochemical studies (McBroom et al. 1999).

The most important manifestations for the pathologist to be familiar with are those of secondary syphilis. Now and then a case unexpectedly appears in the daily routine. The histopathologic pattern, though discreet, is sometimes enough characteristic to alert the pathologist. The involvement of the epidermis and the presence of neutrophils and many plasma cells have been focused on previously (Alessi et al. 1983). It is important to stress the epithelioid cell component of the infiltrate, which in the experience of the author is rather common even in early papular lesions. The number of plasma cells is also variable. Sometimes there may be only a few scattered plasma cells but well-developed epithelioid cell granulomas as in one of the author's cases (not described here).

As in acrodermatitis chronica atrophicans, immunohistochemical investigations have revealed that the lymphocytes are T cells (McBroom et al. 1999). This indicates that plasma cells have not developed in the lesion, but have migrated into the skin (Brehmer-Andersson et al. 1998).

References

1. Alessi E, Innocenti M, Ragusa G (1983) Secondary syphilis. Clinical morphology and histopathology. Am J Dermatopathol 5:11–17
2. Brehmer-Andersson E, Hovmark A, Åsbrink E (1998) Acrodermatitis chronica atrophicans: histopathologic findings and clinical correlations in 111 cases. Acta Derm Venereol 78:207–213
3. Don PC, Rubinstein R, Christie S (1995) Malignant syphilis (lues maligna) and concurrent infection with HIV. Int J Dermatol 34:403–407
4. Engelkens HJ, ten Kate FJ, Vuzevski VD, van der Sluis JJ, Stolz E (1991) Primary and secondary syphilis: a histopathological study. Int J STD AIDS 2:280–284
5. Holzmann H, Hassenpflug K (1962) Tertiary syphilitic lymph node involvement of granulating type in a patient with plate-like gummas of the skin (in German). Arch Klin Exp Dermatol 215:230–245
6. McBroom RL, Styles AR, Chiu MJ, Clegg C, Cockerell CJ, Radolf JD (1999) Secondary syphilis in persons infected with and not infected with HIV-1. A comparative immunohistologic study. Am J Dermatopathol 21:432–441
7. Montgomery H (1967) Dermatopathology. Harper & Row, New York, pp 417–427
8. Sanchez MR (1999) Syphilis. In: Freedberg IM, Eisen AZ, Wolff K, Austen KF, Goldsmith LA, Katz SI, Fitzpatrick TB (eds) Fitzpatrick's dermatology in general medicine. McGraw-Hill, New York, pp 2551–2581
9. Wu SJ, Nguyen EQ, Nielsen TA, Pellegrini AE (2000) Nodular tertiary syphilis mimicking granuloma annulare. J Am Acad Dermatol 42:378–380

18 Lyme Borreliosis

Lyme borreliosis is the collective term for a spectrum of diseases caused by *Borrelia* spirochetes. “Lyme” refers to one of three communities in Connecticut, USA, where, in the 1970s, there was an epidemic outbreak of arthritis in children and adults combined with one or several other symptoms such as skin lesions, fever, headache, stiff neck, myalgia, and lymphadenopathy. The disease was called Lyme disease (Steere et al. 1977). It was discovered that the cause of the disease was a *Borrelia* spirochete, isolated and cultured from both patients and the vector, the tick (*Ixodes dammini*), by Willy Burgdorfer, and after him named *Borrelia burgdorferi* (Burgdorfer 1993). *Borrelia burgdorferi* was then thought to be the cause of all manifestations of Lyme borreliosis. However, Baranton et al. (1992) found that *B. burgdorferi* included three species: *B. burgdorferi sensu stricto*, *B. garinii*, and VS461 later named *B. afzelii*. Together these three species are called *B. burgdorferi sensu lato*. All three of them appear in Europe and Asia, but in North America only *B. burgdorferi sensu stricto*, the cause of Lyme disease, has been found.

18.1 Pathogenesis

The *Borrelia* organism is a straight or curved, and irregularly coiled, spirochete measuring 10 to 30 µm in length and 0.18 to 0.25 µm in width (Burgdorfer et al. 1982). Spirochetes are transmitted to humans by bites from infected ticks. Wild animals serve as reservoirs of spirochetes (Anderson and Magnarelli 1993).

Lyme borreliosis is a multisystem disease, manifestations of which may be early or late. Early borreliosis includes the skin lesions *erythema migrans* and *borrelial lymphocytoma*. Usually only one of these manifestations appears. However, sometimes a lymphocytoma occurs after a short period of time or even before the lesion of erythema migrans has completely disappeared. Spirochetemia and early dissemination may follow the initial lesion. Indications of spread are the appearance of multiple erythema migrans-like lesions, symptoms in the joints, or in the cardiovascular and nervous systems.

Dissemination and manifestations, appearing 12 months or more after the spirochetal inoculation, are regarded as late borreliosis. Different organ systems such as the nervous and cardiovascular systems, the joints and the skin may be affected. The late manifestation in the skin, known as *acrodermatitis chronica atrophicans* (ACA), is prevalent in Scandinavia and central and eastern Europe, and is linked to *B. afzelii* (Canica et al. 1993).

18.2 Erythema Migrans

Erythema migrans lesions appear at the site of the tick bite usually 8–9 days after inoculation of the spirochetes (Berger 1993). The most common sites are the trunk and the lower extremities. Spirochetes may be cultivated from punch biopsy specimens taken from lesions of erythema migrans (Åsbrink and Hovmark 1985). Elevated values of serum antibodies to *Borrelia* spirochetes are usually not present.

18.2.1 Clinical Appearance

The lesion consists of a usually nonscaling erythematous to bluish-red patch or plaque, which grows centrifugally and, if regressing in the center, gives rise to an annular figure. Sometimes a target-like configuration develops. Vesicular and crusted eruptions have also been described. The size is highly variable. Mostly there are no symptoms, but some patients complain of itching or pain. Without treatment the lesions disappear spontaneously.

18.2.3 Histopathologic Appearance

Mostly the epidermis is normal, but may show slight spongiosis, exocytosis, and focal parakeratosis. Usu-

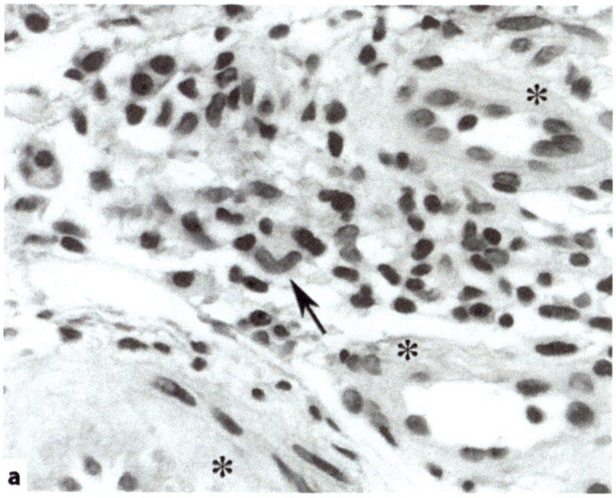

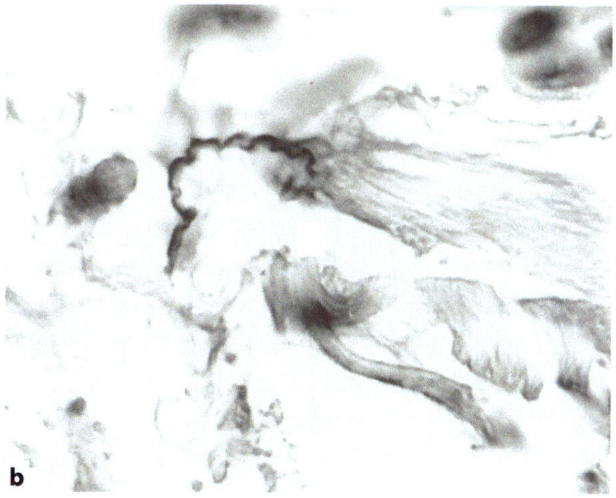

Fig. 18.1 Erythema migrans. **a** In the deep dermis and close to three thick-walled venules with protruding endothelial cells (*asterisks*) there is a mixed cell infiltrate. This is composed of lymphocytes and plasma cells, two of which have two nuclei (*left upper corner*). There are also scattered epithelioid cells, one of which is typically banana-like (*arrow*); H&E. **b** A single distinct, curved, and unevenly waved *Borrelia* spirochete, identified in frozen material from the same lesion as shown in **a**. Immunohistochemical staining with the monoclonal antibody H5332 (gift from Dr. Alan Barbour, San Antonio, Texas); ×1250

ally there is slight edema in the papillary dermis. The main changes are superficial and deep perivascular and interstitial infiltrates of lymphocytes with or without admixture of plasma cells and eosinophils. Sometimes there are also a few neutrophils, mast cells, and histiocytes (Berger 1993).

18.2.3.1 Comment

The above-described nonspecific histopathologic pattern is in accordance with the author's experience. However, in one of the author's cases there was a widespread and deep inflammatory cell infiltrate that contained many plasma cells and diffusely spread epithelioid cells (Fig. 18.1). The pattern was more like that seen in ACA (see below). The patient, a 65-year-old man, had a typical erythema migrans lesion in the hollow of the knee. Six years earlier he had been successfully treated for ACA, and now had a reinfection. This could be the reason for the more prominent and more granulomatous reaction observed in this case, although, as in syphilis, successfully treated borreliosis does not give rise to immunity from reinfection.

18.3 Borrelial Lymphocytoma

The borrelial lymphocytoma appears as a solitary lesion on the site of the inoculation or close to it. The incubation time is usually longer than for erythema migrans. In adults the predilection sites are areola, mammae, nipples, nose and scrotum, in children the ear lobes. The phenomenon has been described previously as Spiegler-Fendt sarcoid and lymphadenosis benigna cutis (Bäfverstedt 1960). Elevated values of IgG antibodies against *Borrelia* spirochetes in the serum are found in about 50% of patients. Spirochetes have been cultured from some lesions (Hovmark et al. 1986).

18.3.1 Clinical Appearance

A typical lesion is a bluish-red tumor-like infiltration about 10–50 mm in diameter. Swelling of the local lymph nodes is common (Hovmark 1993). Without treatment the lesion may remain for several months, but eventually disappears.

18.3.2 Histopathologic Appearance

In the dermis and subcutis there are widespread and dense inflammatory cell infiltrates which consist of small lymphocytes, mainly B lymphocytes, with an admixture of plasma cells and eosinophils. Well-developed typical lesions include one or several germinal centers. These contain centroblasts (stimulated B cells), centrocytes, starry sky cells, and mitotic

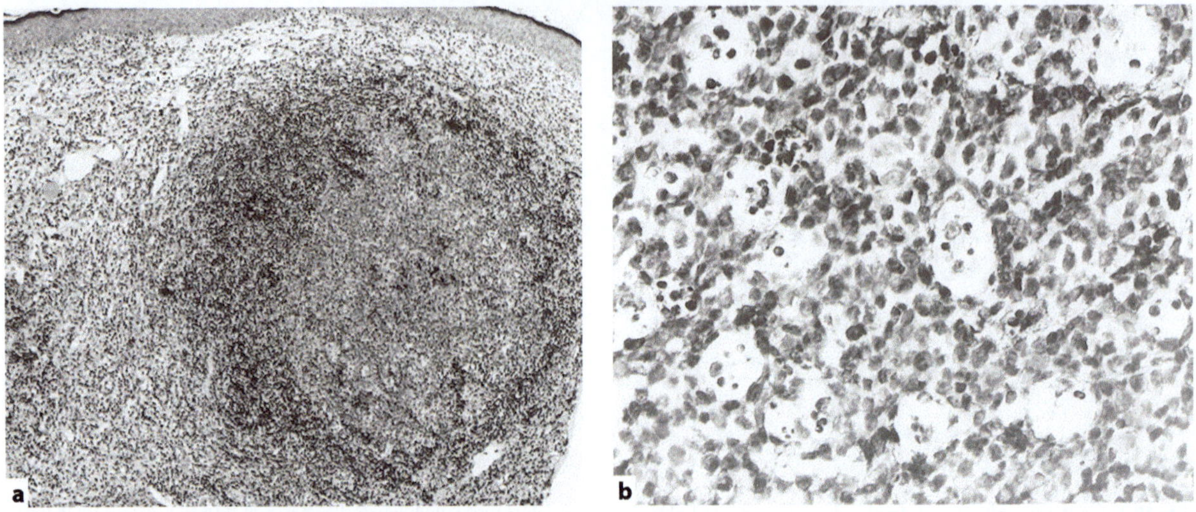

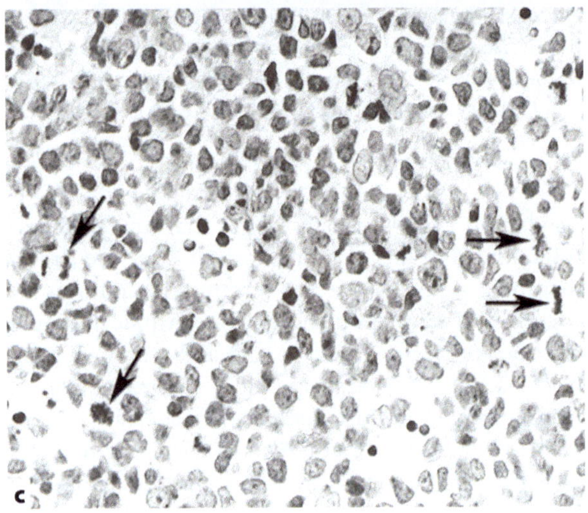

Fig. 18.2 Borrelial lymphocytoma. **a** Well-developed germinal center surrounded by a ring of small lymphocytes. **b** Close-up of the center shows many starry sky cells, the abundant and light cytoplasm of which contains nuclear fragments from phagocytosed cells. **c** Another area of the same center is mainly composed of stimulated B cells (centroblasts) and contains many mitotic figures; at least seven can be identified. The *arrows on the right* indicate two in metaphase, the *upper left arrow*, one in anaphase, and the *lower left arrow*, one in prophase. H&E

Fig. 18.3 ACA. **a** Erythematous lesion on the heel. There are many dilated vessels, both venules and lymphatics, and a dense inflammatory cell infiltrate. **b** Close-up of the dermis shows a dilated and rather thick-walled venule with protruding endothelial cells (*arrow*), and in the right lower corner two dilated lymphatics. In the left upper corner there is a longitudinally cut capillary. The cell infiltrate consists mainly of lymphocytes. However, there are also many plasma cells; H&E. **c** Bluish-red lesion on the elbow. There are widespread, dense inflammatory cell infiltrates throughout the dermis and in the superficial part many dilated vessels and "vacuoles". The dermis is thickened due to fibrosis, which is most marked in the deeper part. At the dermal–subcutaneous interface are two groups of atrophic sweat glands, tightly surrounded by fibrotic connective tissue (*arrow*). **d** Erythematous lesion on the knee. There are numerous plasma cells in the inflammatory cell infiltrate in the dermis. **e** Immunohistochemical staining with the monoclonal antibody H5332 on frozen sections from the same lesion reveals scattered spirochetes; ×1250 (**d** reproduced from Brehmer-Andersson et al. 1998, with permission)

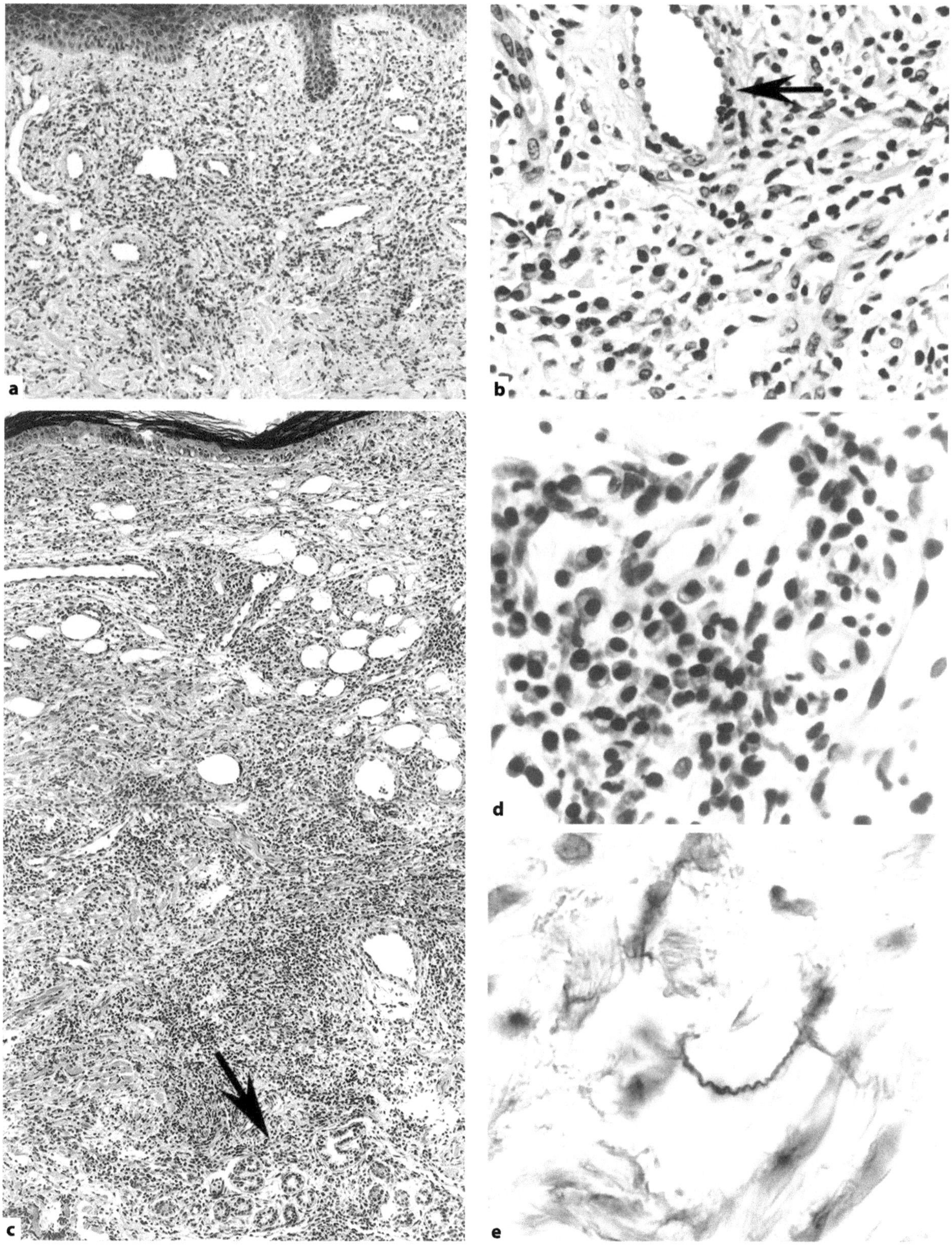
a
b
c
d
e

figures. Reaction centers are surrounded by a ring of small lymphocytes, more closely packed than cells in the rest of the infiltrate. However, like other lesions, the lymphocytoma has a life cycle. In the prime of the lesion the histopathologic pattern is distinctive and characteristic (Fig. 18.2). In the early and late phases of the cycle, germinal centers may lack starry sky cells and mitotic figures, and thus can be difficult to identify.

18.3.3 Differential Diagnosis

- *Infections caused by other kinds of organisms.* Lymphocytomas are a kind of immune response in non-lymphoid tissue (Sect. 4.1.4) and may be caused by different kinds of agents, for example *Leishmania* (Fig. 19.1). Also this type of lymphoid tissue is observed now and then in the oral and genital mucous membranes and is probably provoked by some less serious and passing infection.
- *Lymphomas.* If typical germinal centers are lacking, or in failure of treatment, primary cutaneous B cell lymphomas, which progress slowly and may contain abortive germinal centers, are important differential diagnoses (LeBoit et al. 1994; Willemze et al. 1997).

18.4 Acrodermatitis Chronica Atrophicans

ACA is a chronic disease, which untreated can go on for more than a decade. The patients are often elderly; females predominate. Elevated serum titers of IgG antibodies against *B. burgdorferi* are always present (Åsbrink 1993). Spirochetes have also been isolated from skin lesions and cultured (Åsbrink and Hovmark 1985).

18.4.1 Clinical Appearance

Lesions may be located anywhere, but preference sites are the feet, knees, elbows, and the dorsal aspects of hands. One or more limbs can be involved simultaneously. Active inflammatory lesions are erythematous or bluish-red, nonscaling, and sometimes edematous. They slowly increase in size and eventually cover a large part of an arm or a leg. Usually the borders are indistinct.

In addition to inflammatory lesions there are also occasionally fibrous lesions, such as fibrous nodules situated close to the elbows, knees or big toes, and ulnar bands. Ivory-colored sclerodermatous plaques and lesions impossible to differentiate from lichen sclerosus et atrophicus may also occur. Areas with marked atrophy are seen in patients, who have had untreated ACA for a long time. (Åsbrink et al. 1986; Åsbrink and Hovmark 1993).

18.4.2 Histopathologic Appearance

The following histopathologic description of ACA is based on the microscopic investigation of skin lesions from two series of patients with serologically proven untreated ACA seen in Sweden (Åsbrink et al. 1986; Brehmer-Andersson et al. 1998). Together, the studies comprised 143 patients, and 90 biopsy specimens including a substantial part of the subcutis showed that in nearly 75% the subcutaneous tissue was affected as well as the skin (Figs. 18.3c and 18.7a).

The epidermis is usually normal, but it may be either thin or slightly acanthotic and hyperkeratotic. It does not display signs of dermatitis (eczema). Rarely small areas of thinned epidermis show a lichenoid pattern such as liquefaction degeneration, apoptotic bodies, saw-tooth rete ridges, and subepidermal infiltrates

Fig. 18.4 ACA. **a** The epidermis is normal for the region (central face). The upper dermis shows a markedly dilated lymphatic. To the left of the vessel, there is a conglomerate of large macrophages with abundant hazy cytoplasm. The best discernible is indicated (*arrow*). Note also the plasma cell with two nuclei in the middle of the macrophages. The *arrowhead* indicates a multinucleated macrophage. **b** Aggregates of typical plasma cells with one or two eccentrically located nuclei and a crescent-like perinuclear halo. **c** A group of multinucleated giant cells located in conspicuously edematous tissue. The cytoplasm contains vacuoles and the remains of phagocytosed material. **d** A small and loosely arranged epithelioid cell granuloma surrounded by lymphocytes and scattered plasma cells. The *arrow* indicates a plasma cell with two nuclei. The large cell in the right lower corner is also a plasma cell with two nuclei. **e** Distinct subendothelial lymphocytic cell infiltrate in a thick-walled vein at the dermal–subcutaneous border. **f** A peripheral nerve, recognizable by its wavy appearance, is tightly surrounded and slightly infiltrated by lymphocytes. H&E (**e** reproduced from Brehmer-Andersson et al. 1998, with permission)

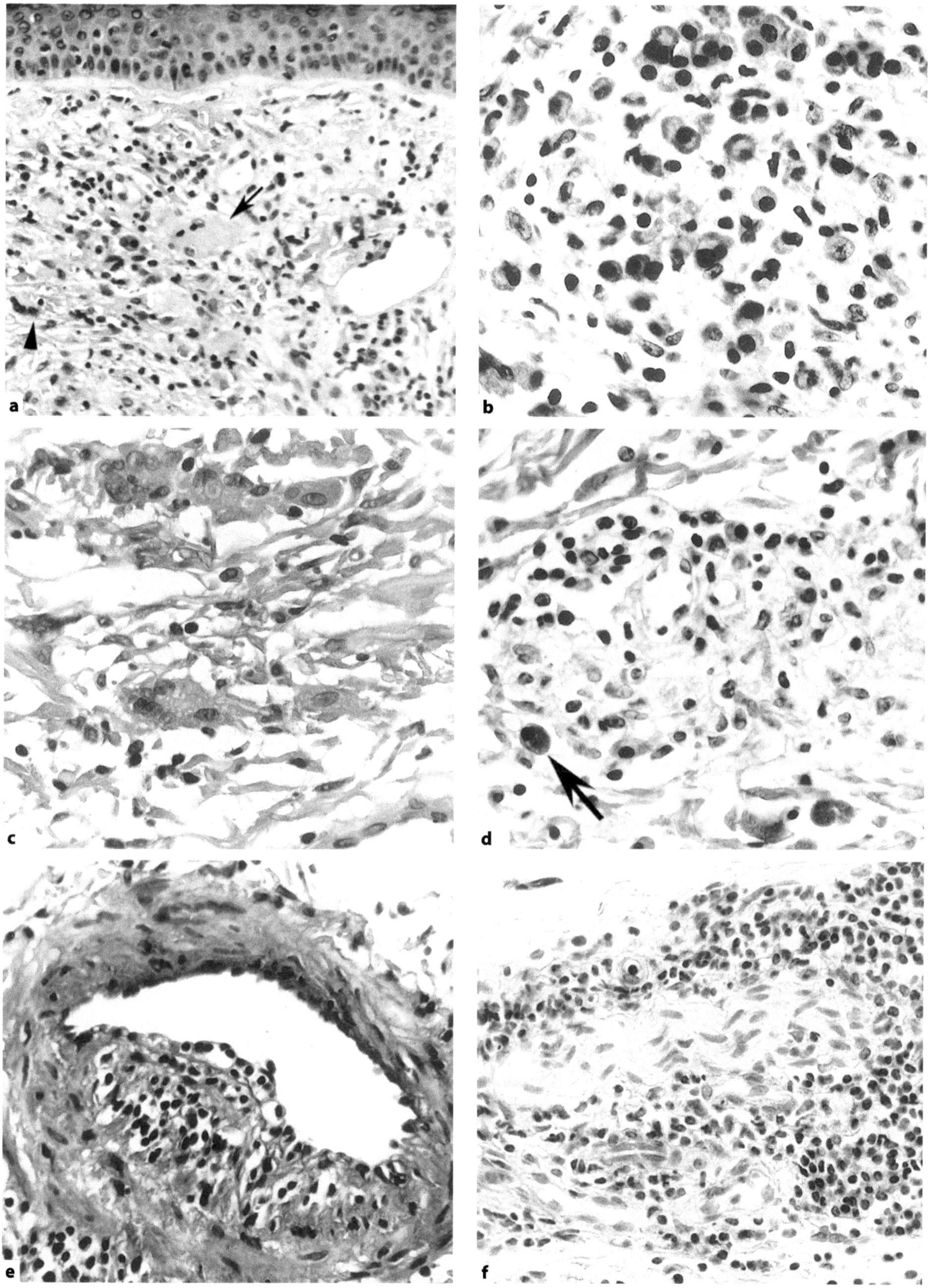
a
b
c
d
e
f

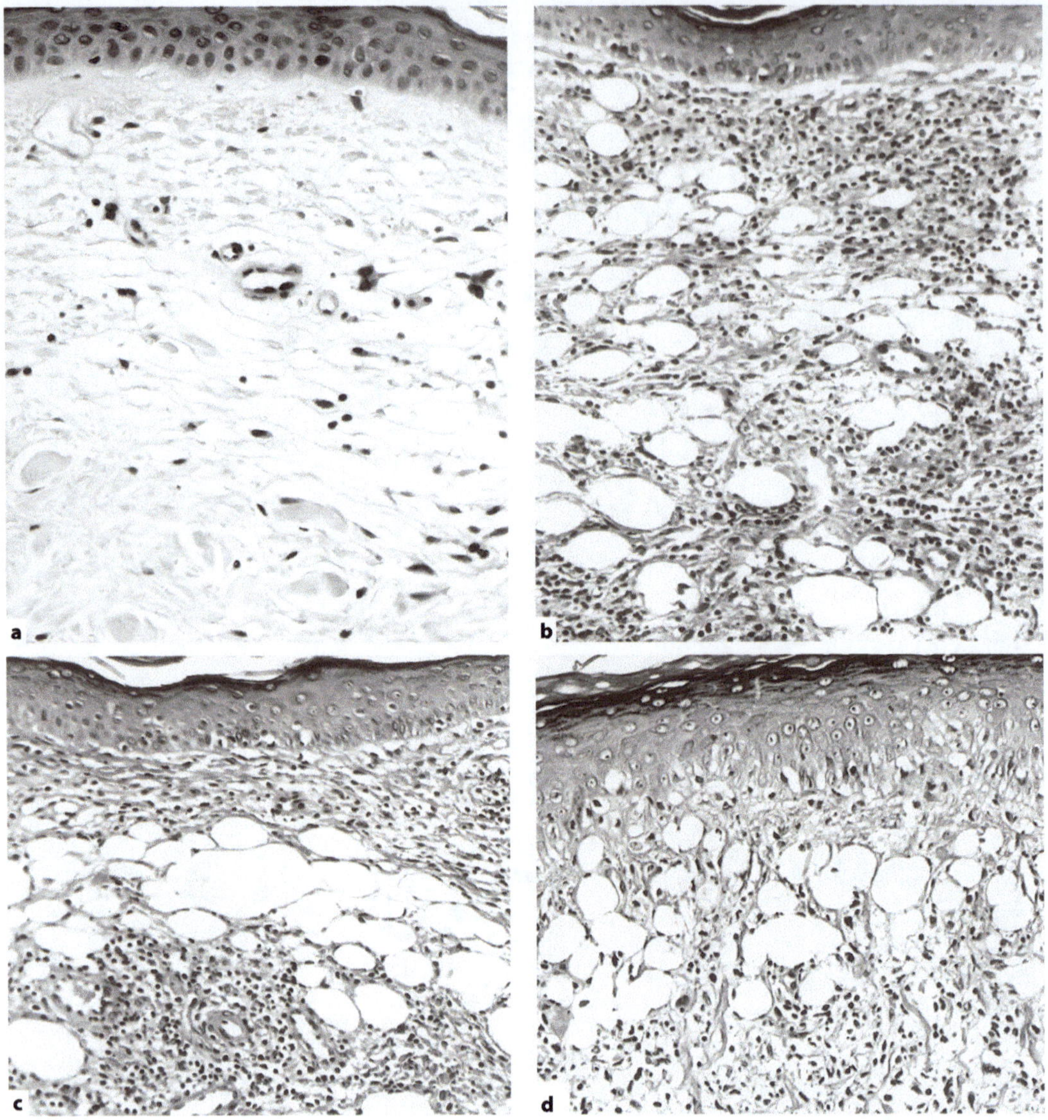

Fig. 18.5 ACA. **a** Erythematous lesion on the knee. Below a flat but otherwise normal epidermis there is a prominent dermal edema that in the mid-dermis splits up the collagen bundles and reduces them to thin threads. **b** Bluish-red lesion on the elbow. Throughout the dermis there are a high number of "vacuoles" and a dense inflammatory cell infiltrate. **c** Some "vacuoles" are oval and cannot be differentiated from thin-walled dilated lymphatics. **d** A band of "vacuoles" is located very close to the epidermis, the lower part of which shows intracellular edema. H&E (**d** reproduced from Brehmer-Andersson et al. 1998, with permission)

of lymphocytes in close contact with the epithelium. However, in contrast to lichen planus, the cell infiltrates are not confined to the subepidermal compartment and usually contain plasma cells.

In active lesions, the inflammatory cell infiltrates vary in density, but are often massive in both the dermis and the subcutis (Fig. 18.3). They may be diffuse, patchy or band-like and often tightly encircle vessels, sweat glands, sebaceous glands, hair follicles, and nerves. Inflammatory cells are rarely observed in the walls of vessels or in nerves (Fig. 18.4e,f). The infiltrates consist mainly of lymphocytes. However usually there is a fair or conspicuous admixture of plasma cells (Figs. 18.3d and 18.4b). The plasma cells often appear in clusters and differ in number from one compartment to the next. Frequently there are more plasma cells in the deep dermis and subcutis than in the superficial dermis. In addition to lymphocytes and

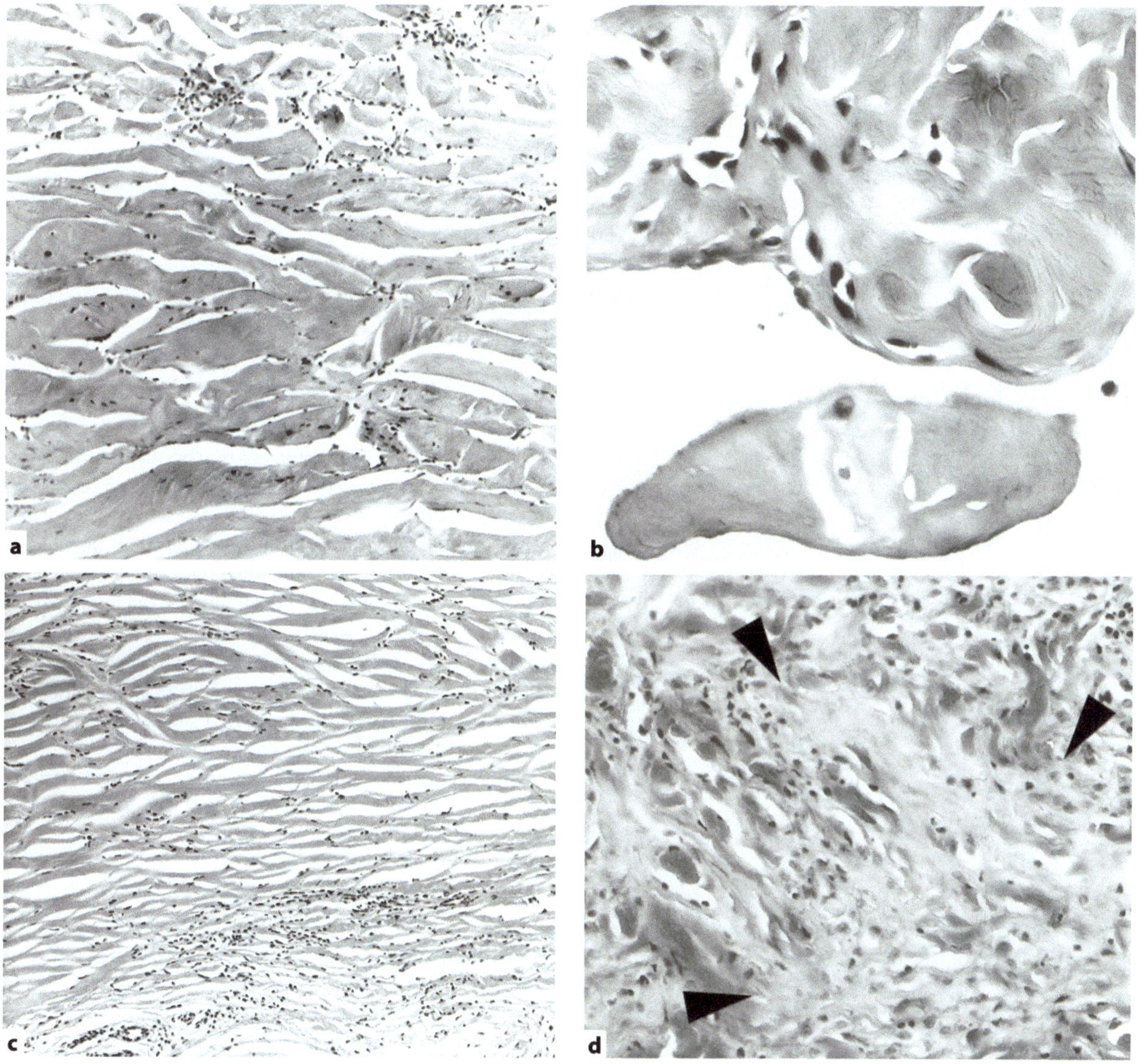

Fig. 18.6 ACA. **a** Sclerodermatous plaque on the back. Dermal sclerosis, which is most conspicuous in the deep part; H&E, ×100. **b** Bluish-red nodule on the elbow. Large sheets of sclerotic collagen tissue are located in subcutis; H&E, ×400. **c** Bluish-red lesion on the dorsal aspect of the hand. The thickened and sclerotic subcutaneous tissue is composed of interlacing bundles of collagen, oriented parallel to the epidermis; H&E, ×100. **d** Fibrous nodules on the elbow. The *arrowheads* demonstrate fibrotic connective tissue with a triangular area of fibrinoid necrosis; vG

plasma cells there are in most cases an increased number of fibroblasts and histiocytes, and in many cases also multinucleated giant cells (Fig. 18.4c), epithelioid cells, and mast cells. As a rule, epithelioid cells are diffusely scattered, although epithelioid cell granulomas may occur (Fig. 18.4d). Now and then neutrophils and eosinophils are seen, but usually they are not numerous.

Dilated venules and/or lymphatic capillaries are observed in nearly all cases and can be a conspicuous phenomenon (Fig. 18.3a–c). Sometimes there are also groups of newly formed blood vessels. Leukocytoclastic vasculitis is not seen.

Marked diffuse edema is sometimes observed in both the dermis and subcutaneous tissue. The edema splits up the collagen bundles and reduces them to thin threads (Fig. 18.5a). In a fair number of cases there are "vacuoles", diffusely scattered throughout the dermis,

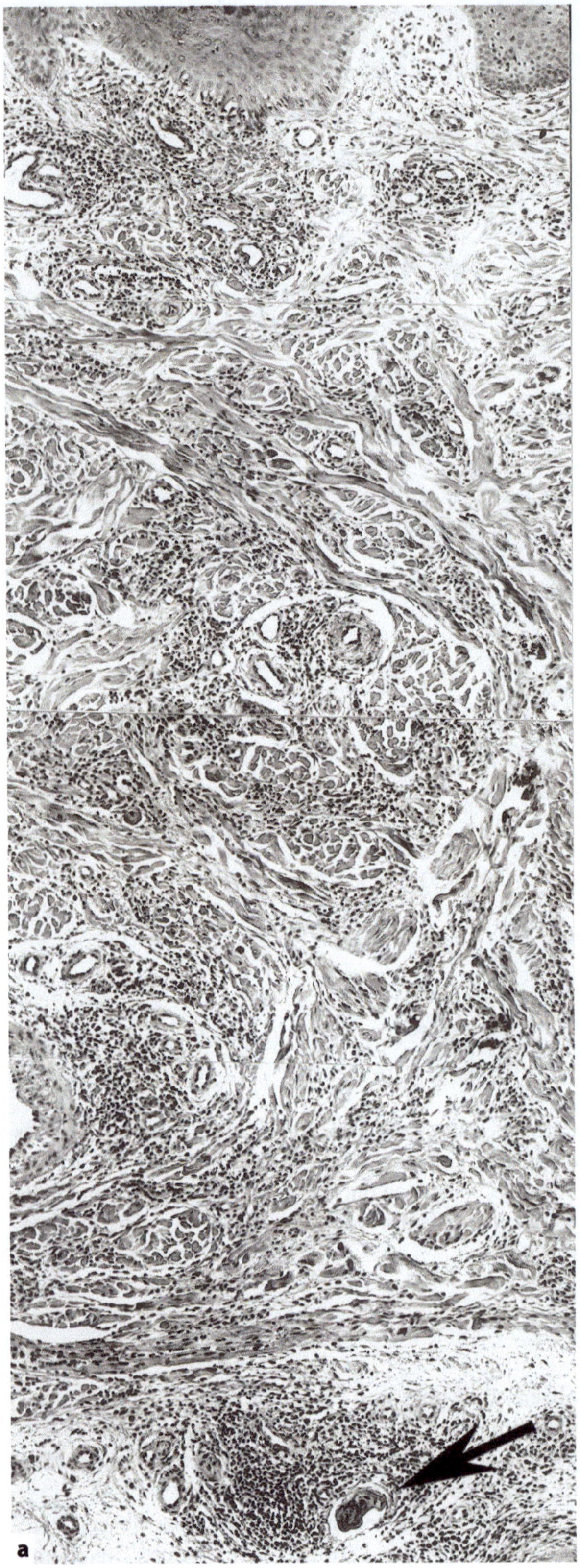

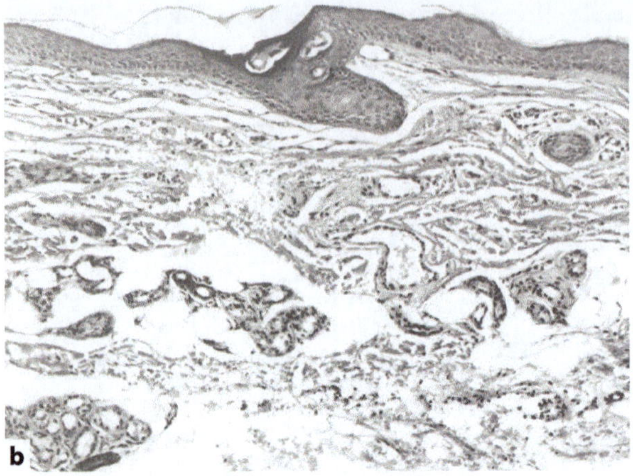

Fig. 18.7 ACA. a Bluish-red tumefaction on the heel. The subepidermal compartment contains dilated vessels and perivascular cell infiltrates. The rest of the dermis and superficial subcutis are fibrotic and conspicuously thickened. It is not possible to identify the dermal–subcutaneous interface. Deep in the subcutis there is a large and dense inflammatory cell infiltrate that includes a peripheral nerve (*arrow*); H&E, ×100. b Atrophic lesion on the knee. The epidermis is flat and contains a sweat gland duct (acrosyringium). The dermis is markedly thin and made up of threads of collagen arranged parallel to the surface. There are a few dilated vessels, but no inflammatory cells. The dermal–subcutaneous interface with groups of sweat gland is very close to the epidermis; vG, ×100

lying singly, or in small groups. They are mostly empty, but occasionally seem to contain a small amount of fluid, have no walls, and are surrounded by connective tissue or inflammatory cell infiltrates. These structures are very much like fat cells, but have a more irregular form. If they are followed in serial sections some of them become oval (Figs. 18.5b–d). Occasionally "vacuoles" lie as a massive band very close to the epidermis. In such cases intracellular edema may also be observed in the basic part of the epidermis (Fig. 18.5d). "Vacuoles" probably represent lymphatic capillaries or prelymphatics (see Sect. 18.4.2.1).

Considerable fibrosis–sclerosis is found in biopsy specimens from fibrous nodules, ulnar bands and sclerodermatous plaques, but also in samples from lesions without clinical signs of fibrosis. By fibrosis is meant a markedly increased number of fibroblasts and collagen bundles. Sclerotic tissue contains a sparse number of fibroblasts, and is thought to be the result of fibrosis. In ACA fibrosis–sclerosis appears in three different forms:

1. Thickened and closely packed collagen bundles

2. Large sheets of sclerotic collagen
3. Thick layers of thin, interlacing collagen bundles

Fibrosis–sclerosis involves both the subcutaneous tissue and dermis (Figs. 18.3c and 18.7a). However, it is more common and usually more conspicuous in the subcutis than in the dermis; thus the process seems to start in the subcutis and successively progresses towards the surface (Fig. 18.6a–c). Groups of atrophic sweat glands tightly surrounded by fibrotic connective tissue are sometimes observed (Fig. 18.3c). In fibrous areas fibrinoid necrosis can be found (Fig. 18.6d). It is not possible histopathologically to differentiate between fibrous nodules, ulnar bands, and sclerodermatous lesions. Nor is it possible to differentiate between scleroderma-like lesions and lesions of scleroderma. Lesions clinically described as lichen sclerosus et atrophicus also show the histopathologic pattern of this disease.

Atrophy of the skin is observed in biopsy specimens from areas with clinically advanced atrophy. The epidermis is flat. However, the most conspicuous changes are seen in the dermis, which is very thin and built up of slender collagen bundles arranged parallel to the surface. Figure 18.7b demonstrates an atrophic lesion in a patient who had had ACA for two decades.

18.4.2.1 Comment

The observation of dilated vessels and inflammatory cell infiltrates with an admixture of plasma cells below an essentially normal epidermis should alert the pathologist to the possibility of ACA. However, ACA can occur in an area already affected with eczema (dermatitis) or with psoriasis. Also the number of plasma cells may be sparse, and can vary considerably in biopsy specimens taken from different lesions on the same occasion.

Immunohistochemical investigations performed on samples with dense inflammatory cell infiltrates containing many plasma cells have revealed that practically all lymphocytes are T cells. This indicates that plasma cells have not developed at the site, but have migrated into the skin, in contrast to the course of events in borrelial lymphocytoma where the most of the lymphocytes are B cells capable of producing plasma cells. Cutaneous B-cell lymphomas have been described in association with ACA (Garbe et al. 1991). There was no such occurrence in the two Swedish series.

In the older literature fat cell-like vacuoles in the upper half of the dermis have been described in lesions of ACA. They were interpreted as fat cells and droplets of fat caused by fatty degeneration (Benjamowitsch and Maschkilleisson 1933; Montgomery and Sullivan 1945). More recently this phenomenon has been reported as fatty infiltration in a patient with psoriasis (Lee et al. 1995) and as pseudolipomatosis cutis in biopsy specimens from different kinds of skin lesions (Trotter and Crawford 1998). Trotter and Crawford interpreted the vacuoles as artifacts presumably due to injection of air during administration of local anesthetic or to inadequate fixation. Today it is not accepted that fat can appear as the result of some degenerative process (Majno and Joris 1996). Also in frozen material, stained for fat and taken from lesions with a large number of vacuoles, fat was observed only in peripheral nerves and subcutaneous tissue and no vacuoles were seen (Åsbrink et al. 1986). This proves that there is no abnormal fat in the dermis, but says nothing about the presence or absence of vacuoles; certainly, freezing destroys these delicate structures. In our cases artifacts such as those mentioned above are highly unlikely, and the author's suggestion is that the vacuoles represent some kind of lymphedema or lymphostasis. The organization of the dermal lymphatic vasculature, and the existence of prelymphatics support this thinking (Sect. 3.3). The author's experience is that this phenomenon appears focally and occasionally may be observed in other kinds of skin lesions.

Fibrosis–sclerosis has been found in all biopsy specimens from clinically observed fibrous or sclerotic lesions, but has also been noted in many specimens taken from lesions where fibrosis–sclerosis was not suspected clinically. This was the case in the samples taken from ACA lesions overlying small joints showing the nonarthritic and nontraumatic subluxation that sometimes occurs in ACA. Presumably fibrosis–sclerosis is the cause of this kind of subluxation.

The occurrence of sclerodermatous (scleroderma-like) lesions and lesions similar to lichen sclerosus et atrophicus besides typical lesions of ACA is the reason why the *Borrelia* spirochete has been suspected to be the cause also of scleroderma and lichen sclerosus et atrophicus. However, recent investigations do not prove this statement (Wienecke et al. 1995; Alonso-Llamazares et al. 1997).

18.4.3 Differential Diagnosis

- *Acne rosacea.* Lesions in the face, as demonstrated in Fig. 4a, may simulate acne rosacea. In acne rosacea there are thin-walled dilated vessels, plasma cells, and sometimes epithelioid cells, but usually also follicular pustules.

- *Secondary syphilis.* ACA containing many plasma cells and epithelioid cells may be mistaken for secondary syphilis. However, usually thin-walled vessels are more conspicuous in ACA than in syphilis and epidermal changes more prominent, at least in early secondary syphilis, than in ACA.

18.5 Methods to Prove the Presence of Spirochetes in Borrelial Skin Lesions

The number of spirochetes in skin lesions of Lyme borreliosis is very low (Hansen 1993). It is therefore difficult to identify spirochetes in histologic sections. However, to prove their presence is of interest in suspected lesions of erythema migrans and borrelial lymphocytoma when serum antibodies have not yet developed. For this purpose different staining methods, culture and the PCR technique are used.

Silver stain (Warthin-Starry, Steiner, Bosma-Steiner) is the time-honored means to prove the presence of *T. pallidum* causing syphilis, and has also been used to visualize spirochetes in lesions of erythema migrans (Berger et al. 1983; De Koning 1993). In lesions of primary and secondary syphilis, aggregates of *T. pallidum* at the epidermal–dermal interface give rise to a local inflammatory reaction and are therefore relatively easy to identify. This is in contrast to spirochetes in erythema migrans and ACA lesions, in which they are very few, often scattered, and lie free without close contact with inflammatory cells. This makes it very difficult to differentiate with certainty a single spirochete from other argentophilic structures in the dermis. Contamination with bacteria including nonpathogenic spirochetes may also happen (author´s own experience). Possible sources of nonpathogenic spirochetes are unclean glass slides, water-bath used for processing, and droplets of saliva. Little is known about nonpathogenic spirochetes in our surroundings.

Immunohistochemical staining with monoclonal or polyclonal antibodies against *B. burgdorferi* (Figs. 18.1a and 18.3e) is preferable, but seems to work well only on frozen material (own experience). The search for stained spirochetes in sections is, like culture, a laborious task, which is why the PCR technique has been tried. Von Stedingk et al. (1995) investigated skin biopsy specimens from patients with erythema migrans and from patients with ACA with this technique. In their investigation 18/26 (69%) of the specimens from erythema migrans and 22/36 (61%) of the specimens from ACA were positive for borrelial DNA.

Lebech et al. (1995) evaluated the diagnostic sensitivity of the immunohistochemical staining technique, culture, and PCR technique in an experimental trial. They used rodents infected with *B. burgdorferi* and applied the three techniques to infected internal organs. They found that culture was positive in 96%, immunohistochemical staining in 33%, and PCR performed on fresh tissue in 71%. The authors considered that the PCR technique was the best diagnostic tool and applied it to patients with erythema migrans and neuroborreliosis (Lebech et al. 2000). In this investigation, 97% of samples from lesions of erythema migrans were positive by PCR, while 41% were positive by serologic testing and 29% were positive by culture.

References

1. Alonso-Llamazares J, Persing DH, Anda P, Gibson LE, Rutledge BJ, Iglesias L (1997) No evidence for Borrelia burgdorferi infection in lesions of morphea and lichen sclerosus et atrophicus in Spain. Acta Derm Venereol 77:299–304
2. Anderson JF, Magnarelli LA (1993) Epizootiology of Lyme disease-causing Borreliae. Clin Dermatol 11:339–351
3. Åsbrink E (1993) Acrodermatitis chronica atrophicans. Clin Dermatol 11:369–375
4. Åsbrink E, Hovmark A (1985) Successful cultivation of spirochetes from skin lesions of patients with erythema chronicum migrans Afzelius and acrodermatitis chronica atrophicans. APMIS 93:161–163
5. Åsbrink E, Hovmark A (1993) Atlas. Clin Dermatol 11:331–334
6. Åsbrink E, Brehmer-Andersson E, Hovmark A (1986) Acrodermatitis chronica atrophicans. A spirochetosis. Clinical and histopathological picture based on 32 patients. Course and relationship to erythema chronicum migrans Afzelius. Am J Dermatopathol 8:209–219
7. Bäfverstedt B (1960) Lymphadenosis benigna cutis (LABC) its nature, course and prognosis. Acta Derm Venereol 40:10–18
8. Baranton G, Postic D, Saint Girons I, Boerlin P, Piffaretti J-C, Assous M, Grimont PAD (1992) Delineation of Borrelia burgdorferi sensu stricto, Borrelia garinii sp. nov., and group VS461 associated with Lyme borreliosis. Int J Syst Bacteriol 42:378–383
9. Benjamowitsch E, Maschkilleisson LN (1933) Weitere Beiträge zur Frage über die Atrophie der Haut. III. Acrodermatitis chronica atrophicans und ihre Beziehung zur Sclerodermia. Acta Derm Venereol 14:313–341
10. Berger BW (1993) Erythema migrans. Clin Dermatol 11:359–362
11. Berger BW, Clemmensen OJ, Ackerman AB (1983) Lyme disease is a spirochetosis. A review of the disease and evidence for its cause. Am J Dermatopathol 5:111–124

12. Brehmer-Andersson E, Hovmark A, Åsbrink E (1998) Acrodermatitis chronica atrophicans: histopathologic findings and clinical correlations in 111 cases. Acta Derm Venereol 78:207–213
13. Burgdorfer W (1993) How the discovery of Borrelia burgdorferi came about. Clin Dermatol 11:335–338
14. Burgdorfer W, Barbour AG, Hayes SF, Benach JL, Grunwaldt E, Davis JP (1982) Lyme disease. A tick-borne spirochetosis? Science 216:1317–1319
15. Canica MM, Nato F, du Merle L, Mazie JC, Baranton G, Postic D (1993) Monoclonal antibodies for identification of Borrelia afzelii sp. nov. associated with late cutaneous manifestations of Lyme borreliosis. Scand J Infect Dis 25:441–448
16. De Koning J (1993) Histopathologic patterns of erythema migrans and borrelial lymphocytoma. Clin Dermatol 11:377–383
17. Garbe C, Stein H, Dienemann D, Orfanos CE (1991) Borrelia burgdorferi-associated cutaneous B cell lymphoma: clinical and immunohistologic characterization of four cases. J Am Acad Dermatol 24:584–590
18. Hansen K (1993) Laboratory diagnostic methods in Lyme borreliosis. Clin Dermatol 11:407–414
19. Hovmark A (1993) Role of Borrelia burgdorferi in lymphocytomas and sclerotic skin lesions. Clin Dermatol 11:363–367
20. Hovmark A, Åsbrink E, Olsson I (1986) The spirochetal etiology of lymphadenosis benigna cutis solitaria. Acta Derm Venereol 66:479–484
21. Lebech A-M, Clemmensen O, Hansen K (1995) Comparison of in vitro culture, immunohistochemical staining, and PCR for detection of Borrelia burgdorferi in tissue from experimentally infected animals. J Clin Microbiol 33:2328–2333
22. Lebech A-M, Hansen K, Brandrup F, Clemmensen O, Halkier-Sørensen L (2000) Diagnostic value of PCR for detection of Borrelia burgdorferi DNA in clinical specimens from patients with erythema migrans and Lyme neuroborreliosis. Mol Diagn 5:139–150
23. LeBoit PE, McNutt NS, Reed JA, Jacobson M, Weiss LM (1994) Primary cutaneous immunocytoma. A B-cell lymphoma that can easily be mistaken for cutaneous lymphoid hyperplasia. Am J Surg Pathol 18:969–978
24. Lee J, Bhawan J, Rothman K (1995) Massive papillary dermal fatty infiltration in a patient with psoriasis. J Cutan Pathol 22:182–184
25. Majno G, Joris I (1996) Cells, tissues, and disease: principles of general pathology. Blackwell Science, Cambridge, pp 77–93
26. Montgomery H, Sullivan RR (1945) Acrodermatitis atrophicans chronica. Arch Dermatol Syph 51:32–45
27. Steere AC, Malawista SE, Snydman DR, Shope RE, Andiman WA, Ross MR, Steele FM (1977) Lyme arthritis an epidemic of oligoarticular arthritis in children and adults in three Connecticut communities. Arthritis Rheum 20:7–17
28. Trotter MJ, Crawford RI (1998) Pseudolipomatosis cutis: superficial dermal vacuoles resembling fatty infiltration of the skin. Am J Dermatopathol 20:443–447
29. von Stedingk LV, Olsson I, Hanson HS, Åsbrink E, Hovmark A (1995) Polymerase chain reaction for detection of Borrelia burgdorferi DNA in skin lesions of early and late Lyme borreliosis. Eur J Clin Microbiol Infect Dis 14:1–5
30. Wienecke R, Schlüpen E-M, Zöchling N, Neubert U, Meurer M, Volkenandt M (1995) No evidence for Borrelia burgdorferi-specific DNA in lesions of localized scleroderma. J Invest Dermatol 104:23–26
31. Willemze R, Kerl H, Sterry W, Berti E, Cerroni L, Chimenti S, Diaz-Perés JL, Geerts ML, Goos M, Knobler R, Ralfkiaer E, Santucci M, Smith N, Wechsler J, van Vloten WA, Meijer CJLM (1997) EORTC classification for primary cutaneous lymphomas: a proposal from the Cutaneous Lymphoma Study Group of the European Organization for Research and Treatment of Cancer. Blood 90:354–371

19 Leishmaniasis

Leishmaniasis is endemic in the Middle East, South Asia, and Africa (oriental leishmaniasis) and in Latin America (American leishmaniasis). In non-endemic areas leishmaniasis may now and then be seen in individuals who have visited or emigrated from infested countries. There are four main types of leishmaniasis: *cutaneous*, *diffuse cutaneous*, *mucocutaneous* and *visceral*. Only cutaneous leishmaniasis is discussed here.

19.1 Pathogenesis

The cause of leishmaniasis is the intracellular protozoan parasite *Leishmania*. The parasites are transmitted to humans through the bite of infected sandflies. In the saliva of the sandfly the parasites are slender and flagellated (i.e., endowed with long, thread-like, and mobile projections). In human macrophages they are transformed into round or oval bodies without flagella. At one end of the body there is a deeply basophilic round nucleus associated with a small comma-like paranucleus or *kinetoplast* (Lever and Schaumburg-Lever 1990). *Leishmania* bodies are visible in routinely stained sections using a ×40 objective, and the nucleus and kinetoplast are visible using a ×100 objective, but are better visualized by a Giemsa stain.

19.2 Cutaneous Leishmaniasis

Oriental cutaneous leishmaniasis (oriental sore) is caused by several species (*L. major*, *L. tropica*, *L. aetiopica*, and *L. infantum*) and American cutaneous leishmaniasis by *L. mexicana* complex and *L. braziliensis* complex (Bryceson and Hay 1992). They all give rise to similar clinical lesions and have a similar histopathologic pattern. The severity of the disease is dependent on the cell-mediated immunity of the host.

19.2.1 Clinical Appearance

At the inoculation site a small erythematous papule appears immediately or 2 to 4 weeks after the bite. The papule grows slowly to a bluish-red and centrally ulcerated or crusted nodule, which may become more than 2 cm in diameter. The nodule may remain like that for several months and finally regress and heal with a scar. Sometimes there are multiple lesions.

19.2.2 Histopathologic Appearance

Histologic investigation of an active non-ulcerated part of the lesion usually shows an acanthotic and hyperkeratotic epidermis. The dermal papillae are widened with dilated venules and extravasated erythrocytes, and in the papillae and the rest of the dermis there are dense confluent or patchy cell infiltrates mainly composed of plasma cells, lymphocytes and macrophages. The macrophages contain a variable, often large, number of *Leishmania* organisms. Later the organisms become less numerous or disappear and instead of macrophages, epithelioid cell granulomas with giant cells develop.

19.2.3 Example

Case 1. Cutaneous Leishmaniasis with Lymphocytoma

The patient was a 22-year-old man of unknown nationality and background. For 7 months he had noticed a tumefaction on the left upper arm. Puncture biopsy of the lesion was followed by excision. Both microscopy of the puncture material and the gross appearance of the excised lesion were indicative of lymphoid tissue and the proposed diagnosis was lymphocytoma.

The excised material comprised skin and a fair amount of subcutaneous tissue. At the dermal–subcutaneous interface and in the upper subcutis there were widespread large and dense aggregates of macrophages surrounded by plasma cells and lymphocytes. The macrophages had abundant, light, foamy or vacuolated cytoplasm, and contained a variable number of *Leishmania* organisms. In addition there were extensive infiltrates of lymphocytes containing

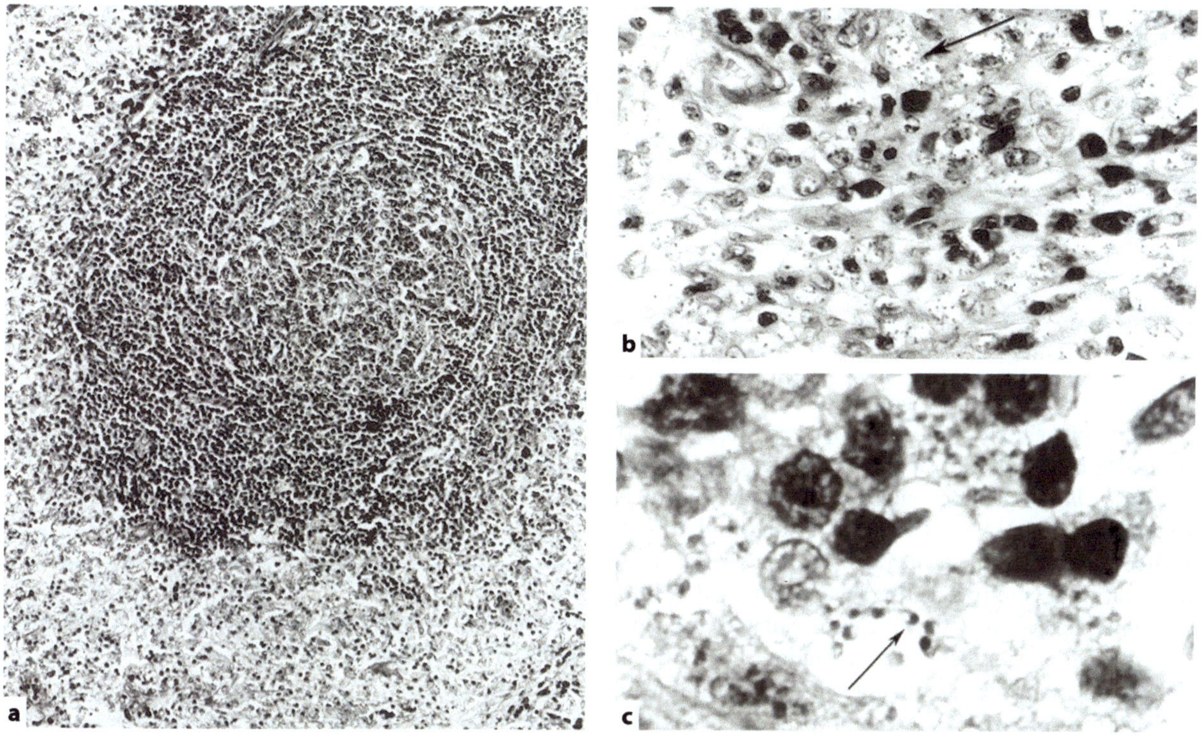

Fig. 19.1 Leishmaniasis with lymphocytoma. **a** A dense infiltrate of small lymphocytes contains a reaction center and is surrounded by a broad band of light macrophages. Giemsa staining. **b** Close-up shows macrophages containing numerous *Leishmania* organisms. Two well-stuffed macrophages are indicated (*arrow*); Giemsa. **c** Close-up of a vacuole in the cytoplasm of a macrophage displays a group of organisms. The body of the organism is a clear oval. It has an eccentric, round, dark nucleus, to which is attached a comma-like kinetoplast. The latter is discernible in one organism (*arrow*); H&E, ×1000

reaction centers. In the dermis infiltrates, composed of lymphocytes, plasma cells and some macrophages, surrounded vessels and adnexa. The epidermis was normal (Fig. 19.1).

19.2.3.1 Comment

In the demonstrated case the lesion was not ulcerated and the inflammatory infiltrates were confined to the dermal–subcutaneous interface, which is unusual. Also the infection had provoked a lymphocytoma (Sect. 4.1.4). The reaction centers were not as well developed as in the lymphocytoma demonstrated in Lyme borreliosis (Fig. 18.2) and starry sky cells and mitotic figures were not observed.

19.2.4 Differential Diagnosis

- *Early syphilis* if there are many plasma cells, but no *Leishmania* organisms
- *Lupus vulgaris* and other diseases with epithelioid granulomas if *Leishmania* organisms are not present

References

1. Bryceson ADM, Hay RJ (1992) Leishmaniasis. In: Champion RH, Burton JL, Ebling FJG (eds) Rook/Wilkinson/Ebling textbook of dermatology. Blackwell Scientific Publications, Oxford, pp 1251–1264
2. Lever WF, Schaumburg-Lever G (1990) Histopathology of the skin. J.B. Lippincott Company, Philadelphia

20 Herpes Simplex, Herpes Zoster/Varicella, and Cytomegalovirus Infections

Viruses are cell parasites. For the propagation (reproduction) of new virus particles, *virions*, they depend on living cells in the host. The virion is composed of the *nucleoid*, the genetic material (nucleic acid), which may be either DNA or RNA, and is surrounded by a protecting protein shell, the *capsid*. Some viruses have an additional outer protecting layer composed of lipoproteins, the *envelope*; they are encapsulated. A virion can survive outside cells in a crystalline form and is able to infect appropriate living cells (different for different kinds of viruses). An appropriate cell has specific surface receptors for a specific virus protein, but must also be permissive (i.e., permit propagation for this virus inside the cell).

To infect a cell, the virus must penetrate into the cell. With respect to encapsulated viruses this is achieved in two steps. First a specific viral protein binds to a specific receptor on the host cell and thereafter the outer leaflet of the virus envelope fuses with the outer leaflet of the cell membrane (White and Blobel 1989). Inside the cell the nucleoid is released from its capsid and becomes functionally active. New parts of the virus (i.e., nucleic acids and proteins) are synthesized in the nucleus of the host cell (Gibson 1994). Newly formed nucleoids and/or capsid proteins are sometimes visualized in routinely processed slides as intranuclear or intracytoplasmic inclusions. New virions are released through the cell membrane. If the virus is encapsulated the virion becomes coated with the envelop when it buds through the cell membrane. The lipids are derived from the host cell and the virus encodes the protein.

Propagation of new virus particles usually results in destruction and death (lysis) of all infected cells. However, there are exceptions. Thus in herpes virus infections the virus may remain in some kinds of cells in a latent state. The virus does not propagate and there are no symptoms (see below). In abortive virus infections, virus DNA forms a stable association with the host cell genome and the process of propagation becomes deficient. This occurs in infections with human papilloma virus (HPV) and Epstein-Barr virus (EBV). Persistent infection means that virions are synthesized continuously with or without altered cell function. This is the case in hepatitis B virus infection (Samuelson 1999).

20.1 Herpes Simplex and Herpes Zoster/Varicella Virus Infections

Herpes simplex viruses (HSVs) and varicella/zoster virus (VZV) are encapsulated DNA viruses and belong to the family *Herpes viridae.*

20.1.1 Clinical Appearance and Pathogenesis

HSVs are of two kinds, HSV-1 and HSV-2. They infect damaged skin and mucous membranes and locally cause vesicular lesions. HSV-1 preferentially affects the facial area (mouth, lips, nose and eyes) and HSV-2 the genital area. The primary infection may be serious and even fatal in the neonatal period and in immunocompromised patients, but is in otherwise healthy individuals mostly subclinical or mild and the lesions disappear without trace. However, the virus may also infect cells in the sensory ganglia of the spinal cord and cranial nerves, which innervate the affected area and remain there in a latent state. Reactivated, the virus gives rise to recurrent spells of vesicles in the area of the primary infection.

VZV is the cause of chickenpox (varicella) and shingles (herpes zoster). Varicella represents the primary infection. It may appear at any age, but mostly affects children and young adults. VZV is airborne and enters the body via the upper respiratory tract. After 2–3 weeks of incubation it gives rise to viremia and a widespread vesicular eruption on the skin and mucous membranes of the mouth and throat. As in HSV infection, the VZV may survive in a latent state in cells in sensory root ganglia and, later in life when for some reason the immunocompetence of the indi-

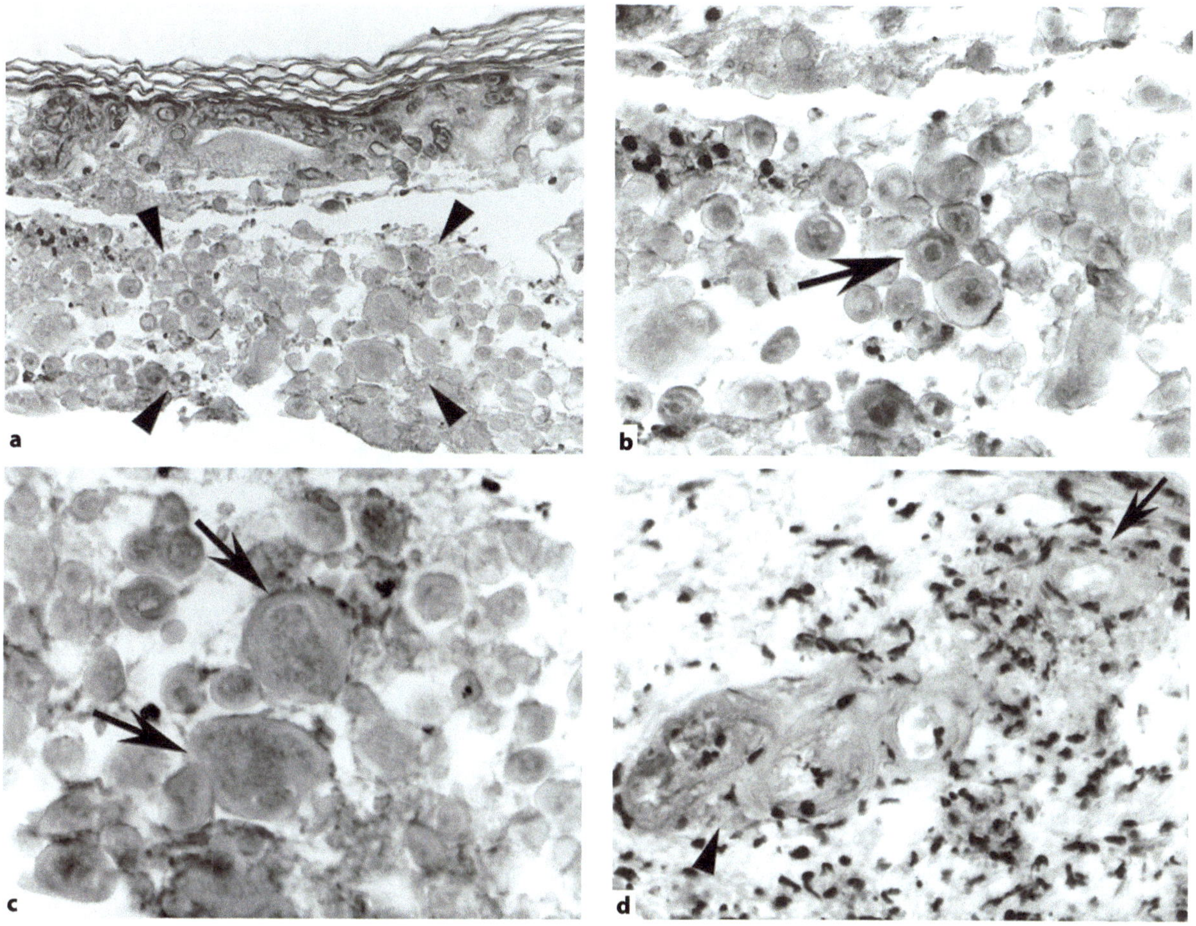

Fig. 20.1 Herpes zoster. **a** The detached epidermis comprises the necrotic remains of a vesicle. **b** Close-up of the left part of the area indicated (*arrows*) in **a** shows faded acantholytic cells of different size and appearance: some are large and ballooned, some lack a nucleus, others have a shadow nucleus. The *arrow* indicates a typical intranuclear inclusion body surrounded by a light halo. **c** Close-up of the right part of the area indicated (*arrows*) in **a**. The arrows indicate two faded giant cells. **d** Vasculitis in the upper dermis. The vessel in the right upper corner is necrotic and surrounded by erythrocytes, neutrophils, and nuclear fragments (*arrow*). In the left lower corner are two venules stuffed with erythrocytes (*arrowhead*). H&E

vidual declines, may be reactivated and cause herpes zoster. In herpes zoster the outbreak is unilateral and confined to a dermatome, but may be more or less generalized in immunocompromised patients.

The primary efflorescence is similar in eruptions due to HSV and VZV, and consists of painful and/or itching, small, often clustered vesicles on a reddish and edematous and sometimes hemorrhagic base. Vesicles may be umbilicated. The fluid in the vesicles is first clear, but soon becomes purulent, and then encrusted before healing. Sometimes a lesion ulcerates; this is most common on mucous membranes. LeBoit et al. (1992) reported on a chronic verrucous variant of lesions caused by VZV infection in patients with AIDS.

20.1.2 Histopathologic Appearance

The vesicles of HSVs and VZV cannot be differentiated histologically. Discrimination requires culture or immunohistochemical investigation. The virus propagates inside the cells, giving rise to *secondary acantholysis* (see Glossary) and cell death. Thus the typical herpes vesicles are composed mainly of acantholytic different-sized keratinocytes in various stages of disintegration. Many cells are swollen or ballooned. Usually there are also a number of so-called virus giant cells, the presence of which is an important clue to the diagnosis. The viral protein, which was inserted in the cell membrane during fusion of the virus with the epithelial cell, promotes infected cells to coalesce and

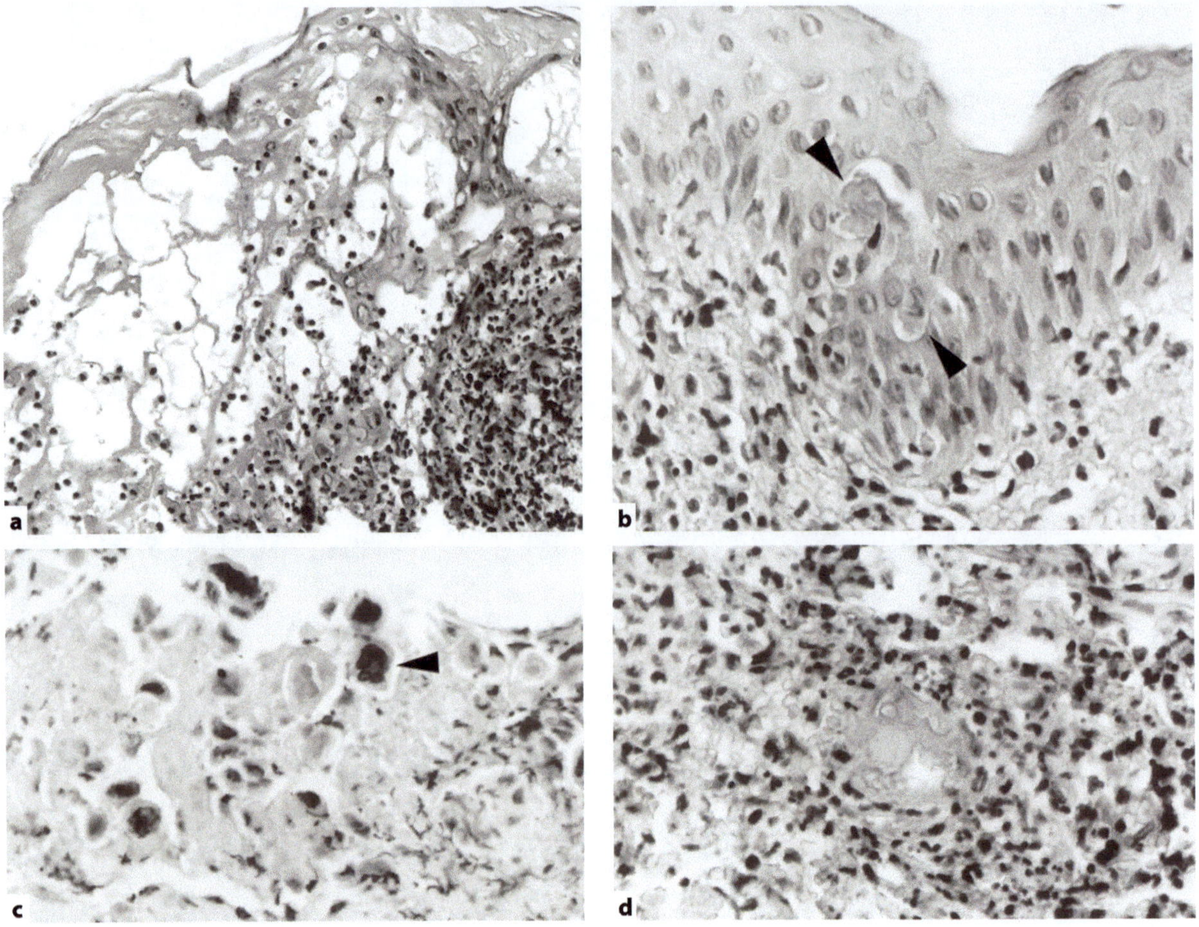

Fig. 20.2 Herpes zoster. **a** Vesicle with marked reticular degeneration. In the right lower corner there is a dense inflammatory cell infiltrate composed mainly of neutrophils. **b** A group of apoptotic bodies in the epidermis outside the vesicle (*arrowheads*). **c** Degenerated epithelial cells with some giant cells at the floor of the vesicle. The best-preserved giant cell is indicated (*arrowhead*). **d** A dense infiltrate of neutrophils surrounds a venule obliterated by an erythrocyte thrombus. H&E

form giant cells. A single intranuclear, round, glossy, eosinophilic inclusion body may be observed in scattered cells. The inclusion is surrounded by a light ring, which in turn is encircled by a dark ring of condensed chromatin at the cell margin, forming a target-like figure. This phenomenon is not as common as is the presence of giant cells. Pyknotic or faded nuclei in disintegrating keratinocytes and giant cells should not be mistaken for virus inclusion bodies.

In lesions of VZV virus infection dermal hyperemia and hemorrhages are common. Also vasculitis with erythrocyte thrombi, wall necrosis and infiltrates of neutrophils are observed. Hair follicles and sebaceous glands are often, and sometimes the only structures, affected. The kind and density of inflammatory cells differ considerably from one case to another. Mostly there are infiltrates of both neutrophils and lymphocytes with predominance of one of them. In the dermis histiocytes and sometimes eosinophils are also present. In immunocompromised patients inflammatory cells may be sparse and sometimes absent.

20.1.3 Examples

Case 1. Herpes Zoster

A 56-year-old man presented with hemorrhagic, indurated papules on the medial aspect of the right lower leg. The lesion was thought to be due to vasculitis.

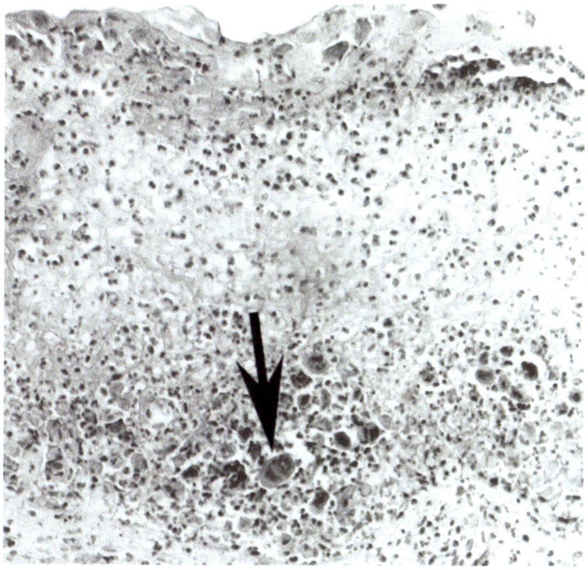

Fig. 20.3 Herpes zoster. Biopsy specimen from the trunk. The vesicular epidermis is penetrated by inflammatory cells. The *arrow* indicates highly degenerated epithelial cells and a distinct virus giant cell. H&E

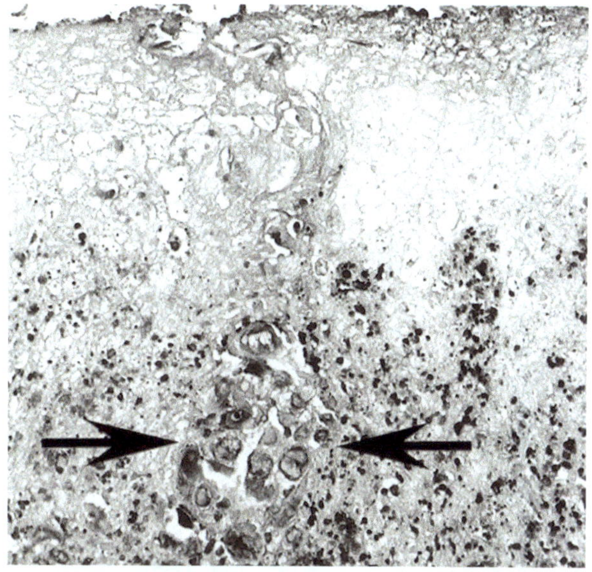

Fig. 20.4 Herpes simplex. Biopsy from the hard palate. The epithelium is totally necrotic and detached from the lamina propria. The *arrows* indicate a group of virus giant cells. H&E

Histologic investigation disclosed a typical herpes virus vesicle. The epidermis was detached from the dermis and consisted of closely packed acantholytic epithelial cells in different stages of disintegration. Two faded giant cells and scattered cells with typical intranuclear inclusion bodies were identified. Neutrophils were sparse. In the upper dermis venules with erythrocyte thrombi surrounded by erythrocytes and infiltrates of neutrophils were observed (Fig. 20.1).

Case 2. Generalized Herpes Zoster

A 54-year-old man had zoster-like efflorescences on the right side of the head and widespread red macules with central vesicles on the trunk.

A biopsy specimen from the trunk disclosed a wide vesicle, which comprised the entire epidermis and had a variegated appearance. Areas with conspicuous reticular degeneration (see Glossary) alternated with dense aggregates of neutrophils and densely packed eosinophilic epithelial cells without inner structures. A few virus giant cells were seen. Small clusters of apoptotic bodies were observed outside the vesicle. In the upper dermis venules with erythrocyte thrombi, wall necrosis, hemorrhages and dense infiltrates of neutrophils and nuclear fragments were noted (Fig. 20.2).

Case 3. Generalized Herpes Zoster

A 71-year-old woman had been treated continuously for several years with a low dose of oral corticosteroids because of arthritis. Grouped and crusted lesions developed on the chin and somewhat later small erythematous maculae with central vesicles were observed on the trunk. She also complained of pain in the right auditory meatus.

A biopsy specimen from the trunk disclosed a disintegrating and edematous epidermis, densely infiltrated by neutrophils and nuclear fragments. At the vesicular–dermal interface, aggregates of highly degenerated epithelial cells and scattered virus giant cells were observed. (Fig. 20.3).

Case 4. Oral Herpes Simplex

A 65-year-old woman presented with small vesicles, one of which was ruptured, on the hard palate.

Histologic investigation showed a detached and completely necrotic epithelium, the base of which was densely permeated with neutrophils and nuclear fragments. The clue to the diagnosis was an accumulation of typical virus giant cells. (Fig. 20.4).

Case 5. Herpes Zoster

A 45-year-old man presented with itching vesicles on the lateral aspect of the neck. Suggested possible diag-

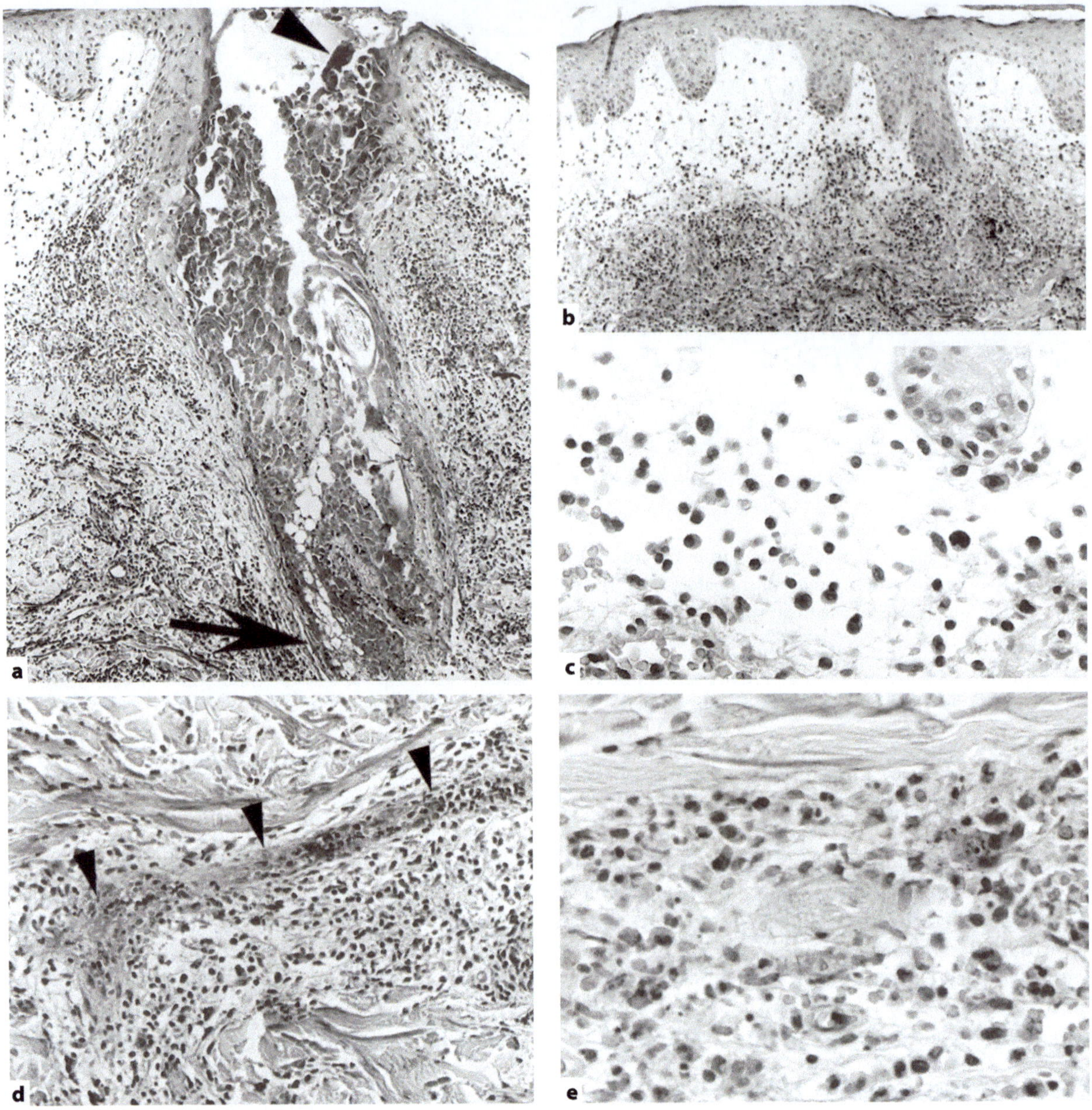

Fig. 20.5 Herpes zoster. **a** The micrograph shows a necrotic hair follicle and its sebaceous gland (*arrow*). A few giant cells lie in the orifice (*arrowhead*). **b** Around the follicle there is a conspicuous subepidermal edema, but no signs of herpetic infection in the epidermis. **c** Close-up of the edematous area demonstrates inflammatory cells with scattered large atypical (stimulated) lymphocytes. **d** A venule can be followed through the dermis (*arrowheads*): to the left the wall is necrotic and surrounded by fibrinous exudate. **e** Another vessel is obliterated by an erythrocyte thrombus and encircled by a mixed inflammatory cell infiltrate and nuclear dust. H&E

noses were folliculitis, herpes zoster, and fungal infection.

The biopsy specimen was investigated at several levels. It reached down to the dermal–subcutaneous interface. Changes typical of herpes virus infection were observed only in a large, deep-seated hair follicle. Nearly the entire follicle including a sebaceous gland was composed of acantholytic, necrotic epithelial cells of different size and form. A few giant cells were seen in the orifice and in the bulb. The adjacent parts of epidermis were normal. The vesicle was caused by a conspicuous subepidermal edema, which extended at both sides of the follicle. It contained lymphocytes, some of which were atypical (stimulated) and had a

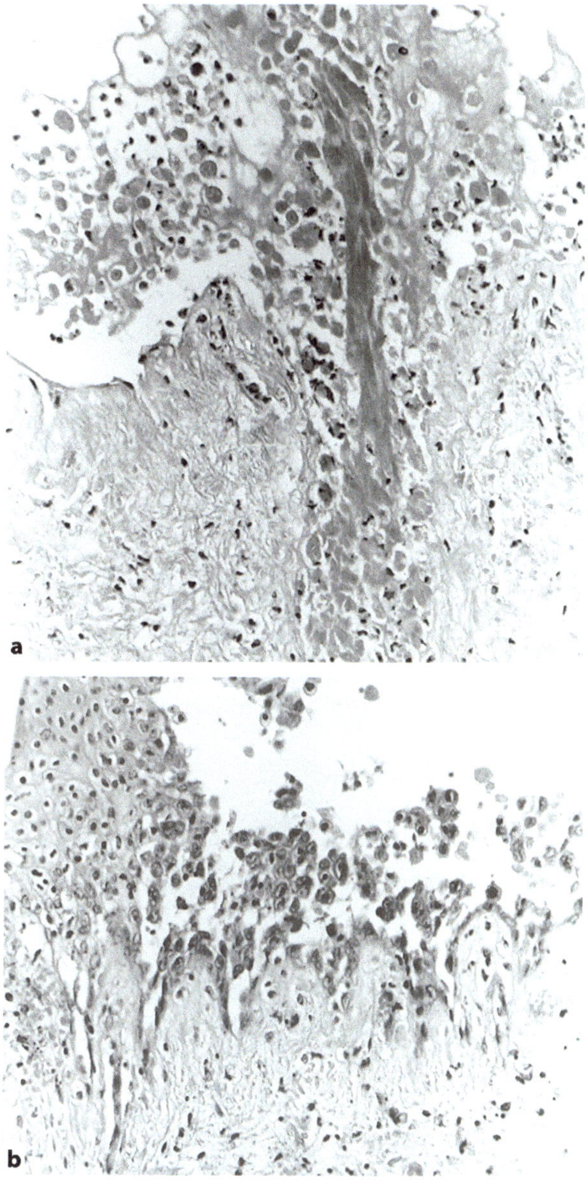

Fig. 20.6 Varicella. **a** Advanced vesicular lesion with a shadow hair follicle. **b** The end of a vesicle. There are sheets of acantholytic cells above elongated dermal papillae, to which some basal cells are still attached. H&E

larger, more hyperchromatic, and somewhat irregular nucleus than ordinary small lymphocytes (Sect. 5.1.3). Throughout the dermis there were perivascular and diffuse mixed inflammatory cell infiltrates composed of lymphocytes, eosinophils, neutrophils, and histiocytes. Small venules were filled with erythrocytes, some of them contained erythrocyte thrombi and showed wall necrosis and perivascular hemorrhages (Fig. 20.5).

Case 6. Varicella

A 48-year-old woman had suffered for at least 7 years from eczematous skin lesions associated with unbearable itching. During this period she had received repeated courses of irradiation treatment up to what was considered to be her maximum dose. When she finally presented with tumors typical of mycosis fungoides, she was given a combination cytostatic treatment. The skin lesions disappeared and did not return. However, a few months later she died of varicella with widespread vesicular and hemorrhagic skin lesions associated with zoster virus pneumonia. VZV was isolated from skin lesions.

Histologic investigation of skin lesions, taken at the autopsy, showed vesicles due to epidermal necrosis. The lumen contained sheets of acantholytic and severely degenerated epithelial cells, and single virus giant cells, but no inflammatory cells. In areas, the floor of the vesicles was made up of dermal papillae covered with a row of acantholytic cells, a pattern similar to that seen in pemphigus vulgaris (Fig. 25.2d). Hair follicles were also involved. The upper dermis was edematous and contained a sparse number of inflammatory cells, dilated vessels and hemorrhages, but no vasculitis (Fig. 20.6).

Case 7. Varicella

A 27-year-old man had undergone cytostatic treatment for Hodgkin disease and shortly after that contracted varicella. He developed a conspicuous general eruption of densely set small vesicles and suddenly died a few days after the outbreak of the skin lesions. Autopsy revealed that the herpetic infection also involved the liver and lungs.

A skin biopsy showed a mainly intraepidermal vesicle that contained virus giant cells without signs of regressive changes and very few inflammatory cells. Outside the vesicle groups of giant cells, presumably in the making, were observed. In upper dermis there was a sparse number of lymphocytes. Vasculitis was not seen (Fig. 20.7).

Case 8. Herpes Zoster

The patient suffered from Hodgkin disease and shortly after treatment with cytostatic drugs and irradiation developed a typical herpes zoster.

Two biopsy specimens showed vesicles, which were mainly intraepidermal and contained many virus giant cells. In the upper dermis vessels filled with erythrocytes and extravasated red blood cells, but

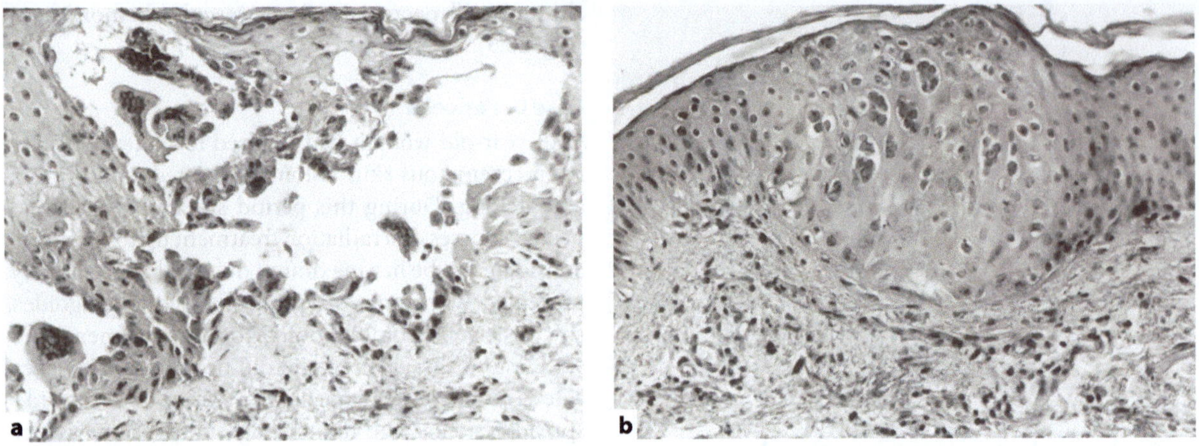

Fig. 20.7 Varicella. **a** Intraepidermal vesicle with many giant cells, but very few inflammatory cells. **b** Thickened area of epidermis with faded epithelial cells and giant cells in the making. Inflammatory cells are sparse in the dermis. H&E

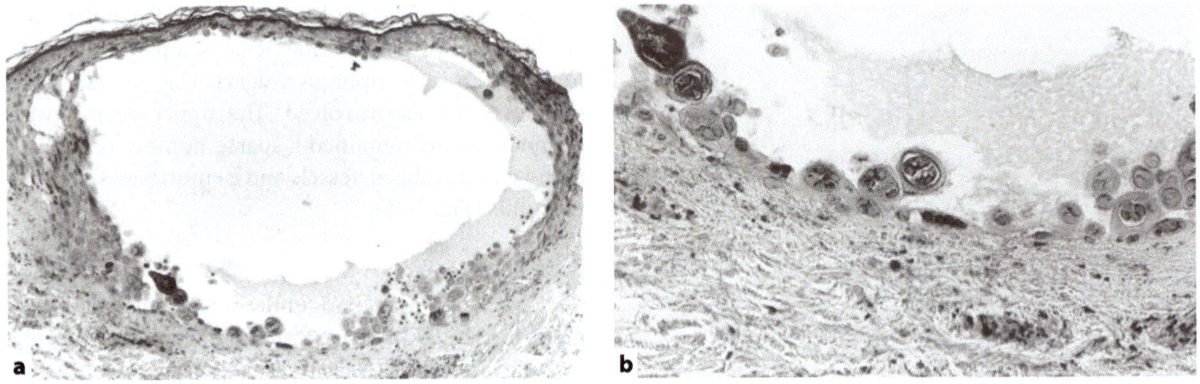

Fig. 20.8 Herpes zoster. **a** Mainly intraepidermal and nearly empty vesicle with a row of giant cells at the floor. **b** Close-up of the giant cells. Note the sparse number of inflammatory cells both in the vesicle and in the dermis. H&E

only a sparse number of lymphocytes, were observed (Fig. 20.8).

20.1.4 Comment

In a selected series of 16 patients with herpes virus vesicles, 2 had herpes simplex, 12 herpes zoster, and 2 varicella. In 4 patients with herpes zoster the lesions were more or less generalized.

In four cases small clusters of apoptotic bodies were observed in the epidermis at a short distance from the vesicles (Fig. 20.2b). It is possible that these apoptotic bodies were the result of the cell-mediated immune response against the virus, and were due to interaction between cytotoxic T cells and epithelial cells, which on their surface express both class I HLA antigen and the specific viral antigen (Sect. 4.1.2.2) The moment to attack and kill the virus-infected cell together with the virus is presumably when the virus has bound to the cell surface but before the virus envelope has fused with the cell membrane.

In ten cases hair follicles were involved. In two of these no signs of herpetic lesions or inflammation could be detected in the epidermis in spite of many investigated sections (Fig. 20.5a). Isolated herpetic lesions in sweat gland ducts were not observed, but have been described by others (Sangueza et al. 1995). In two cases the vesicles were mainly intraepidermal and contained many distinct and well-preserved giant cells (Figs. 20.7a and 20.8b). Presumably they represented very early lesions, not so often observed. Both patients were under treatment for Hodgkin disease and thus in close contact with the medical service, which allowed observation of the herpetic lesions at an early stage.

In all cases except one, marked extravasation of erythrocytes was noted. Vasculitis affecting venules in the upper and middle dermis was seen in 7 of the 12 cases with herpes zoster (Figs. 20.1d, 20.2d, and 20.5d,e). Erythrocyte thrombi, fibrinoid wall necrosis, perivascular cell infiltrates mainly composed of neutrophils, and nuclear dust were observed. Endothelial cells with signs of viral infection were not detected. Thus the histopathologic pattern was the same as that described as leukocytoclastic vasculitis (Sect. 7.1). By means of electron microscopic investigations, Hasegawa (1971) observed the presence of herpes zoster virions in endothelial cells in VZV lesions. Later Cohen and Trapuckd (1984) and Erhard et al. (1995) made the same observation. The virus has also been found in pericytes of the vascular wall and in perivascular fibroblasts (Cohen and Trapuckd 1984). The proven presence of virus in endothelial cells and stroma cells of lesional skin in herpes zoster and the spread of lesions outside the primary dermatome in some cases indicate viremia.

A prominent feature was the near absence of inflammatory cells in three immunocompromised patients (Figs. 20.6–20.8). In one case the presence of atypical lymphocytes was evident (Fig. 20.5c); very likely these cells were stimulated (activated) T cells proliferating at that location.

20.1.5 Differential Diagnosis

The variegated appearance of disintegrating epithelial cells of different form and size, for example as demonstrated in Fig. 20.1, is diagnostic of HSV and VZV infection even without the presence of typical intranuclear inclusions or distinct virus giant cells. However, in advanced lesions the changes are nonspecific and may be misinterpreted as:

- Toxic epidermal necrolysis (Sect. 28.4)
- Various kinds of chemical or mechanical damage (Sect. 29.7)
- Necrolytic migratory erythema (Sect. 27.2)
- Recurrent erythema multiforme (Sect. 26.1)

20.1.5.1 Comment

A smear from herpes vesicles by means of the Tzanck test (see Glossary) can be used to rapidly arrive at the diagnosis in suspected cases of HSV and VZV infections (Fig. 20.9). The goal is to obtain diagnostic virus giant cells (Brehmer-Andersson 1965).

20.2 Cytomegalovirus Infection

Cytomegalovirus belongs to the herpes family and like HSVs and VZV has an envelope, and when propagating kills the cell. It is ubiquitous and affects animals as well as humans, but is strictly species-specific. Humans are believed to be the only reservoir for the human cytomegalovirus (HCMV).

20.2.1 Pathogenesis and Clinical Appearance

The virus is transmitted by close contact between individuals and infected body secretions. Contamination also occurs from organ transplants and blood transfusions containing cells infected with latent virus. The fetus may be infected in the uterus or in the neonatal period by breast-feeding.

HCMV infections are common and appear early in life. The primary infection is in most cases subclinical, but is followed by a lifelong latent infection. Repeated recurrences without clinical symptoms associated with shedding of HCMV may occur. In most developed countries 40–80% of children are infected before puberty. In early life the infection may be serious, and even fatal. In adults serious generalized infections, usually due to reactivation of latent disease, are seen in patients with advanced HIV infection and in bone marrow and heart–lung transplant recipients (Mocarski 1994).

Infection in the skin and mucous membranes is uncommon, but has been described in immunosuppressed patients (Lee and Peel 1989; Smith et al. 1991; Resnik et al. 2000; Kanas et al. 1987), and after severe burns and severe tissue destruction without immunosuppression (Swanson and Feldman 1987).

Skin lesions do not have a characteristic gross appearance, while the histopathologic pattern is typical and therefore important to be familiar with.

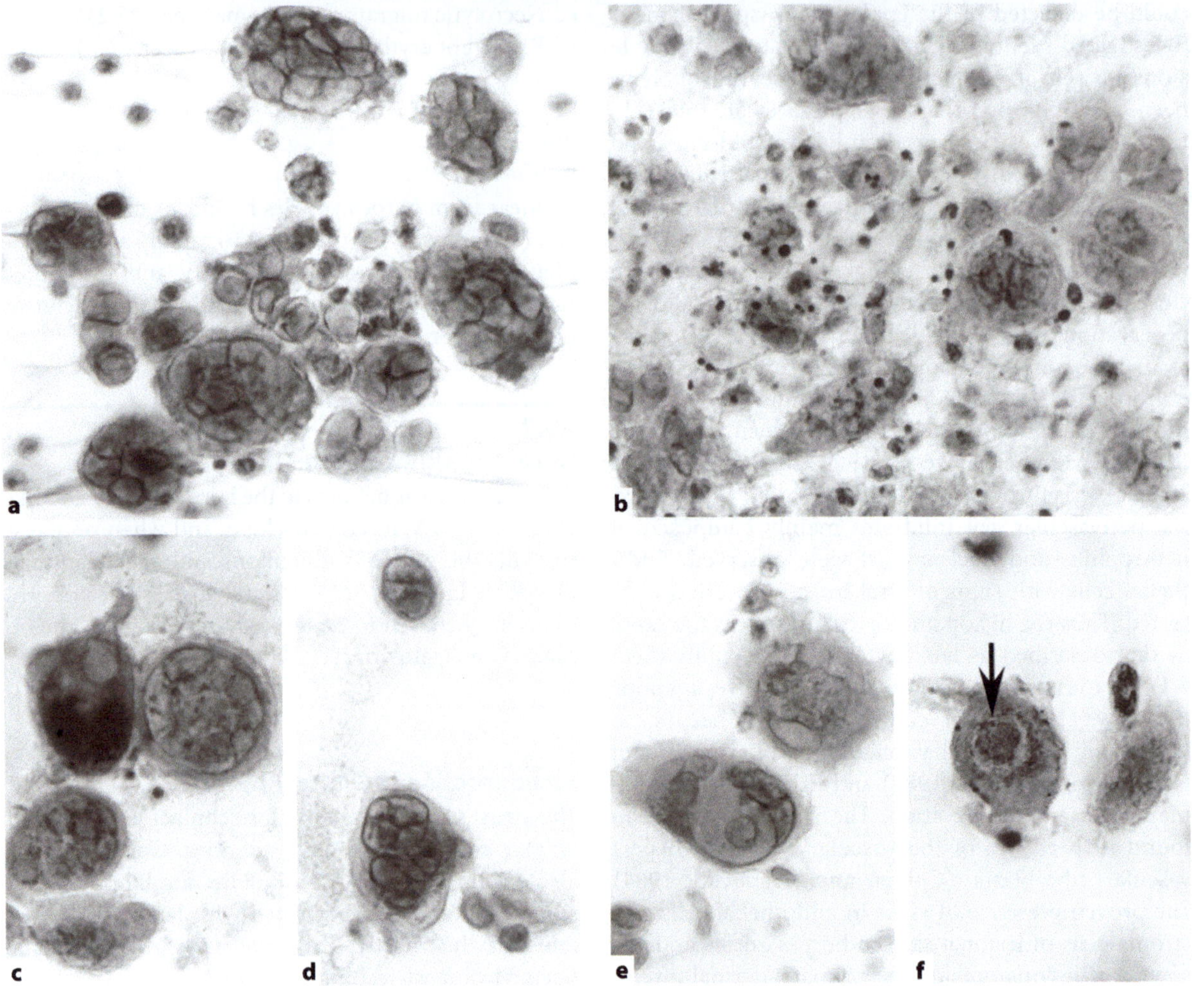

Fig. 20.9 Smears from herpes simplex and herpes zoster vesicles. **a–e** Virus giant cells, shadow cells and nuclear fragments. In **b** there are also many inflammatory cells; ×500. **f** A ballooned keratinocyte with an intranuclear inclusion body surrounded by a light halo (*arrow*); ×1000. Mayer staining

20.2.2 Histopathologic Appearance

In inner organs epithelial and endothelial cells are the cells most often infected, but also other cells such as stroma cells and blood cells may be affected. Common locations are the salivary gland ductal epithelium and the tubular epithelium of the kidney. In the mucous membranes and the skin, affected cells have been observed in vessels, and in the skin also in sweat gland ducts (Resnik et al. 2000).

Virus-affected cells are swollen and may be several times their normal size. Also the nucleus is large and often elongated. Both the nucleus and the cytoplasm may contain virus inclusion bodies. These are of different size and form. The color is variously described as purple, eosinophilic, basophilic, or amphophilic (Resnik et al. 2000).

Because of the lack of material from infected skin, a specimen from the small intestine is presented here as an example.

20.2.3 Example

Case 9. Cytomegalovirus Infection

A 34-year-old HIV-infected man was operated upon because of a hemorrhage from the small intestine. On the mucous membrane of the excised part several dispersed ulcers (10–20 mm in diameter) were observed.

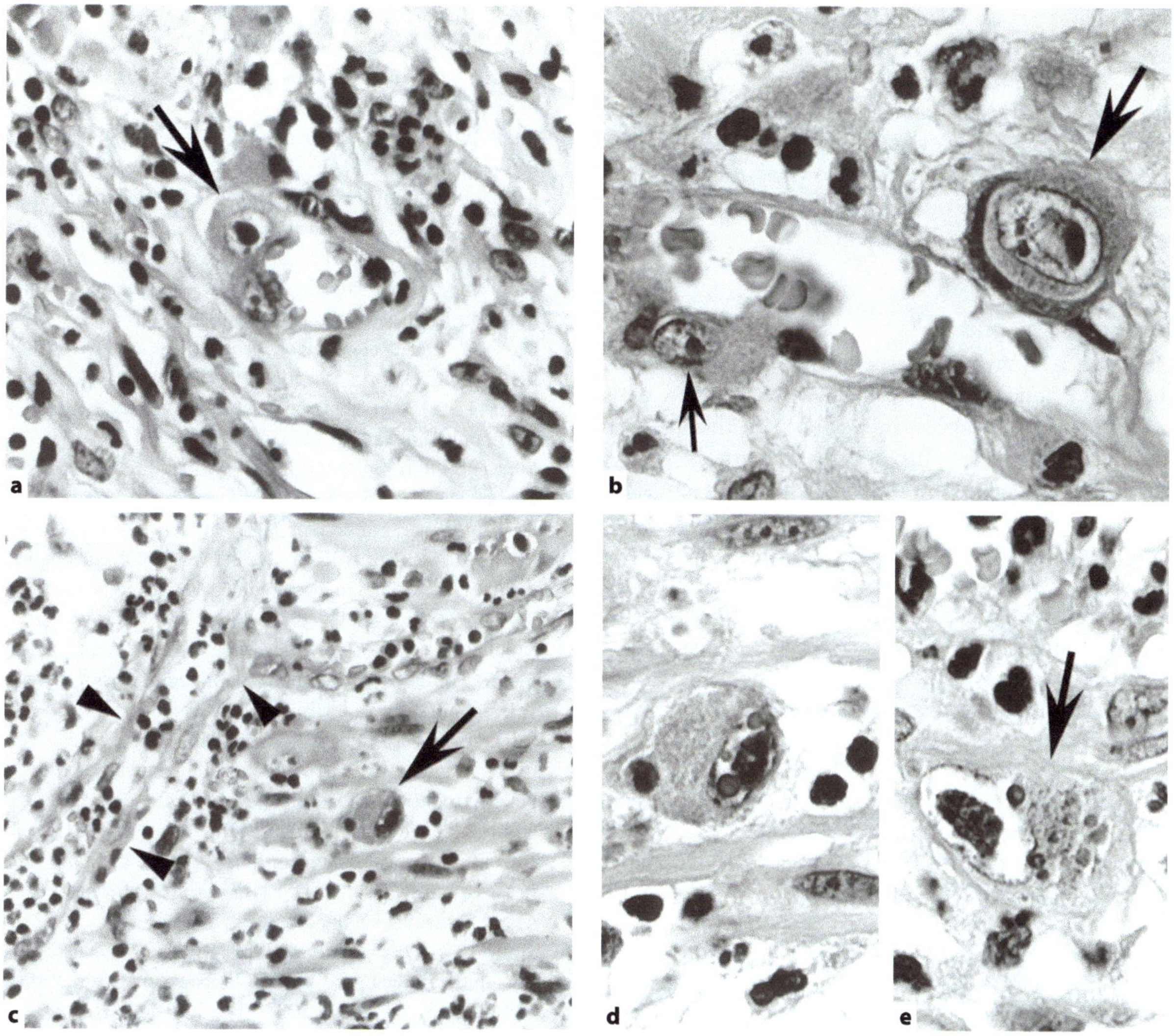

Fig. 20.10 CMV infection in the small intestine. **a** A transversely cut venule contains a ballooned endothelial cell with a large intranuclear inclusion surrounded by a clear halo (*arrow*); ×600. **b** Venule with two affected endothelial cells (*arrows*), the larger of which has a clear nucleus with several different-sized irregular inclusions and granules. Opposite the larger cell two disintegrating endothelial cells are seen; ×1000. **c** To the left there is a longitudinally cut venule giving off a branch to the right (*arrowheads*). In the angle between the vessels there is a row of disintegrating smooth muscle cells. One of these cells contains a large elongated nucleus (*arrow*); ×400. **d** Close-up of the cell indicated in **c** shows several different-sized intranuclear inclusions. The rounded black body in the cytoplasm is probably also a virus inclusion body; ×1000. **e** An infected and disintegrating stroma cell contains many small rounded inclusions both in the nucleus and in the cytoplasm. Note the granular cytoplasm and the blurred cell membrane (*arrow*); ×1000. H&E

Histologic investigation of sections stained with H&E showed a small ulcer which included the mucosa, muscularis mucosae, and the uppermost part of the submucosa. Below the center of the cavity there were several small thrombosed vessels. The entire wall of the gut showed signs of acute inflammation with marked edema, dilated venules, extravasated erythrocytes, and conspicuous infiltrates of inflammatory cells (neutrophils, lymphocytes, eosinophils). Many endothelial cells, pericytes, smooth muscle cells and scattered fibroblasts were infected with CMV. These cells were several times their normal size, had rich, slightly basophilic, slightly granular cytoplasm, and a large nucleus. One or several inclusion bodies were observed in the nucleus only, in the cytoplasm only, or in both locations in the same cell. Intranuclear inclusions prevailed. The inclusions varied in size and color (eosinophilic to slightly basophilic). The most characteristic were distinct, round, eosinophilic bodies, in the nucleus often surrounded by a clear halo. Many infected cells displayed signs of advanced disintegration (lysis) such as fading of the nucleus and cytoplasm or loss of substance. Affected vessels showed fibrinoid wall necrosis. No virus-infected cells were observed in the mucosal epithelium (Fig. 20.10).

20.2.4 Differential Diagnosis

HSV and VZV infections show similarities. However, in HCMV lesions, affected cells are larger and may contain several inclusion bodies both in the nucleus and in the cytoplasm. Also, mostly, the target cells are different. A problem may occur when concurrent skin infections with CMV and HSV appear (Lee and Peel 1989; Smith et al. 1991). However, a suspected CMV infection can be verified or screened out by means of immunohistochemical investigation using monoclonal antibodies.

References

1. Brehmer-Andersson E (1965) Diagnostic importance of punch biopsy and cytologic examination in herpes zoster and herpes simplex. Acta Derm Venereol 45:262–271
2. Cohen C, Trapuckd S (1984) Leukocytoclastic vasculitis associated with cutaneous infection by herpesvirus. Am J Dermatopathol 6:561–565
3. Erhard H, Rünger TM, Kreienkamp M, Müller J, Müller-Hermelink H-K, Bröcker E-B (1995) Atypical varicella-zoster virus infection in an immunocompromised patient: result of virus-induced vasculitis. J Am Acad Dermatol 32:908–911
4. Gibson W (1994) Cytomegaloviruses: molecular biology (human). In: Webster RG, Granoff A (eds) Encyclopedia of virology. Academic Press, Harcourt Brace, London, pp 299–304
5. Hasegawa T (1971) Further electron microscopic observations of herpes zoster virus. Arch Dermatol 103:45–49
6. Kanas RJ, Jensen JL, Abrams AM, Wuerker RB (1987) Oral mucosal cytomegalovirus as a manifestation of the acquired immune deficiency syndrome. Oral Surg Oral Med Oral Pathol 64:183–189
7. LeBoit PE, Límová M, Yen TSB, Palefsky JM, White CR, Berger TG (1992) Chronic verrucous varicella-zoster virus infection in patients with the acquired immunodeficiency syndrome (AIDS). Histologic and molecular biologic findings. Am J Dermatopathol 14:1–7
8. Lee JY-Y, Peel R (1989) Concurrent cytomegalovirus and herpes simplex virus infections in skin biopsy specimens from two AIDS patients with fatal CMV infection. Am J Dermatopathol 11:136–143
9. Mocarski ES Jr (1994) Cytomegaloviruses. In: Webster RG, Granoff A (eds) Encyclopedia of virology. Academic Press, Harcourt Brace, London, pp 292–298
10. Resnik KS, DiLeonardo M, Maillet M (2000) Histopathologic findings in cutaneous cytomegalovirus infection. Am J Dermatopathol 22:397–407
11. Samuelson J (1999) Infectious diseases. In: Cotran RS, Kumar V, Collins T (eds) Robbins pathologic basis of disease. W.B. Saunders, Philadelphia, pp 340–344
12. Sangueza OP, Gordon MD, White CRJ (1995) Subtle clues to the diagnosis of herpesvirus by light microscopy. Herpetic syringitis. Am J Dermatopathol 17:163–168
13. Smith KJ, Skelton HG, James WD, Angritt P (1991) Concurrent epidermal involvement of cytomegalovirus and herpes simplex virus in two HIV-infected patients. J Am Acad Dermatol 25:500–506
14. Swanson S, Feldman PS (1987) Cytomegalovirus infection initially diagnosed by skin biopsy. Am J Clin Pathol 87:113–116
15. White JM, Blobel CP (1989) Cell-to-cell fusion. Curr Opin Cell Biol 1:934–939

Chapter 21

Langerhans Cell Histiocytosis in Skin and Mucous Membranes

21

In Langerhans cell histiocytosis accumulations of a special kind of Langerhans cells give rise to granulomas, which may appear in any tissue or organ. In the old literature the disease was described as three diseases of different severity and different histopathologic pattern with the ability to change from one kind of disease to one of the others: Letterer-Siwe disease (the most serious form), Hand-Schüller-Christian disease, and eosinophilic granuloma (the most benign). Lichtenstein (1953) asserted that the three diseases were manifestations of the same nosologic entity and coined the concept histiocytosis X. However, Nezelof et al. (1973) found histogenetic arguments for a Langerhans cell origin of the disease, which led to the more appropriate designation Langerhans cell histiocytosis (LCH).

The disease may appear at any age, but is most common in childhood. There is a prevalence for males. It is regarded as a benign reactive process with a variable course and morbidity depending on the site of the lesions and, most important, on whether the disease is unifocal or multifocal (Lieberman et al. 1996; Titgemeyer et al. 2001). However, in some patients with multisystem disease the outcome is fatal, most often due to circulatory failure or infections. Rare complications are diabetes insipidus, which is due to granulomas located in the posterior part of the pituitary gland or hypothalamus, exophthalmia due to retroorbital granulomas, and otitis media caused by infiltrate in the temporal bone. In both unifocal and multifocal disease, bones are the most common sites with preference for (in order) skull, femur, pelvic bones, ribs and vertebrae (Lieberman et al. 1996). The most common soft-tissue organs that may be involved in unifocal or multifocal disease are lungs, lymph nodes and skin.

21.1 Clinical Appearance

Skin lesions are most common in the neonatal period and in small children, but also occur in older children, young adults and the elderly. In small children the lesions appear as vesicular or pustular papules, occasionally as nodules, or as dermatitis (eczema). In the latter case they may be mistaken for diaper dermatitis or seborrheic dermatitis. Commonly affected regions are the trunk, groin, armpits, scalp, the area behind the ears, and the auditory meatus. Sometimes the oral mucosa, including the gingiva, is affected with loosening of the teeth. The disease may be unifocal, but in many patients there are, or later develop, lesions even in other organs (Stein et al. 2001). In old patients the disease appears as scattered hemorrhagic infiltrated lesions, papules, or nodules (Aoki et al. 1998; Stefanato et al. 1998).

21.2 Histopathologic Appearance

As already mentioned, Langerhans cells are bone-marrow-derived dendritic cells normally present in the skin and mucous membranes. They cannot be identified in routinely stained sections, but may be visualized by means of histochemical staining with S-100 and CD1a antibodies (Sect. 4.4.2). The granulomas in LCH consist of polymorphic histiocyte-like cells, which like normal Langerhans cells, are S-100- and CD1a-positive, and also contain Birbeck granules (see Glossary). They are here called LCH cells.

LCH cells are of different sizes, but usually have a rich well-demarcated and finely granular cytoplasm. The nuclei are usually clear, sometimes vacuolated, and vary conspicuously in shape. They may be rounded, oval, kidney-shaped, lobulated or deeply cleaved and contain one or several non-prominent nucleoli. Usually there is only one nucleus, but scattered or several multinucleated giant cells may be present. A few mitotic figures may be observed. In addition to LCH cells, there is a variable admixture of eosinophils, neutrophils and lymphocytes. The granulomas are loosely composed, often not well demarcated. They are mostly confined to the upper dermis, but may be

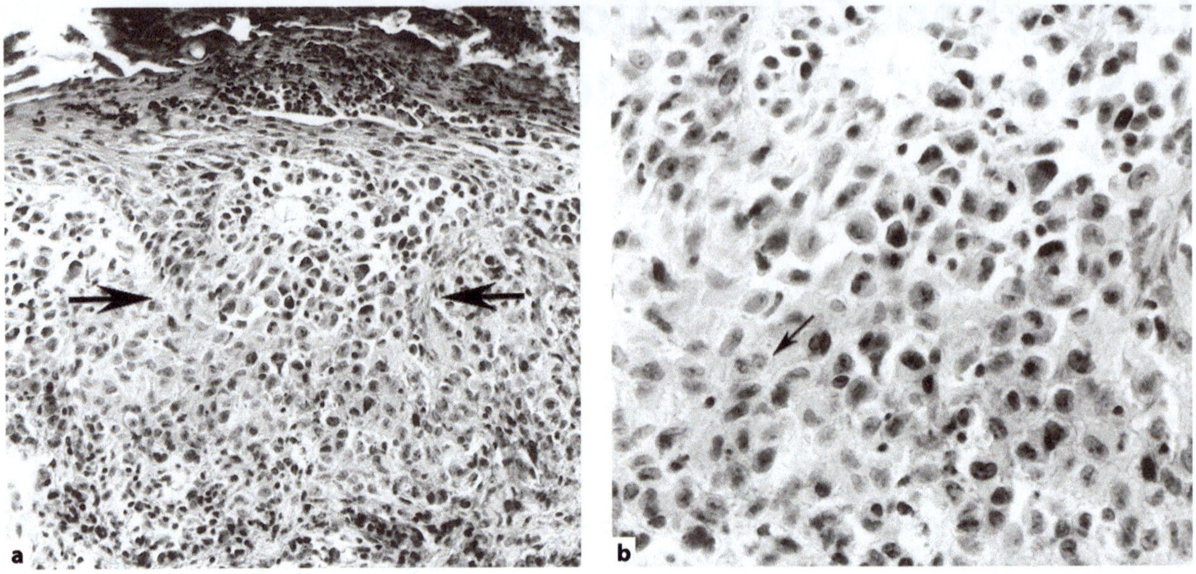

Fig. 21.1 Langerhans cell histiocytosis. **a** A dense infiltrate of LCH cells in the papillae and upper dermis invade and destroy the epidermis giving rise to saw-tooth rete ridges and a superficial crusted pustule. **b** Close-up of the area indicated (*arrows*) in **a** shows LCH cells with abundant cytoplasm and different-shaped nuclei. The *arrow* indicates a mitotic figure in anaphase. H&E

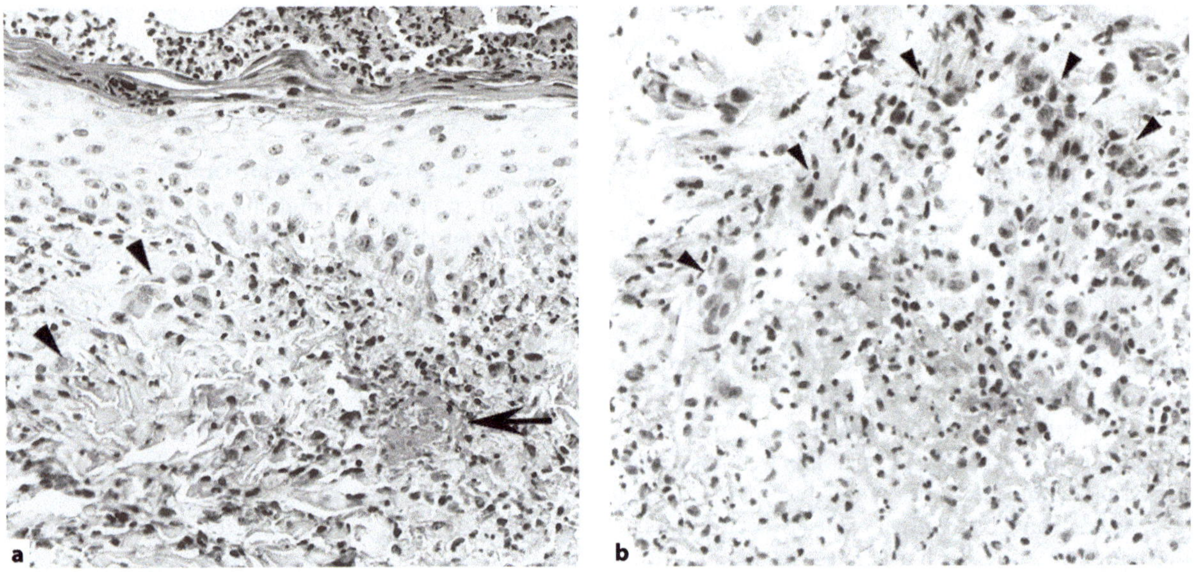

Fig. 21.2 Langerhans cell histiocytosis. **a** The *upper arrowhead* indicates a small accumulation of LCH cells and the *lower arrowhead* an area of fibrinoid necrosis. At the *arrow* there is a small venule with fibrinoid wall necrosis, hemorrhage and nuclear dust. The epidermis is covered with a crust. **b** Fibrinoid necrosis with disintegrating neutrophils and nuclear dust in the middle of the dermis. The area is partly walled of by a band of LCH cells (*arrowheads*). H&E

massive and reach down to the dermal–subcutaneous interface. Characteristically the LCH cells invade the epidermis and in the center of the lesion give rise to a small ulcer covered by a crust. In some settings the inflammatory cells prevail and the true character of the disease could be missed as in genital and oral lesions. Extravasation of erythrocytes is a prominent feature. Sometimes neutrophilic venular vasculitis may occur, affecting only scattered vessels.

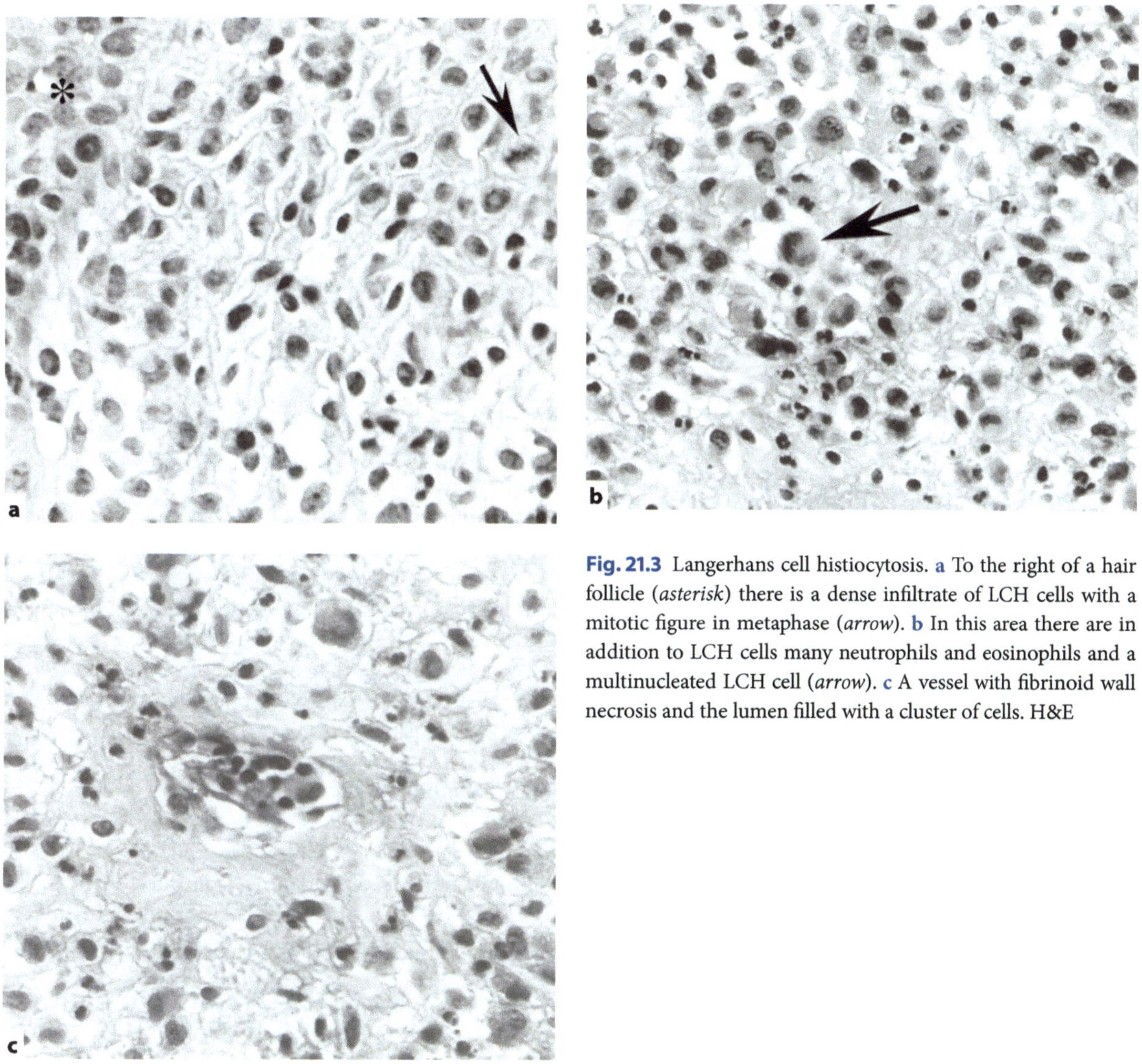

Fig. 21.3 Langerhans cell histiocytosis. **a** To the right of a hair follicle (*asterisk*) there is a dense infiltrate of LCH cells with a mitotic figure in metaphase (*arrow*). **b** In this area there are in addition to LCH cells many neutrophils and eosinophils and a multinucleated LCH cell (*arrow*). **c** A vessel with fibrinoid wall necrosis and the lumen filled with a cluster of cells. H&E

21.3 Examples

Case 1. Langerhans Cell Histiocytosis

The patient had from the neonatal period suffered from a severe and therapy-resistant dermatitis in the groin and on the scalp and auricles. At 6 months a nodule in the right temporal area with underlying bone destruction was also detected, and at the age of 10 months the left tonsil was affected.

Histologic investigation of two skin lesions from the abdominal wall showed in the papillae and upper dermis dense infiltrates of LCH cells, which in the center of the lesion invaded and ulcerated the epidermis. A few mitotic figures, but no giant cells were observed. There was a moderate admixture of eosinophils, neutrophils, lymphocytes, and extravasated erythrocytes.

A biopsy from the bone lesion revealed a granuloma which consisted of LCH cells and a high number of eosinophils. In the tonsil, aggregates of LCH cells but only a moderate number of eosinophils were observed (Fig. 21.1).

Case 2. Langerhans Cell Histiocytosis

This 1-year-old boy for some time had had scattered papulopustules all over the body and spells of fever. Investigation revealed a high ESR (85 mm/h), palpable lymph nodes, and multiple bone lesions. The disease became generalized and the patient died about 18 months later due to circulatory failure. A biopsy specimen was taken from a lesion on the back.

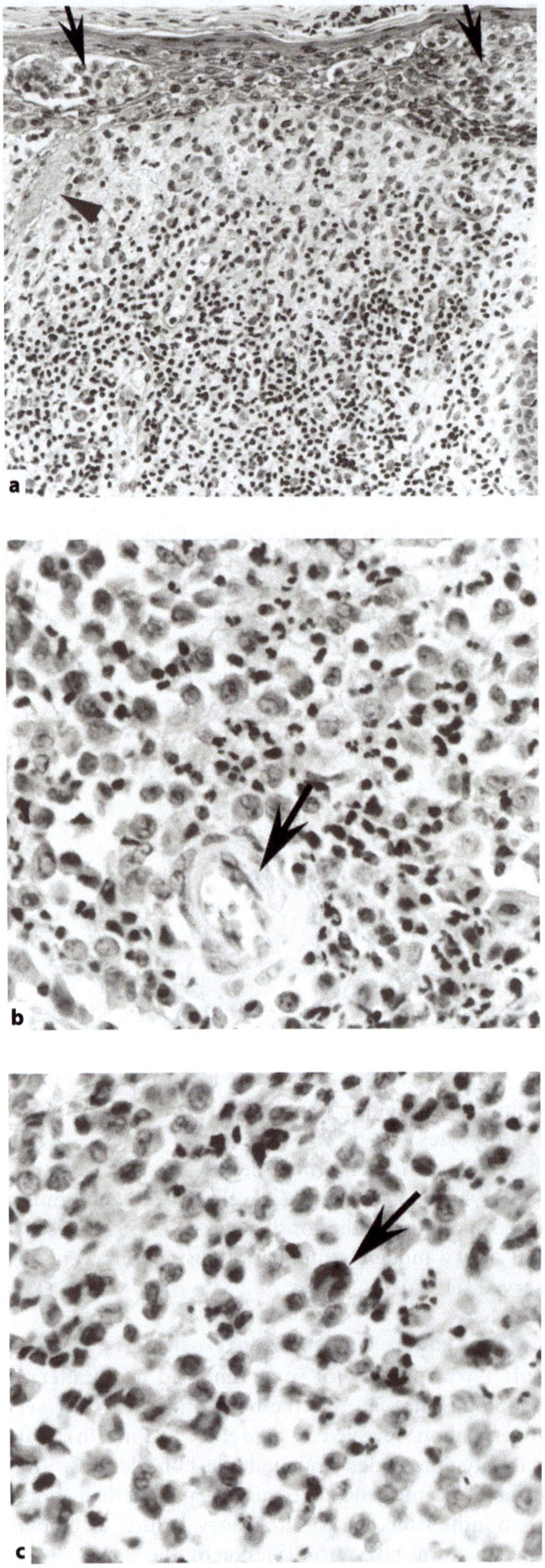

Fig. 21.4 Langerhans cell histiocytosis. **a** Biopsy specimen from the axilla. There is a dense cell infiltrate in the dermis. The upper half is composed of LCH cells, which have also migrated into the epidermis and form intraepidermal abscesses (*arrows*); the lower part consists of lymphocytes. The *arrowhead* indicates a venule with fibrinoid wall necrosis. **b** Specimen from the inner aspect of the lower lip. A partly necrotic venule (*arrow*) is surrounded by a compact infiltrate of LCH cells and inflammatory cells, mainly neutrophils. **c** The arrow indicates a multinucleated LCH cell. H&E

Histologic investigation revealed at all levels of the dermis large infiltrates of LCH cells, a fair number of which were multinucleated. No mitotic figures were seen. In and between the infiltrates there were areas of fibrinoid necrosis with accumulation of neutrophils. In the upper dermis a single small vessel with fibrinoid wall necrosis was noted; extravasation of erythrocytes was prominent. The cell infiltrate appeared to gnaw at the epidermis, which in the central part showed a small ulceration. There were many lymphocytes, but only sparse eosinophils (Fig. 21.2).

Case 3. Langerhans Cell Histiocytosis

A 17-year-old girl had been bothered for a long time by large genital ulcers. She also had diabetes insipidus and later developed lung infiltrates. At the age of 41 years she was in good health and, with the exception of remaining diabetes insipidus, she had no symptoms.

Histologic investigation showed widespread infiltrates of LCH cells that reached from the epidermis to the dermal–subcutaneous interface. A fair number of these cells were large and had two or three nuclei. Scattered mitotic figures were noted. Scattered LCH cells invaded the epidermis. Eosinophils were numerous. The tissue was edematous and contained a single totally necrotic venule which was filled with LCH cells and lymphocytes and surrounded by nuclear fragments and neutrophils. Many venules were stuffed with erythrocytes, but only a sparse number were observed outside vessels (Fig. 21.3).

Case 4. Langerhans Cell Histiocytosis

A 25-year-old woman had suffered from the age of 15 years from itching and oozing lesions in the vulva, perianal region, axilla, and scalp with periods of spontaneous healing. For about a year she had also had vesicular and granulomatous lesions on the gingiva and loosening teeth. She presented with erythematous, scaling and pustular lesions in the areas named above

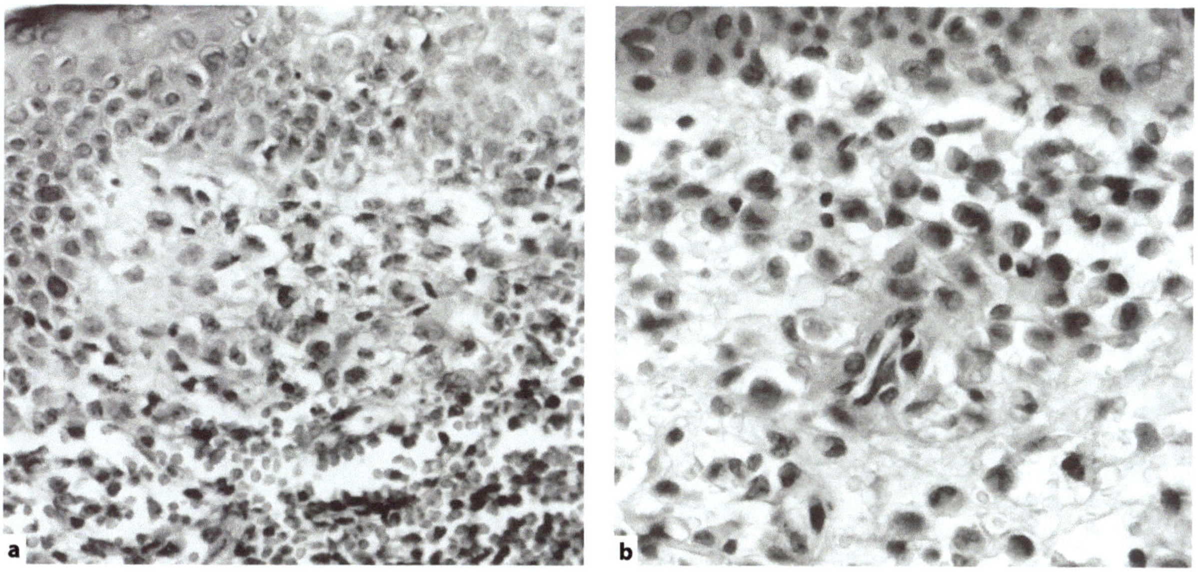

Fig. 21.5 Langerhans cell histiocytosis. a A small infiltrate of LCH cells is located close to a rete ridge in the papillary dermis. Below are aggregates of erythrocytes (light cells) and lymphocytes. b Close-up of LCH cells surrounding a venule. H&E

and in the auricles. The patient returned 3 years later with a lesion on the inner aspect of the lower lip.

At the first visit a biopsy specimen was taken from the axilla. This showed a dense subepidermal cell infiltrate mainly composed of LCH cells and lymphocytes. Several mitotic figures were noted. Eosinophils were sparse. In areas the LCH cells invaded and accumulated in the epidermis. There were many extravasated erythrocytes and scattered venules with fibrinoid wall necrosis. In the specimen taken from the lip there was a massive and deep infiltrate composed of LCH cells with scattered giant cells and scattered mitotic figures. There were many neutrophils, some lymphocytes, but few eosinophils. Many small vessels were dilated and filled with neutrophils and small fibrinoid wall necrosis was observed. In the central part of the lesion the epithelium was ulcerated (Fig. 21.4).

Case 5. Langerhans Cell Histiocytosis

An 88-year-old woman presented with purpuric and slightly infiltrated lesions on the back and purpura in intertriginous areas. The lesions had developed during the last few days.

Histologic investigation showed widespread and massive hemorrhages and perivascular infiltrates of lymphocytes in the mid-dermis, but no vasculitis. In the edematous and hemorrhagic subepidermal area small infiltrates of LCH cells were observed. These cells were S-100-positive (Fig. 21.5).

Case 6. Langerhans Cell Histiocytosis

An 84-year-old woman had for 2 months noticed scattered, bluish, infiltrated lesions over the sternal area. Lesions were observed also in the vulva and perianal region. A thorough investigation did not reveal lesions in other organs or tissues. A biopsy specimen was taken from a lesion on the breast.

Histologic investigation showed massive accumulation of LCH cells in the subepidermal area. These cells invaded and destroyed the epidermis, and were observed even in lymphatics. Multinucleated cells, mitotic figures or eosinophils were not observed. Below the polymorphic cell infiltrates there were hemorrhages and infiltrates of lymphocytes. Vasculitis was not observed. The polymorphic cells were strongly positive for S-100. A battery of immunohistochemical markers excluded lymphoma and leukemia (Fig. 21.6).

21.4 Comment

The patients discussed above represent all age groups. Four of them were encountered before the era of the routine use of immunohistochemical markers, but showed typical clinical and histopathologic patterns of LCH. The number of eosinophils, neutrophils and lymphocytes differed from one case to another. A high number of eosinophils were noted only in Case 3 and in a bone lesion in Case 2. There were no es-

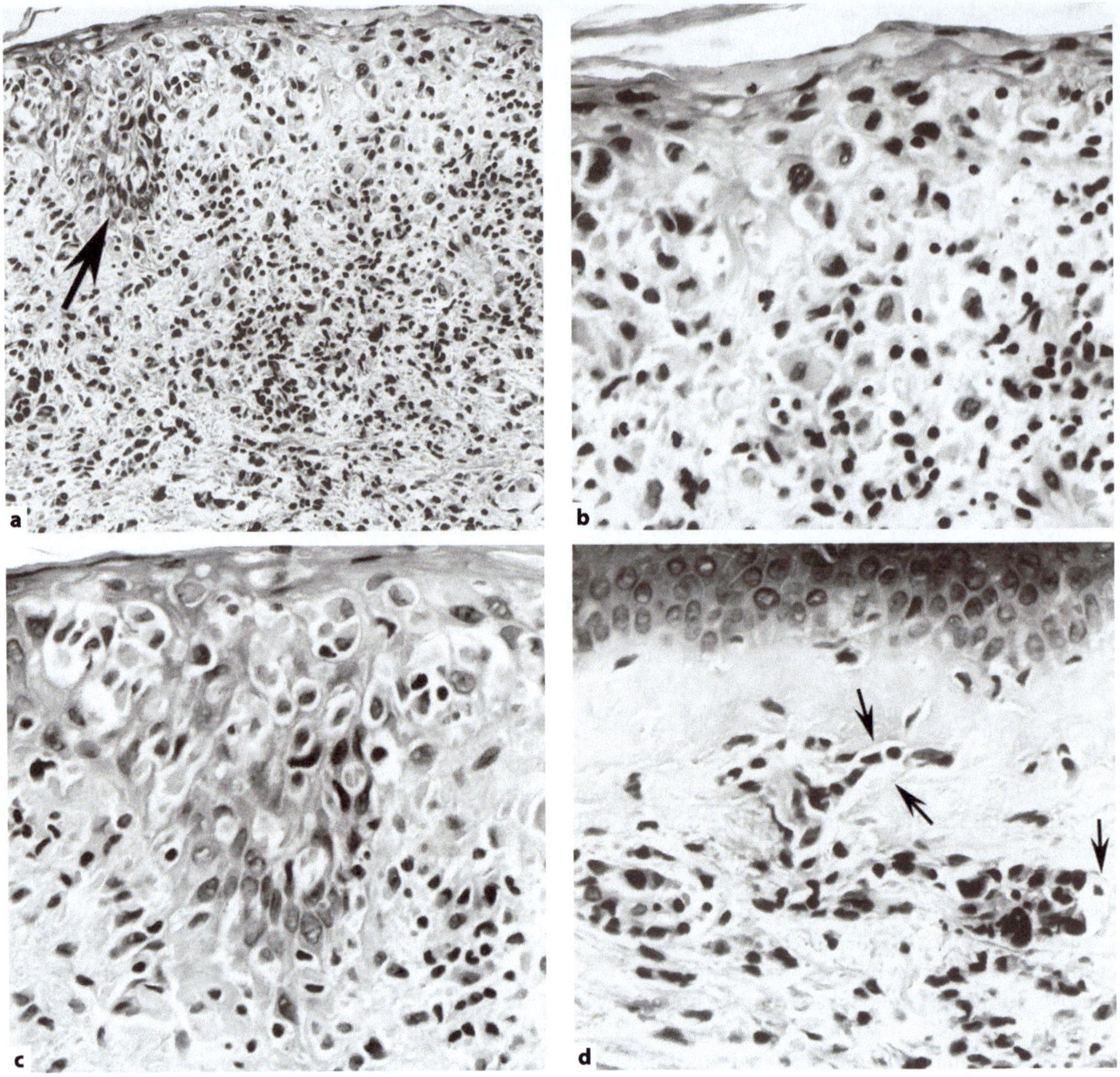

Fig. 21.6 Langerhans cell histiocytosis. **a** Below a thinned epidermis and to the right of a thickened rete ridge (*arrow*) there are aggregates of large LCH cells; beneath are infiltrates of erythrocytes and lymphocytes. **b** Close-up of the area to the right of the rete ridge shows that the LCH cells have a rich and well-defined cytoplasm and a nucleus that differs in size and form from one cell to another. **c** Close-up of the ridge demonstrates that many LCH cells have invaded the epidermis. **d** In this area LCH cells lie in thin-walled vessels, presumably lymphatics (*arrows*). H&E

sential differences in the features of the LCH cells in the six described cases. Giant cells with two or three nuclei were found in three cases (Figs. 21.2–21.4). Scattered mitotic figures were observed in three cases (Fig. 21.3a). In all but one case extravasated erythrocytes were prominent. Also leukocytoclastic vasculitis was observed in scattered venules in three cases, in one of which the necrotic vessel contained LCH cells and lymphocytes (Fig. 21.3c). In one case some LCH cells seemed to lie in lymphatics (Fig. 21.6d). Xanthoma cells were not observed.

Extravasation of erythrocytes is noted in some textbooks as a rather common phenomenon (Lever and Schaumburg-Lever 1990; McKee 1989), but vasculitis, as far as the author is aware, has not been described before. The vasculitis has the character of leukocytoclastic vasculitis, and seems, like the lymphocytic vasculitis in pityriasis et varioliformis acuta (Fig. 26.3d), to appear only sporadically.

In 1996, Lieberman et al. presented their experiences of LCH based on 238 patients and called it Langerhans cell (eosinophilic) granulomatosis. They emphasized that the old concepts Letterer-Siwe disease and Hand-Schüller-Christian disease are based on case reports of several kinds of diseases which are today difficult to analyze and therefore should be disregarded. They also stressed that xanthoma cells have nothing to do with LCH. Both assertions are in agreement with the experience of the author. It was not possible to discriminate different kinds of diseases or foresee the outcome of the disease based on the histopathologic pattern in the six cases described above, or in five other cases in the author's record. Nor were xanthoma cells observed in any case.

Lieberman et al. (1996) also emphasized the usually benign character of the disease, but malignant LCH with clonal proliferation of cells has been described in elderly patients (Itoh et al. 2001).

21.5 Pathogenesis

The pathogenesis of the disease is unknown. A viral agent has been suspected. Herpes virus 6 has been found in lesional skin in LCH, but its causal role in this disease has not yet been proved (Leahy et al. 1993). Investigations with immunohistochemical markers have revealed that Langerhans cells in bone and other chronic forms of the disease have an immature profile (Geissmann et al. 2001).

21.6 Differential Diagnosis

- *Congenital self-healing reticulohistiocytosis* (CSHRH). This is a rare and controversial concept, first described in a baby girl by Hashimoto and Pritzker (1973) and by them separated from LCH because of the favorable outcome. By electron microscopy they observed cells which in the cytoplasm contained Birbeck granules together with laminated dense bodies, the latter of which were more numerous in resolving than in fresh lesions. They did not observe laminated dense bodies in LCH and regarded the concurrent presence of Birbeck granules and dense bodies in the infiltrating cells as diagnostic for CSHRH (Hashimoto et al. 1986). In recent years possible cases of CSHRH have been described and discussed by Alexis et al. (1991), Schaumburg-Lever et al. (1994), Longaker et al. (1994), Larralde et al. (1999), and Stein et al. (2001). However, so far it has not been possible to conclude whether it is justified or not to regard CSHRH as a separate disease.
- *Mastocytoma*. Mastocytoma may appear in the neonatal period and in small children. There may be one or several tumor-like lesions with a central crust or vesicle. In mastocytoma, mast cells accumulate in the upper and papillary dermis and, like LCH cells, invade and destroy the epidermis. A special staining for mast cells easily solves the diagnostic problem and should be routine for biopsy material taken from skin lesions appearing at early ages (Sect. 5.1.5).
- *Dermatitis*. The presence of LCH cells may be overlooked if inflammatory cells prevail.
- *Lymphoma/leukemia*. LCH cells may be mistaken for lymphoma/leukemia cells especially in elderly patients. Atypical cell infiltrates in the subepidermal area, gnawing at or invading the epidermis in combination with many extravasated erythrocytes should evoke suspicion of LCH. Immunohistochemical investigations are decisive.
- *Benign cephalic histiocytosis*. This is a rare disease, which belongs to the group non-Langerhans cell histiocytoses. It was first described by Gianotti et al. in 1971 (Gianotti et al. 1993). During the first three years of life, eruptions of small pinkish or brownish-yellow papules occur on the head, preferentially on the face. New eruptions may continue to appear for several months, but finally subside and disappear without sequelae. Mucous membranes and other organ systems are not involved. Histologically, accumulations of histiocytes occupy the superficial or the whole dermis, but do not invade the epidermis. The infiltrates contain a variable number of foamy cells (xanthoma cells). The histiocytes are S-100- and CD1a-negative and contain no Birbeck granules (Gianotti et al. 1993). The eruption is thought to be an abortive form of juvenile xanthogranuloma (Jih et al. 2002).

References

1. Alexis JB, Poppiti RJ, Turbat-Herrera E, Smith MD (1991) Congenital self-healing reticulohistiocytosis. Report of a case with 7-year follow-up and a review of the literature. Am J Dermatopathol 13:189–194
2. Aoki M, Aoki R, Akimoto M, Hara K (1998) Primary cutaneous Langerhans cell histiocytosis in an adult. Am J Dermatopathol 20:281–284

3. Geissmann F, Lepelletier Y, Fraitag S, Valladeau J, Bodemer C, Debré M, Leborgne M, Saeland S, Brousse N (2001) Differentiation of Langerhans cells in Langerhans cell histiocytosis. Blood 97:1241–1248
4. Gianotti R, Alessi E, Caputo R (1993) Benign cephalic histiocytosis. A distinct entity or a part of a wide spectrum of histiocytic proliferative disorders of children? A histopathological study. Am J Dermatopathol 15:315–319
5. Hashimoto K, Pritzker MS (1973) Electron microscopic study of reticulohistiocytoma. An unusual case of congenital, self-healing reticulohistiocytosis. Arch Dermatol 107:263–270
6. Hashimoto K, Bale GF, Hawkins HK, Langston C, Pritzker MS (1986) Congenital self-healing reticulohistiocytosis (Hashimoto-Pritzker type). Int J Dermatol 25:516–523
7. Itoh H, Miyaguni H, Kataoka H, Akiyama Y, Tateyama S, Marutsuka K, Asada Y, Ogata K, Koono M (2001) Primary cutaneous Langerhans cell histiocytosis showing malignant phenotype in an elderly woman: report of a fatal case. J Cutan Pathol 28:371–378
8. Jih DM, Salcedo SL, Jaworsky C (2002) Benign cephalic histiocytosis. A case report and review. J Am Acad Dermatol 47:908–913
9. Larralde M, Rositto A, Giardelli M, Gatti CF, Santos Munoz A (1999) Congenital self-healing histiocytosis (Hashimoto-Pritzker). Int J Dermatol 38:693–696
10. Leahy MA, Krejci SM, Friednash M, Stockert SS, Wilson H, Huff JC, Weston WL, Brice SL (1993) Human herpesvirus 6 is present in lesions of Langerhans cell histiocytosis. J Invest Dermatol 101:642–645
11. Lever WF, Schaumburg-Lever G (1990) Histopathology of the skin. J.B. Lippincott, Philadelphia
12. Lichtenstein L (1953) Histiocytosis X. Integration of eosinophilic granuloma of bone, "Letterer-Siwe disease", and "Schüller-Christian disease" as related manifestations of a single nosologic entity. Arch Pathol 56:84–102
13. Lieberman PH, Jones CR, Steinman RM, Erlandson RA, Smith J, Gee T, Huvos A, Garin-Chesa P, Filippa DA, Urmacher C, Gangi MD, Sperber M (1996) Langerhans cell (eosinophilic) granulomatosis. A clinicopathologic study encompassing 50 years. Am J Surg Pathol 20:519–552
14. Longaker MA, Frieden IJ, LeBoit PE (1994) Congenital "self-healing" Langerhans cell histiocytosis. The need for long-term follow up. J Am Acad Dermatol 31:910–916
15. McKee PH (1989) Pathology of the skin with clinical correlations. J.B. Lippincott, Philadelphia
16. Nezelof C, Basset F, Rousseau MF (1973) Histiocytosis X. Histogenetic arguments for a Langerhans cell origin. Biomedicine 18:365–371
17. Schaumburg-Lever G, Rechowicz E, Fehrenbacher B, Möller H, Nau P (1994) Congenital self-healing reticulohistiocytosis. A benign Langerhans cell disease. J Cutan Pathol 21:59–66
18. Stefanato CM, Andersen WK, Calonje E, Swain FA, Borghi S, Massone L, Kowalski JV, Bhawan J (1998) Langerhans cell histiocytosis in the elderly: a report of three cases. J Am Acad Dermatol 39:375–378
19. Stein SL, Paller AS, Haut PR, Mancini AJ (2001) Langerhans cell histiocytosis presenting in the neonatal period. A retrospective case series. Arch Pediatr Adolesc Med 155:778–783
20. Titgemeyer C, Grois N, Minkov M, Flucher-Wolfram B, Gatterer-Menz I, Gadner H (2001) Pattern and course of single-system disease in Langerhans cell histiocytosis data from the DAL-HX 83- and 90-study. Med Pediatr Oncol 37:108–114

Chapter 22

Dermatitis (Eczema) 22

Ackerman and Ragaz (1982) started a major debate about the term "eczema". Because of the difficulty in shortly and exactly defining what eczema really is they wanted the term to be expunged from the vocabulary of dermatology and dermatopathology and replaced by "dermatitis". Eczema, a word with tradition, is to the author a clinical concept that encompasses a group of different skin conditions which, for the experienced eye, have a common characteristic trait making it possible to discriminate them from other dermatoses. Hebra (Austrian dermatologist, 1816–1880) ingeniously expressed it: "eczema is which looks like eczema" (Ackerman and Ragaz 1982). In modern literature the terms eczema and dermatitis are used as synonyms. However, histopathologically, all kinds of eczema principally show the pattern of what pathologists call dermatitis. Thus it is not possible to distinguish different kinds of eczema by means of the histopathologic pattern, nor does the histopathologic pattern of dermatitis always represent a kind of eczema.

22.1 Clinical Appearance

As already mentioned there are clinically different types of dermatitis (eczema): *allergic contact dermatitis, irritant contact dermatitis, atopic dermatitis, nummular dermatitis, seborrheic dermatitis* and *stasis dermatitis*. Even mucous membranes may be affected.

22.1.1 Allergic Contact Dermatitis

Allergic contact dermatitis may be caused by a large number of allergens dealt with in the occupational sphere or in private life. It is a type IV delayed hypersensitivity reaction, the mechanism of which has been described in more detail (Sect. 4.5). Often allergens are haptens such as nickel, components of a locally applied remedy or cosmetics, or some kind of chemical added to clothing and shoes. The eruption may be acute to chronic. Acute lesions consist of local or widespread erythematous and edematous areas, on which papules, vesicles and, occasionally, bullae appear. Vesicles and bullae burst and give rise to an oozing surface; later on, when the inflammation subsides, crusts cover the lesions. Chronic lesions are scaling and may also be fissured or thickened (lichenified) due to repeated rubbing or scratching. Eruptions sometimes show a mixed acute and chronic pattern. Often lesions are severely itching.

22.1.2 Irritant Contact Dermatitis

This kind of dermatitis is due to repeated contact with non-immunologic irritants and is a common cause of eczema on the hands of those involved in wet work. Rather often the patient suffers from both contact dermatitis and irritant dermatitis.

22.1.3 Atopic Dermatitis

Atopic dermatitis occurs in genetically disposed individuals when they are subjected to one or several environmental factors, of which climate is the most important. Also food allergens or aeroallergens may be of significance. Many of these patients also suffer from allergic rhinitis, and/or asthma. The eruptions vary in intensity and change with the age of the patient. The disease is most common during early infancy and childhood. In small children the lesions are located on the face, scalp and extensor aspects of the extremities and have the character of subacute to acute dermatitis with erythema, papules, vesicles and oozing. Severe itch is notorious and scratch marks are common. In older children the flexural folds of the extremities are affected and the pattern is that of a chronic lichenified dermatitis. When the patient grows up the eruptions in most cases disappear; however, patients with an atopic disposition are more sensitive than non-atopic individuals to exogenous irritants. They are inclined to get irritant contact dermatitis and *lichen simplex chronicus*. The latter is a plaque of severely itching dermatitis that most often occurs in adults

22.1.4
Nummular Dermatitis

By nummular dermatitis is meant spells of discrete, coin-shaped, erythematous plaques on the trunk and extremities, which remain for weeks to years. The pattern may be acute, subacute or chronic. The cause of nummular dermatitis is unknown.

22.1.5
Seborrheic Dermatitis

Seborrheic dermatitis appears in seborrheic areas and affects both infants and adults. The lesions are characterized by erythema covered with oily-looking scales. The cause of seborrheic dermatitis is unknown. It is the most common skin lesion in HIV-infected individuals and eruptions are often conspicuous.

22.1.6
Stasis Dermatitis

Stasis dermatitis appears on the lower legs in patients with insufficient return of the venous flow and is usually located above the medial malleolus. Pigmentation due to deposition of iron pigment may be conspicuous.

22.1.7
Allergic Contact Stomatitis

Allergic contact stomatitis is rare, but may be caused for example by flavorings added to toothpastes, mouth washes, candy, chewing gum and food (Rietschel 2001). Stomatitis caused by chemical irritants is discussed in Sect. 29.7).

22.2
Histopathologic Appearance

Histopathologically dermatitis may be described as *acute*, *subacute* or *chronic*; however, often one form merges into another.

22.2.1
Acute Dermatitis

In lesions of acute dermatitis fluid accumulates in the epidermis and gives rise to both *intercellular* and *intracellular* edema. Augmentation of the intercellular fluid increases the distance between the keratinocytes and stretches the desmosomes (i.e., the filaments that serve as links between the keratinocytes). This makes the desmosomes visible in routinely stained sections; the phenomenon is called *spongiosis* (Fig. 22.1a). Intracellular edema is expressed as different-sized, clear spaces (vacuoles) in the cytoplasm. Large vacuoles compress the nucleus and displace it close to the cell membrane; the cell acquires the shape of a signet ring (Fig. 22.1a). The edema is patchy and, if not advanced, is reversible.

Progression results in disintegration of the keratinocytes. Intercellular edema causes rupture of the desmosomes, and intracellular edema impairs vital intracellular cell structures, or disrupts the cell. In turn this leads to development of small cavities (vesicles), which may coalesce and form larger cavities (bullae). In the fully developed acute dermatitis there are tightly set vesicles and/or bullae (Fig. 22.1b). The vesicles/bullae contain clear fluid and lymphocytes. There are more or less dense infiltrates of lymphocytes in the dermal papillae and in the subpapillary area and also a conspicuous papillary edema. Sometimes there are, in addition to lymphocytes, a variable number of eosinophils both in the dermis and epidermis. Now and then, so-called reticular degeneration appears, as also seen in herpes virus vesicles (Fig. 20.2a).

If the trigger of the dermatitis is eliminated, the inflammation subsides and the lesions heal without residue. However, an acute stage may pass over into a subacute stage.

Fig. 22.1 Dermatitis. **a** Inter- and intracellular edema and the beginning of vesiculation. The *arrow* indicates a keratinocyte with marked intracellular edema and the nucleus pressed to the cell membrane. To the right of this cell there are stretched desmosomes due to intercellular edema. **b** Acute dermatitis. There are densely set vesicles and papillary edema. **c** Subacute dermatitis. The rete ridges are thickened and irregularly elongated. There is a fresh vesicle to the right and some older, filled with protein-rich exudate to the left (*arrows*). The crust is composed of parakeratotic keratin including exudate and inflammatory cells. **d** Healing lesion. The detached material (*arrows*) indicates earlier vesiculation. **e** Chronic dermatitis. The epidermis shows acanthosis together with hyper- and parakeratosis. **f** Psoriasiform dermatitis. A papilla (*arrowheads*), walled off by slender rete ridges, contains thin-walled dilated vessels and is covered by a thin epidermis and a parakeratotic crust. In the papillary and upper dermis of all variants there are infiltrates of lymphocytes, some of which are migrating into the epidermis. H&E

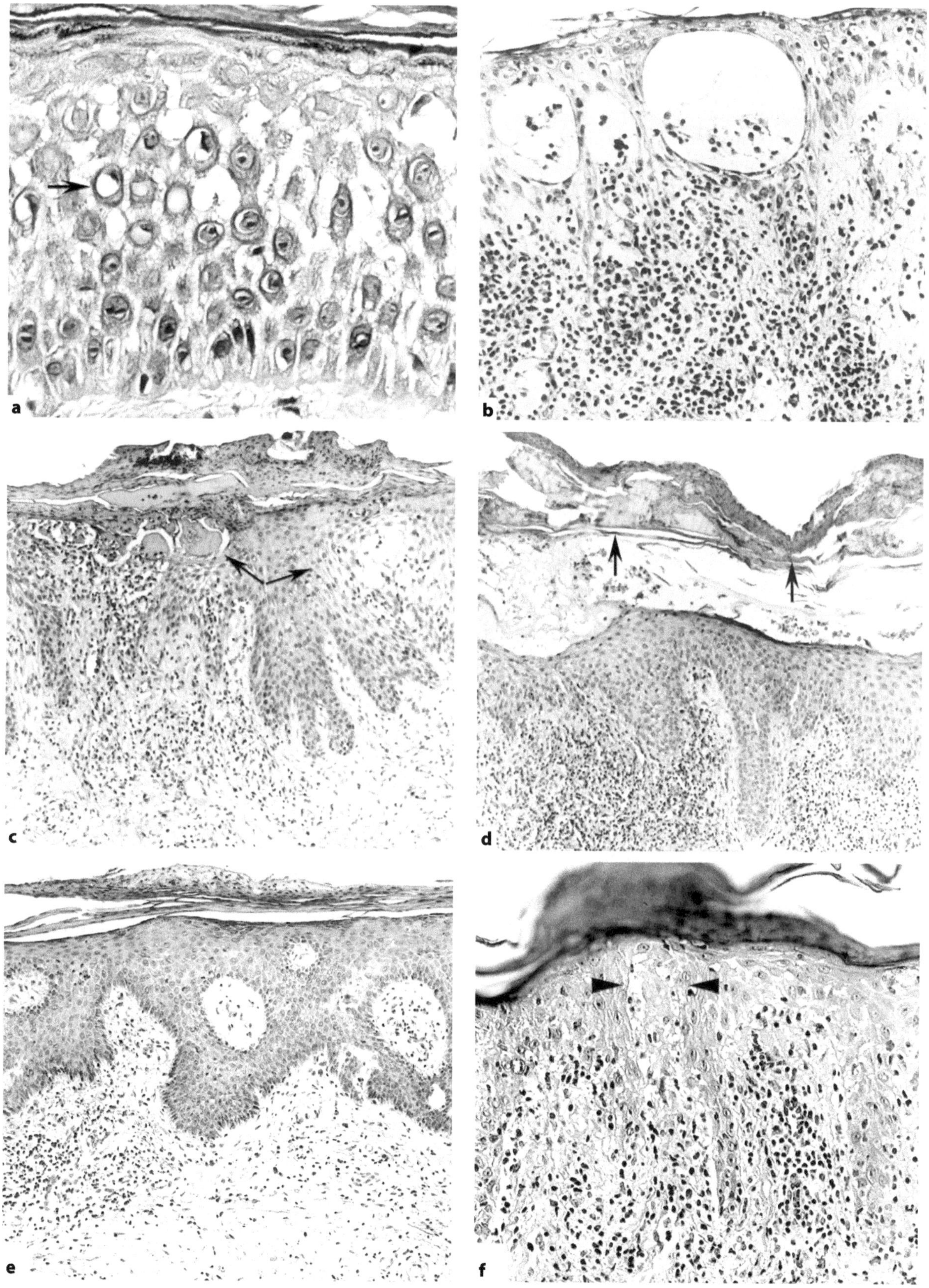
a
b
c
d
e
f

22.2.2. Subacute Dermatitis

Subacute dermatitis may start as such or, as mentioned above, may follow a spell of acute dermatitis. The epidermis is irregularly thickened and has unevenly lengthened and thickened rete ridges. This is called *acanthosis*. There are patches of spongiosis and intracellular edema and scattered vesicles, some of which may contain eosinophilic, protein-rich exudate (Fig. 22.1c). As in acute dermatitis, lymphocytes migrate through the epidermis, a phenomenon called *exocytosis*. The surface is covered with a crust consisting of eosinophilic exudate and *parakeratotic keratin* (i.e., keratin containing nuclear remains). In the papillae and upper dermis there is edema, dilated venules, and sometimes proliferation of new vessels. The inflammatory cell infiltrates mainly consist of lymphocytes, but there may be a fair admixture of eosinophils in both the dermis and epidermis.

Subacute dermatitis may contain vesicles with histiocyte-like cells in addition to small lymphocytes (Fig. 22.2). This phenomenon has been mistaken for Pautrier abscesses (see Glossary), appearing in mycosis fungoides (LeBoit and Epstein 1990). Investigations have shown that these cells are dendritic cells with a histochemical phenotype that is somewhat different from that of Langerhans cells normally present in the epidermis and dermis. They are thought to be precursors of Langerhans cells, immigrated from the circulation and recruited to the site of inflammation by cytokines released by epidermal cells or associated T cells (Candiago et al. 2000).

Healing of vesicular dermatitis starts from the preserved basic part of the epidermis. A more or less normal-looking epidermis sheds a thick horny layer containing remnants of vesicles. Sometimes the presence of these residues is helpful in discriminating dermatitis and psoriasis (Fig. 22.1d).

22.2.3 Chronic Dermatitis

The process starts as a chronic dermatitis or follows an acute or subacute phase of the disease. The course is protracted. The epidermis shows moderate to marked acanthosis and hyper- and parakeratosis (Fig. 22.1e). There may be areas of inter- and intracellular edema, and rarely scattered small vesicles. The inflammatory cell infiltrates mainly consist of lymphocytes. Edema in the dermis is not prominent, but proliferation of new vessels may be seen. Sometimes the pattern is psoriasis-like and shows long, slender rete ridges and papillae, which are covered by a thin epidermis and contain thin-walled dilated venules filled with erythrocytes (Fig. 22.1f; compare Fig. 23.1a).

In stasis dermatitis, there are in addition to a thickened and acanthotic epidermis numerous newly formed vessels, most marked at the level of the sweat glands, where also deposition of iron pigment is a characteristic phenomenon. Abnormal veins, demonstrated below in Case 3 (Fig. 22.3), are rarely observed. Scratching and secondary infections may modify all histopathologic patterns described above (Figs. 29.1 and 29.2). Herpes simplex virus infection may be a serious complication in atopic dermatitis and is called *eczema herpeticum*.

22.3 Examples

Case 1. Subacute Dermatitis

A 38-year-old man presented with two nummular lesions on the back.

Histologic investigation showed the pattern of subacute dermatitis with several small vesicles, which contained lymphocytes as well as a fair number of histiocyte-like cells with pale cytoplasm and one elongated and often indented nucleus. The dermal papillae were edematous and contained scattered histiocytes. In the subpapillary area there were perivascular infiltrates composed mainly of lymphocytes. Immunohistochemical investigations revealed that the histiocyte-like cells in the epidermis were positive for S-100 protein and CD1a and thus were Langerhans cells. Also in the upper dermis many cells were positive for these markers; a few cells were positive for CD68, a marker of monocytes and macrophages (Fig. 22.2).

Case 2. Stasis Dermatitis

This patient presented with a 4×10 cm, well circumscribed, and bluish-red eczematous patch on the medial aspect of the right lower leg. The lesion had slowly increased over 3 years and was resistant to treatment with corticosteroids. There were neither visible varicose veins nor edema, and stasis dermatitis was not suspected. Following surgery for varicose veins the skin lesion healed and did not return.

A biopsy specimen was taken and investigated at three levels with many sections. In two sections at one of the levels a large, tortuous, thick-walled, and dilated venule was observed. Otherwise the pattern was that of chronic stasis dermatitis (Fig. 22.3).

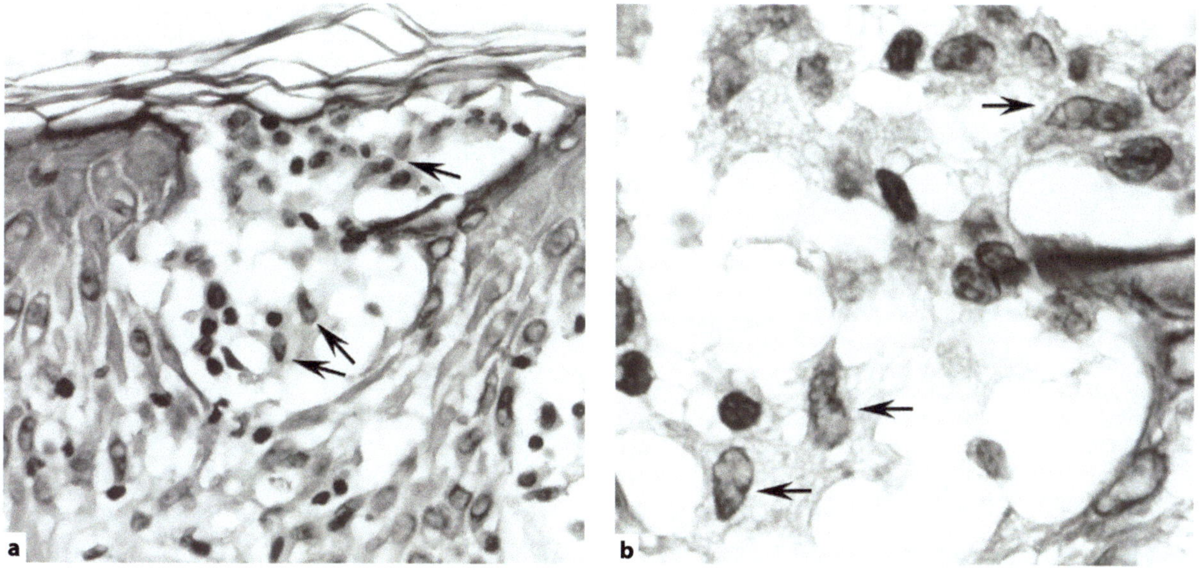

Fig. 22.2 Vesicular dermatitis with Langerhans cells. **a** A small vesicle contains lymphocytes and several histiocyte-like cells (*arrows*); ×400. **b** Close-up of the cells indicated in **a** (*arrows*); ×1000. H&E

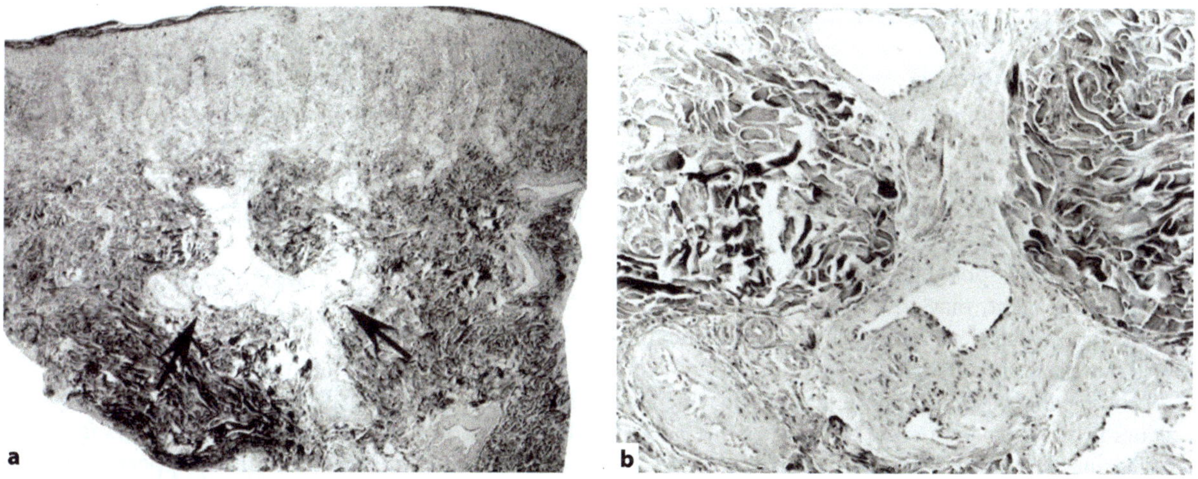

Fig. 22.3 Stasis dermatitis. **a** The overview shows a conspicuously thickened, tortuous and branching vein located in the upper and middle part of the dermis. The epidermis is thickened and acanthotic. **b** Close-up of the part of the vessel located above the *arrows* in **a**. vG

Case 3. Subacute Stomatitis

The patient was 9 years old when a biopsy was taken from the buccal mucosa. From the age of 5 years he had had white lesions on the buccal mucosa and the tongue with no other symptoms. He was allergic to milk and egg.

Histologic investigation disclosed a thickened, but not keratinized epithelium with inter- and intracellular edema and small vesicles. Both epithelium and submucosa were diffusely infiltrated by lymphocytes and eosinophils. PAS staining did not reveal fungal structures (Fig. 22.4).

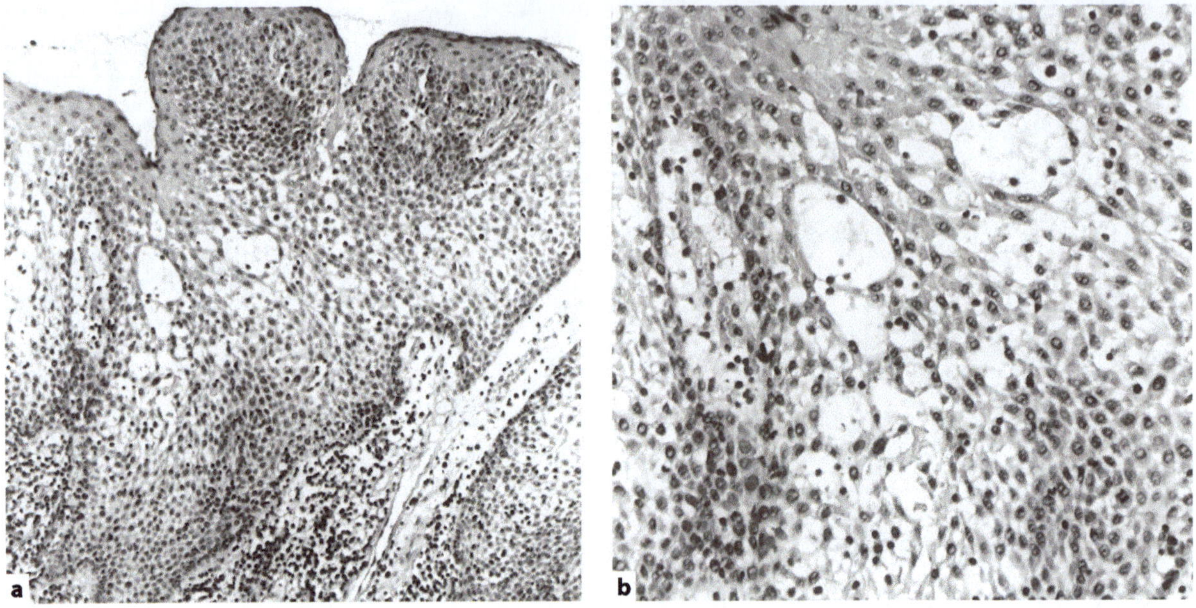

Fig. 22.4 Subacute stomatitis. **a** The epithelium is thickened, but not keratinized. It shows pronounced inter- and intracellular edema and also small vesicles. **b** Close-up of the vesicular area. H&E

22.4 Differential Diagnosis

- *Fungal infections*. Fungal infections may clinically as well as histopathologically be mistaken for chronic, subacute or acute dermatitis (Fig. 13.1d). Stomatitis has to be differentiated from *Candida* infection (Fig. 13.7). PAS staining is mandatory.
- *Pityriasis rosea*, possibly caused by some unknown infectious agent, may show the pattern of spongiotic or vesicular dermatitis, but has a different clinical pattern and course than dermatitis.
- *Incontinentia pigmenti*, the first stage of which occurs in the neonatal period and shows the pattern of acute dermatitis with eosinophilia, is a hereditary disease.
- *Langerhans cell histiocytosis* (Sect. 21.2).

22.5 Erythroderma (Exfoliative Dermatitis)

Erythroderma or exfoliative dermatitis implies a generalized or nearly generalized dermatitis and is a complication that is common for several completely different dermatoses and skin conditions. It may thus develop from various kinds of eczema, other preexisting dermatoses such as psoriasis, lichen planus, pityriasis rubra pilaris, and pemphigus foliaceus. It may also be provoked by drugs and, notably, may represent the early stage of cutaneous T cell lymphoma. If no underlying cause is detected, the condition is called *idiopathic erythroderma* or the *red man syndrome*, a chronic disease, which may extend over years. The disease affects all ages and is most common in men. The pathogenesis is unknown.

22.5.1 Clinical Appearance

From 80% to 90% of the body surface is involved. In the beginning of the disease the skin is highly erythematous and shiny, and sometimes oozing. Later powdery or flaky exfoliation usually appears. The condition is associated with a burning sensation and itching (often severe). Dermatopathic lymphadenopathy may be present as well as systemic symptoms such as fever, elevated ESR, blood eosinophilia and increased levels of IgE antibodies (Sehgal and Srivastava 1986; Thestrup-Pedersen et al. 1988).

22.5.2 Histopathologic Appearance

According to textbooks on dermatopathology and dermatology, the histopathologic pattern of erythroderma is, depending on the phase of the disease, that of an acute, subacute, or chronic dermatitis (Lever

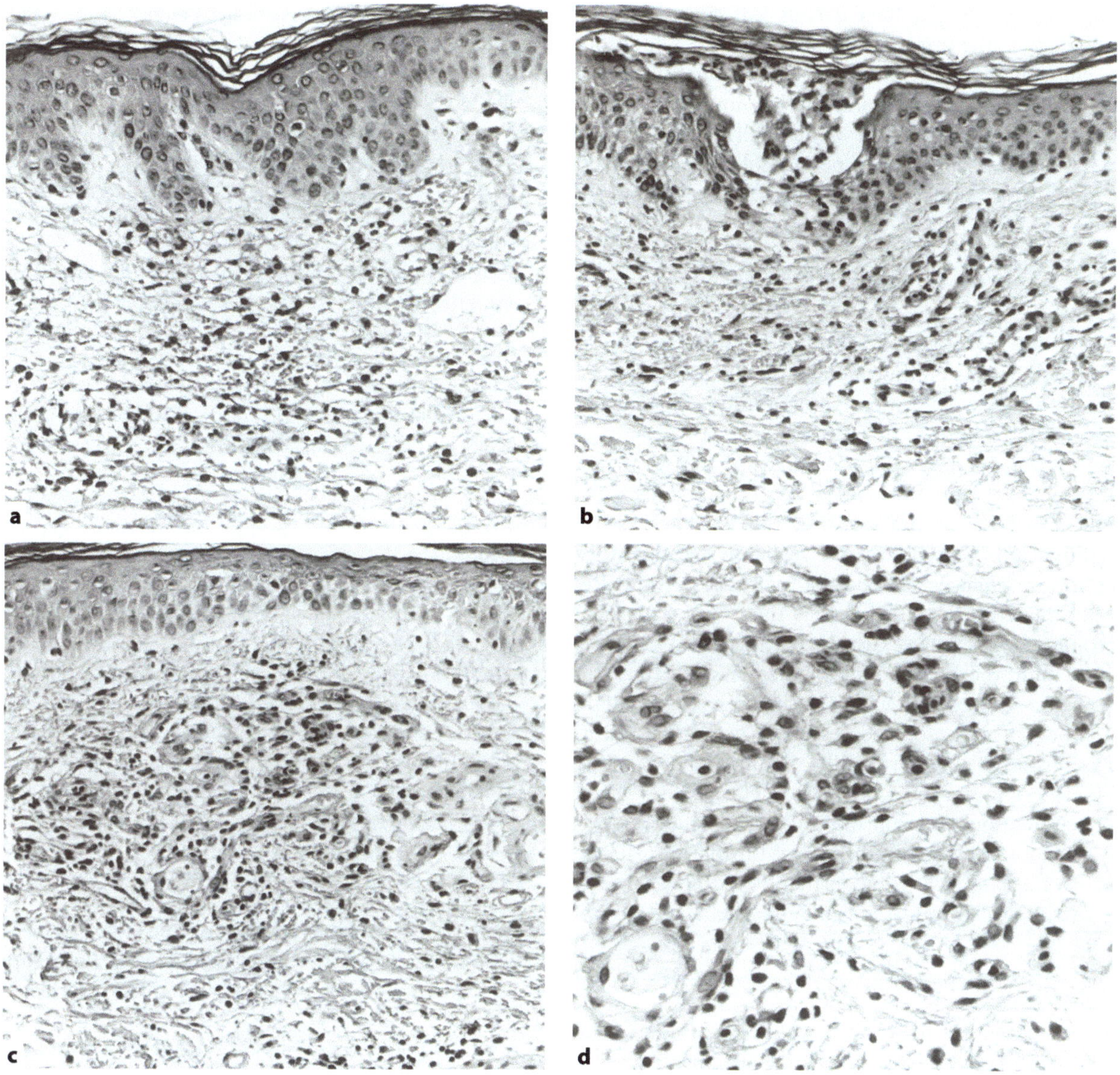

Fig. 22.5 Erythroderma. **a** The epidermis is slightly irregular. In the upper dermis there are dilated lymphatics, many extravasated red blood cells and a moderate number of lymphocytes. **b** The epidermis contains a single small vesicle. In the upper dermis there are red blood cells and newly formed vessels. **c** An area in the upper dermis, which contains a conglomeration of proliferating vessels. **d** Close-up shows both venules and capillaries. H&E

and Schaumburg-Lever 1990; Burton 1992; Freedberg 1999). In investigations of larger series of unknown erythroderma, the discussion on histopathology has mainly dealt with the possibility of tracking the underlying disease (Thestrup-Pedersen et al. 1988; Zip et al. 1993; Walsh et al. 1994; Botella-Estrada et al. 1994). The most common pattern seems to be that of a mild to moderate chronic dermatitis. In cases representing early T cell lymphoma, atypical T cells may be observed in the dermal inflammatory cell infiltrate and/or in the epidermis.

22.5.3 Example

Case 4. Erythroderma

A 71-year-old woman presented with penicillin-induced erythroderma.

A punch biopsy included the dermal–subcutaneous interface. The epidermis was slightly irregular and spongiotic, and contained one single small vesicle. The latter contained a few lymphocytes and histiocyte-like cells (Langerhans cells?) The horny layer was normal. The papillary dermis was conspicuously edematous. The upper dermis contained, in addition to many dilated thin-walled vessels, prominent groups of newly formed vessels, and a rich amount of extravasated erythrocytes. In the upper half of the dermis there were small, mainly perivascular infiltrates of lymphocytes with a slight admixture of eosinophils (Fig. 22.5).

22.5.3.1 Comment

Erythroderma is on the whole a rare diagnosis and to obtain a biopsy specimen is uncommon. The experience of the author is limited; however, in every case the author has been confronted with, the great discrepancy between the clinical and the microscopic appearance has been a surprise. This was the first reaction also in this case, before realizing that the most important changes affected the microvasculature. Besides dilated thin-walled vessels there was a marked proliferation of new vessels. Newly formed vessels are leaky and probably account for the massive extravasation of erythrocytes in Case 4. If the presence of a high number of newly formed vessels in erythroderma is a criterion, it may explain the findings of Groves et al. (1995) indicating significantly elevated levels of the circulating adhesion molecules ICAM-1, VCAM-1 and ELAM-1 (E-selectin) in erythroderma caused by psoriasis as well as by dermatitis (eczema). These CAMs may all be released from endothelial cells.

References

1. Ackerman AB, Ragaz A (1982) A plea to expunge the word "eczema" from the lexicon of dermatology and dermatopathology. Am J Dermatopathol 4:315–326
2. Botella-Estrada R, Sanmartin O, Oliver V, Febrer I, Aliaga A (1994) Erythroderma. A clinicopathologic study of 56 cases. Arch Dermatol 130:1503–1507
3. Burton JL (1992) Eczema, lichenification, prurigo and erythroderma. In: Champion RH, Burton JL, Ebling FJG (eds) Rook/Wilkinson/Ebling textbook of dermatology. Blackwell Scientific, Oxford, pp 584–585
4. Candiago E, Marocolo D, Manganoni MA, Leali C, Facchetti F (2000) Nonlymphoid intraepidermal mononuclear cell collections (pseudo-Pautrier abscesses). A morphologic and immunophenotypical characterization. Am J Dermatopathol 22:1–6
5. Freedberg IM (1999) Exfoliative dermatitis. In: Freedberg IM, Eisen AZ, Wolff K, Austen KF, Goldsmith LA, Katz SI, Fitzpatrick TB (eds) Fitzpatrick's dermatology in general medicine. McGraw-Hill, New York, pp 534–540
6. Groves RW, Kapahi P, Barker JNWN, Haskard DO, MacDonald DM (1995) Detection of circulating adhesion molecules in erythrodermic skin disease. J Am Acad Dermatol 33:32–36
7. LeBoit PE, Epstein BA (1990) A vase-like shape characterizes the epidermal-mononuclear cell collections seen in spongiotic dermatitis. Am J Dermatopathol 12:612–616
8. Lever WF, Schaumburg-Lever G (1990) Histopathology of the skin. J.B. Lippincott, Philadelphia
9. Rietschel RL (2001) Contact stomatitis and cheilitis. In: Rietschel RL, Fowler JF Jr (eds) Fisher's contact dermatitis. Lippincott Williams & Wilkins, Philadelphia, pp 663–685
10. Sehgal VN, Srivastava G (1986) Exfoliative dermatitis. A prospective study of 80 patients. Dermatologica 173:278–284
11. Thestrup-Pedersen K, Halkier-Sørensen L, Søgaard H, Zachariae H (1988) The red man syndrome. Exfoliative dermatitis of unknown etiology: a description and follow-up of 38 patients. J Am Acad Dermatol 18:1307–1312
12. Walsh NMG, Prokopetz R, Tron VA, Sawyer DM, Watters AK, Murray S, Zip C (1994) Histopathology in erythroderma: review of a series of cases by multiple observers. J Cutan Pathol 21:419–423
13. Zip C, Murray S, Walsh NMG (1993) The specificity of histopathology in erythroderma. J Cutan Pathol 20:393–398

Chapter 23

Psoriasis

23

Psoriasis is a worldwide disease with dominance in areas with a cold climate and little sunshine. In Western countries the prevalence is approximately 2% and in Scandinavia slightly higher. The disease is more common among white than among black and Asiatic people. It may appear at any age including small children. Males and females are equally affected. The degree of severity and response to treatment vary considerably. Usually the disease becomes more serious if the onset is early in life. It may be associated with, sometimes disabling, arthritis.

23.1 Clinical Appearance

Psoriasis may appear as a lifelong chronic disease, *psoriasis vulgaris*, as one or several spontaneously resolving occurrences, or as more or less acute eruptions such as *psoriasis guttata*, *pustular psoriasis*, and *erythroderma*.

23.1.1 Psoriasis Vulgaris

The lesions are characteristic and consist of up to palm-sized and distinct demarcated plaques covered with thick silvery scales. When the scales are rubbed off a shiny red surface is displayed, on which in a short while pin-point-sized droplets of blood appear (the bloody dew or *Auspitz* sign). Sometimes the lesions are serpiginous or annular. Predilection sites are elbows, knees, scalp and lumbar region. Any area may be affected, but the face is often spared. Psoriasis located in intertriginous areas is called *inverse psoriasis*; because of the moistness of these regions the lesions are dazzlingly red and lack scales. Nails are often markedly deformed and can even come loose; however slight nail changes may be the only sign of the disease.

23.1.2 Psoriasis Guttata

By guttate psoriasis is meant outbreaks of small lesions, 0.5–1.5 cm in diameter, mostly located on the upper half of the trunk and the proximal part of the extremities. The eruption is in many cases preceded and triggered by a streptococcal throat infection and is often the first sign of the disease in young individuals.

23.1.3 Psoriasis Pustulosa

The occurrence of pustules in psoriatic lesions usually indicates exacerbation of the disease. The pustules are 1–3 mm in diameter and are sterile (i.e., they do not contain bacteria). Generalized pustular psoriasis (von Zumbusch type) is a serious condition associated with fever and general malaise. Also the oral mucosa may be involved. Localized pustular psoriasis exists in two variants: acrodermatitis continua suppurativa (Hallopeau) and pustulosis palmoplantaris (demonstrated in Case 5 and Case 6, respectively).

23.1.4 Psoriatic Erythroderma

Exacerbation of chronic non-pustular psoriasis as well as pustular psoriasis may lead to erythroderma (Sect. 22.5).

23.2 Histopathologic Appearance

In the typical and fully developed psoriatic lesion the epidermis is conspicuously thin over the papillae, and has elongated and slender rete ridges with club-shaped ends (Fig. 23.1a,b). In certain areas, the horny layer is markedly thickened and parakeratotic and the granular layer is lacking (Fig. 23.1c,d). There is conspicuous edema in the papillae and the capillary loop is dilated, elongated and coiled (Ryan 1980); therefore in a histologic section the capillary may be cut more than once in the same papilla (Fig. 23.1b,d). The thin epidermis overlaying the top of the papillae and the capillary changes together cause the Auspitz sign, described above. The inflammatory cells in the papillae and upper dermis consist mainly of lymphocytes, but there are also some neutrophils. Typically, here and there, some neutrophils are seen migrating through the epidermis (Fig. 23.1d). These finally end up in the horny layer as small aggregations of disintegrating neutrophils, called *Munro microabscesses* (Fig. 23.1c,d). Sometimes scattered minute spongiform pustules consisting of microcavities filled with neutrophils are seen in the superficial epidermis (Fig. 23.1e,f).

In macroscopic pustular psoriasis there are large spongiform pustules in the outermost part of the epidermis. Kogoj (1938) described this kind of pustule as characteristic of acrodermatitis continua suppurativa Hallopeau. The same kind of pustule is seen in balanitis circinata, but is mainly lacking in pustulosis palmoplantaris, where only minute areas of spongiosis are observed at the lateral margins of a large unilocular pustule (Fig. 23.5a). The fully developed spongiform pustule is stuffed with neutrophils and has a central large cavity, which is surrounded by a brim of cavities, which towards the periphery become smaller and smaller. The smallest cavity seems to be composed of a single epithelial cell occupied by a single neutrophil (Figs. 23.2 and 23.3).

23.3 Pathogenesis

The pathogenesis is complex and not fully understood. It is clear that a hereditary disposition is basic and involves several genes, the most important of which are located on, or linked to, HLA-Cw6, a part of the major histocompatibility complex (MHC). Which genes and the number and combination of them are of importance for the expression of the disease (Bowcock and Barker 2003). However, several nongenetic factors, such as infections, trauma, "stress", drugs and climate are of importance for the outbreak and manifestation of the disease.

There is increasing evidence that psoriasis is a type IV immunologic disorder. The responsible antigen or antigens are not yet identified. However, TCR rearrangement analysis (see Glossary) has shown that in an individual patient, the same antigen-specific pathogenic T cells are present in lesions appearing several years apart (Vollmer et al. 2001). The activated T cells secrete different kinds of cytokines/chemokines which give rise to further migration of T cells from the blood into the skin and also activate keratinocytes and other local cells such as macrophages and dendritic cells. These secondarily activated cells secrete their own cytokines and thereby maintain the process (Mehlis and Gordon 2003).

In a typical lesion of psoriasis vulgaris the inflammatory cell infiltrate consists mainly of lymphocytes. However, as described above, in contrast to other cell-mediated immunologic reactions, there are also a substantial number of neutrophils in the epidermis, which suddenly may increase in number and give rise to pustular ps=oriasis. Drawing a parallel between pustular psoriasis and drug-induced acute generalized exanthematous pustulosis, Britschgi and Pichler (2002) have suggested that in psoriasis the formation of pustules can also be caused by antigen-specific T cells, which by giving rise to high levels of secretion of IL-8, attract neutrophils (Sect. 28.5).

23.4 Examples

Case 1. Psoriasis Guttata

A 3½-year-old boy presented with closely set psoriasis-like, pea-sized, scaling papules on the trunk, extremities, and face. The eruption had started 4 weeks previously. Culture from the throat grew β-streptococci. The paternal grandmother suffered from psoriasis.

Fig. 23.1 Psoriasis. **a** Lesion on the glans penis. The generally thin epidermis has elongated and slender rete ridges, the ends of which are slightly club-shaped. Note how thin the epidermis is over the dermal papillae (*arrow*). In the papillae and upper dermis there is a dense cell infiltrate consisting mainly of lymphocytes. **b** Chronic psoriasis; lesion on the thigh. There are conspicuous edema and dilated capillaries in the papillae (*arrowheads*). **c** The same specimen as shown in **b**. In this area the horny layer is markedly thickened and parakeratotic and contains a Munro microabscess (*arrow*). There is no granular layer. **d** Guttate psoriasis; lesion on the thigh. The rete ridges are elongated and the papillae markedly edematous with dilated capillaries. The horny layer is thick and includes a Munro abscess (*small arrow*). Below the abscess a sparse number of neutrophils are trickling through the upper epidermis (*large arrow*). **e** The same specimen as shown in **a**. In this area there is a small spongiotic pustule infiltrated by neutrophils (*arrow*). **f** Close-up of the pustule in **e**. H&E

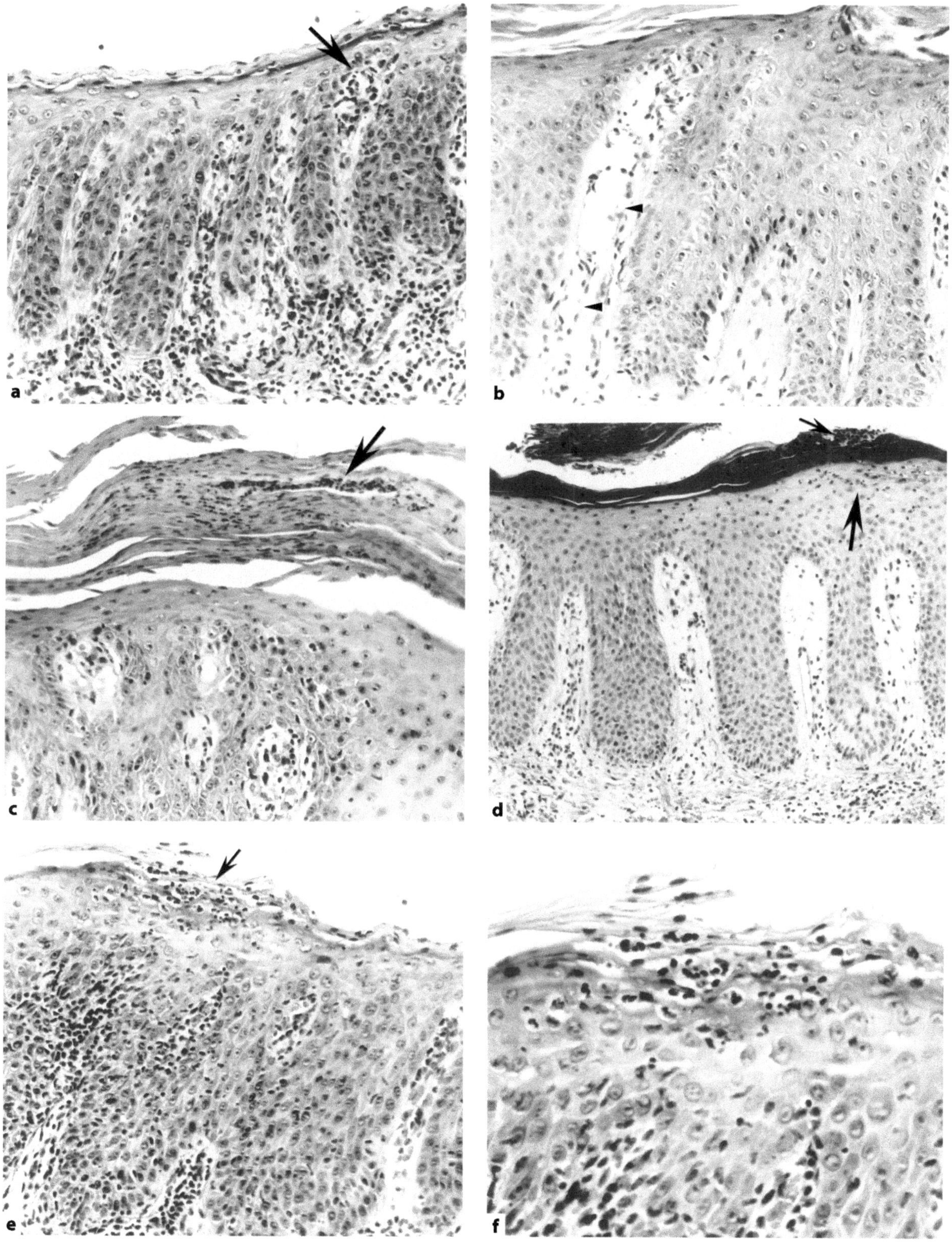

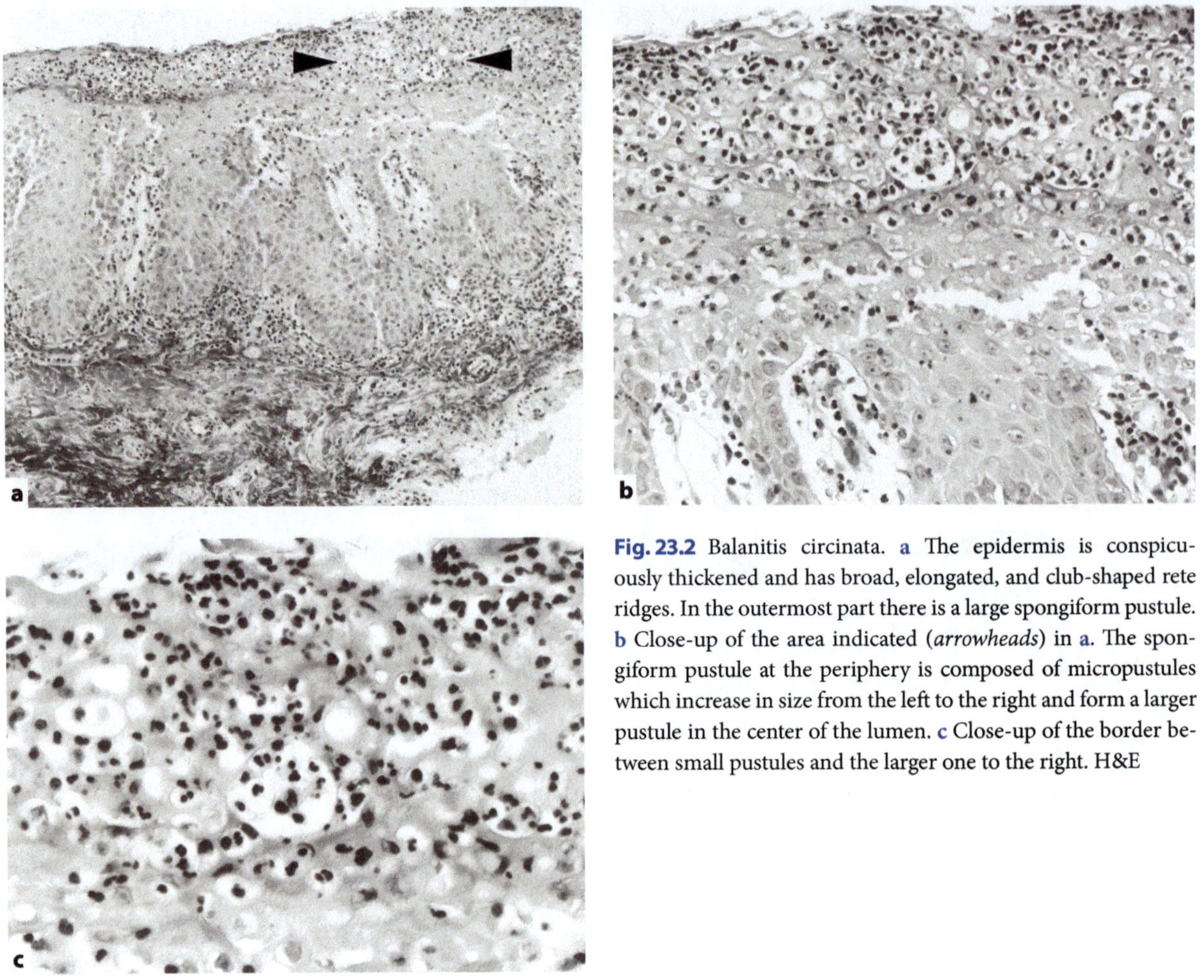

Fig. 23.2 Balanitis circinata. **a** The epidermis is conspicuously thickened and has broad, elongated, and club-shaped rete ridges. In the outermost part there is a large spongiform pustule. **b** Close-up of the area indicated (*arrowheads*) in **a**. The spongiform pustule at the periphery is composed of micropustules which increase in size from the left to the right and form a larger pustule in the center of the lumen. **c** Close-up of the border between small pustules and the larger one to the right. H&E

Histologic investigation revealed changes typical of psoriasis including hyper- and parakeratosis with Munro microabscesses (Fig. 23.1d).

Case 2. Psoriasis on the Glans Penis

The patient suffered from small erythematous papules on the glans, which came and vanished. He was otherwise healthy. Proposed diagnoses were psoriasis and plasma cell balanitis.

Histologic investigation showed epidermal and papillary changes typical of psoriasis and scattered minute spongiform pustules. Plasma cells were sparse. Fungal structures were not observed (Fig. 23.1a,e,f).

Case 3. Balanitis Circinata

A 31-year-old man presented with a raised erythematous plaque on the glans penis and a circinate erythematous lesion in the sulcus coronarius. The clinical consideration was balanitis circinata or psoriasis. Biopsy specimens were taken from the glans penis and the sulcus coronarius.

The specimen from the glans penis showed a conspicuously thickened epidermis with elongated and club-shaped rete ridges and a large superficial spongiotic pustule massively infiltrated by neutrophils. The dermal papillae were edematous and contained dilated venules, but only a few lymphocytes and neutrophils. In the upper dermis there were only sparse infiltrates composed of lymphocytes. Fungal structures were not found. The specimen from the sulcus coronarius showed principally the same picture (Fig. 23.2). For the differentiation between balanitis circinata and pustular psoriasis on the glans penis, see Sect. 23.5.

Case 4. Generalized Pustular Psoriasis (Zumbusch)

A 68-year old man was as an emergency case referred to the hospital because of general debility, fever, and skin eruption that had started 2 weeks previously.

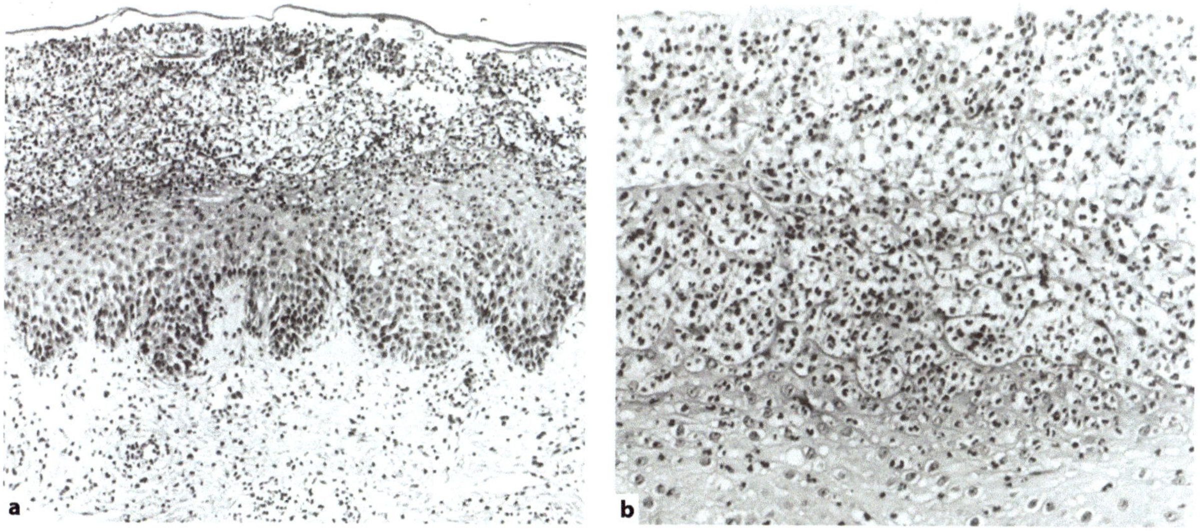

Fig. 23.3 Psoriasis pustulosa Zumbusch. a There is a large spongiform pustule in the upper half of the epidermis which shows a moderate acanthosis. The upper half of the dermis is conspicuously edematous and diffusely infiltrated by inflammatory cells. b Close-up shows that the large central pustule at the base is walled off by a series of different-sized smaller pustules. H&E

Over the whole body erythematous, rather thin and slightly scaling plaques studded with pustules were observed. The lesions in the armpits and groins were oozing. There was conspicuous hyperkeratosis in the palms and soles, and general onycholysis.

Histologic investigation showed a moderately thickened epidermis with a huge spongiotic pustule filled with neutrophils. The pustule comprised the outer half of the epidermis. In the subepidermal area there were edema and a diffuse infiltrate of neutrophils and around vessels a sparse infiltrate of lymphocytes (Fig. 23.3).

Case 5. Acrodermatitis Continua Suppurativa (Hallopeau)

A 48-year-old woman had had lesions extending on the toes of the left foot for about 4 months. The process had started with a pustule at the base of the left big toe. At the first visit a swollen edematous big toe with an oozing well-circumscribed area around the nail and a pustule over the distal joint of the toe were observed. Culture grew β-streptococci, but antibiotics were given without effect. During follow-up the condition became worse and the patient also showed small psoriasis-like lesions on the elbows and thighs. Biopsy specimens were taken from the big toe and from a lesion on the thigh.

Investigation showed the pattern of psoriasis pustulosa in both specimens and the diagnosis acrodermatitis continua suppurativa was considered. (Fig. 23.4) The patient was given etretinate with good effect. At follow-up about 2 years after the first visit the nails were dystrophic, but there were no signs of activity.

Case 6. Pustulosis Palmoplantaris

A 32-year-old man had had vesicles and pustules on the palms and soles for 4 months. A biopsy specimen was taken from the edge of the foot.

Histologic investigation showed a large intraepidermal pustule filled with neutrophils. The roof consisted of the horny layer and the floor of the basic part of epidermis and rete ridges. At the lateral margins there were small spongiotic areas. Other parts of the epidermis showed a psoriasis-like pattern with elongated, club-shaped rete ridges, papillae with dilated capillaries, and a thickened and parakeratotic horny layer (Fig. 23.5).

23.4.1 Comment

In the experience of the author, Case 6 with a mainly unilocular pustule is typical of pustulosis palmoplantaris. Thus, with the exception of small areas at the margins, the pustule is not spongiform.

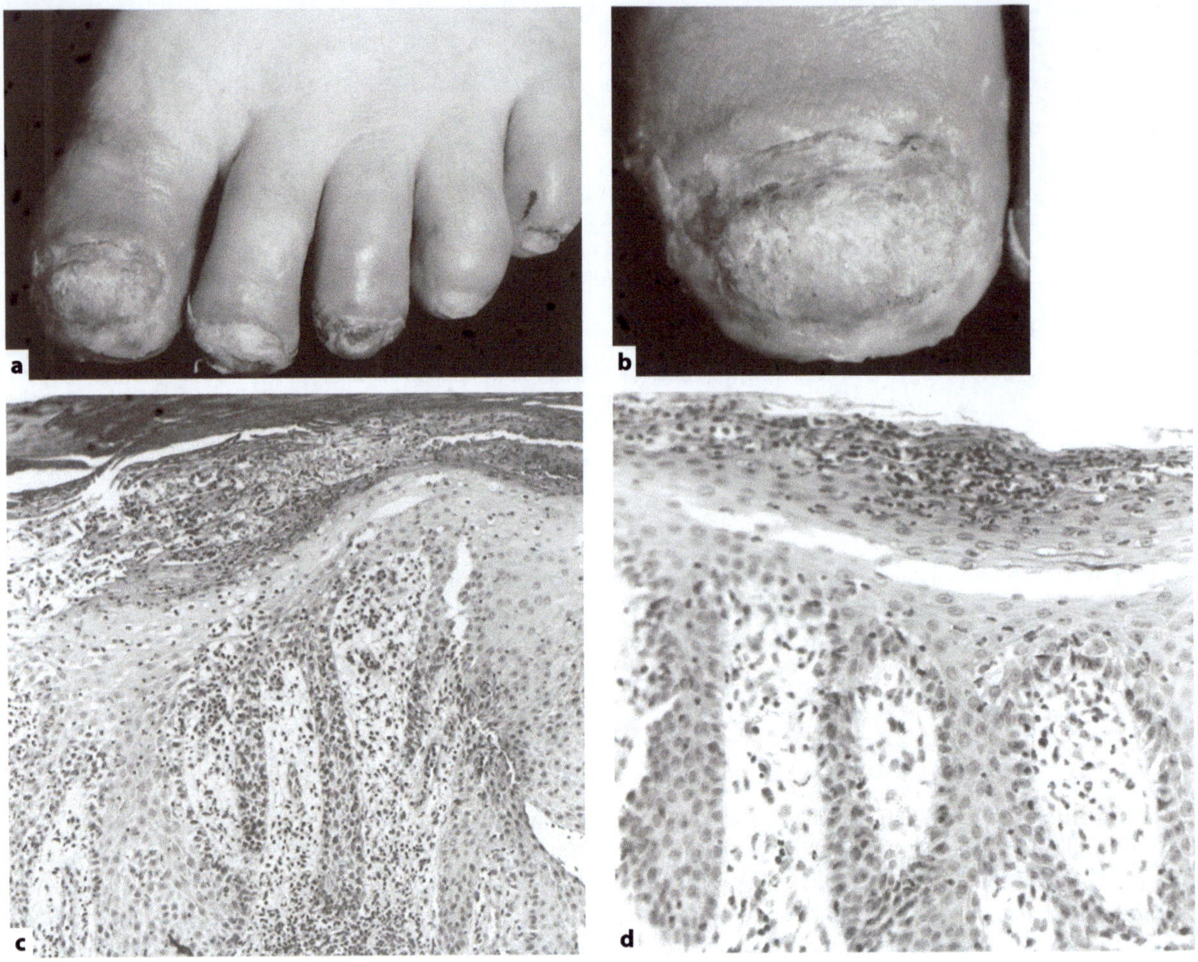

Fig. 23.4 Acrodermatitis continua suppurativa. a, b Active crusted lesion on the toes. c Specimen from the big toe. The epidermis contains a large superficial pustule. The rete ridges are elongated and have club-shaped ends and the dermal papillae are obscured by a dense inflammatory cell infiltrate. d Specimen from a scaling lesion on the thigh displays a similar histopathologic pattern. H&E

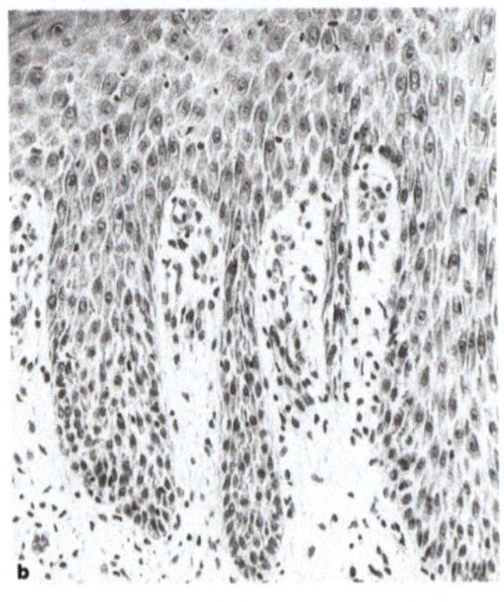

Fig. 23.5 Pustulosis palmoplantaris. a There is a large intraepidermal pustule. The roof consists of the horny layer and the floor of the basal part of the epidermis and rete ridges. The pustule is mainly unilocular and filled with inflammatory cells. However, in the right upper corner there is an area with small cavities (*arrow*). b The area close to the left side of the pustule. The epidermis shows intercellular edema and has elongated and club-shaped rete ridges. The dermal papillae are markedly edematous and contain dilated capillaries. H&E

23.5 Differential Diagnosis

- *Psoriasiform dermatitis* may be very difficult and sometimes impossible to differentiate from lesions of psoriasis vulgaris (Fig. 22.1e).
- *Fungal and bacterial infections* must be considered in vesicular and pustular lesions. PAS staining and culture are mandatory, especially if the lesions are confined to glans penis or palms and soles (Fig. 13.2).
- *Balanitis circinata* may appear as an isolated lesion or as a manifestation of *Reiter disease.* In a typical case of Reiter disease the patient suffers from a combination of urethritis, arthritis and conjunctivitis. Some patients also have balanitis circinata and/or pustular skin lesions in other areas. Considering the histopathologic pattern only, it is not possible to differentiate balanitis circinata from pustular psoriasis on the glans penis.
- *Acute generalized exanthematous pustulosis* (Sect. 28.5).

References

1. Bowcock AM, Barker JN (2003) Genetics of psoriasis: the potential impact on new therapies. J Am Acad Dermatol 49:51–56
2. Britschgi M, Pichler WJ (2002) Acute generalized exanthematous pustulosis, a clue to neutrophil-mediated inflammatory processes orchestrated by T cells. Curr Opin Allergy Clin Immunol 2:325–331
3. Kogoj F (1938) Die spungiforme (schwammartige) Pustel. Dermatol Wochenschr 107:1485–1487
4. Mehlis SL, Gordon KB (2003) The immunology of psoriasis and biologic immunotherapy. J Am Acad Dermatol 49:44–50
5. Ryan TJ (1980) Microcirculation in psoriasis: blood vessels, lymphatics and tissue fluid. Pharmacol Ther 10:27–64
6. Vollmer S, Menssen A, Prinz JC (2001) Dominant lesional T cell receptor rearrangements persist in relapsing psoriasis but are absent from nonlesional skin: evidence for a stable antigen-specific pathogenic T cell response in psoriasis vulgaris. J Invest Dermatol 117: 296–1301

24 Lichen Planus and Lichen Nitidus

24.1 Lichen Planus

Like psoriasis, lichen planus is a worldwide disease. The prevalence is about 1% of the general population. There are no race or sex differences and no genetic disposition. It appears most often between 30 and 60 years of age, but children and older persons may also be affected (Daoud and Pittelkow 1999a).

24.1.1 Clinical Appearance

The disease starts insidiously, progresses slowly and remains delimited. While older lesions resolve and wane, new lesions appear. If no treatment is given, lesions usually recede and vanish after a couple of years. Sometimes one or several lesions become chronic and hypertrophic. Rarely an acute and more or less generalized form may appear.

All parts of the skin, including the palms, soles, scalp, hair and nails, and genital and oral mucous membranes, may be involved; predilection sites are the ventral part of the wrists, ankles, and the buccal mucosa. Usually the lesions are severely, and sometimes unbearably itching. However, occasionally itch is lacking. Oral lesions are most often located on the buccal mucosa, but also the gingiva, tongue and lips may be affected. Ulcerated, erosive, oral lichen is painful and may be disabling.

The primary efflorescence is a flat, polygonal and reddish papule with a violaceous hue. Papules that may be of different sizes coalesce to plaques, the surface of which is crowned with a white and delicate network of lines. Sometimes annular lesions occur due to central clearing of the plaques. Papules can be triggered by mechanical injury, the *Köbner phenomenon*. If scratching is the cause of the injury, the lesion may be linear. Due to different locations and development of the lesions they may become atrophic, vesicular, bullous, ulcerated (erosive) or hypertrophic. In lichen follicularis mainly hair follicles are affected. In the scalp, lichen follicularis may cause patchy hair loss or scarring alopecia as the only sign of the disease (Mehregan et al. 1992)

24.1.2 Histopathologic Appearance

A typical lesion shows a dense, band-like infiltrate of lymphocytes that is strictly confined to the subepidermal area. The lymphocytes attack and destroy the basic part of the epidermis, giving rise to characteristic saw-tooth-like rete ridges and often to deposition of a large number of apoptotic bodies at the epidermal–dermal interface. However, the remaining part of the epidermis is also affected. Here the cells are only slightly stained, are sometimes vacuolated, and many of them have no nucleus; this is in contrast to the usually better preserved cells of the granular cell layer, which may even be hypertrophic. Scattered apoptotic bodies are also seen in the epidermis, but no or only scattered lymphocytes. The horny layer is thickened and never parakeratotic (Fig. 24.1).

If the process advances further, the epidermis gradually disintegrates from the base towards the surface and a cleft appears between the flattened epidermis and dermis. This is atrophic lichen (Fig. 24.1c). Finally, a subepidermal vesicle or bulla, and even ulceration, may occur. The roof of vesicles and bullae consists of a thickened horny layer and scattered disintegrating granular cells, and the floor of lymphocytes and a variable number of apoptotic bodies (Fig. 24.1d).

Apoptotic bodies in the dermis are eosinophilic and slightly PAS-positive; those in the epidermis are PAS-negative. Apoptotic bodies in the dermis may become coated with IgM (Abell et al. 1975; Mehregan et al. 1992; Boyd 1996). This may explain why they are PAS-positive in the dermis but not in the epidermis. The cell infiltrate in the dermis consists of lymphocytes with an admixture of some mast cells and macrophages; there is also a variable amount of melanin pigment which has leaked from the injured epidermis. There are no plasma cells or eosinophils.

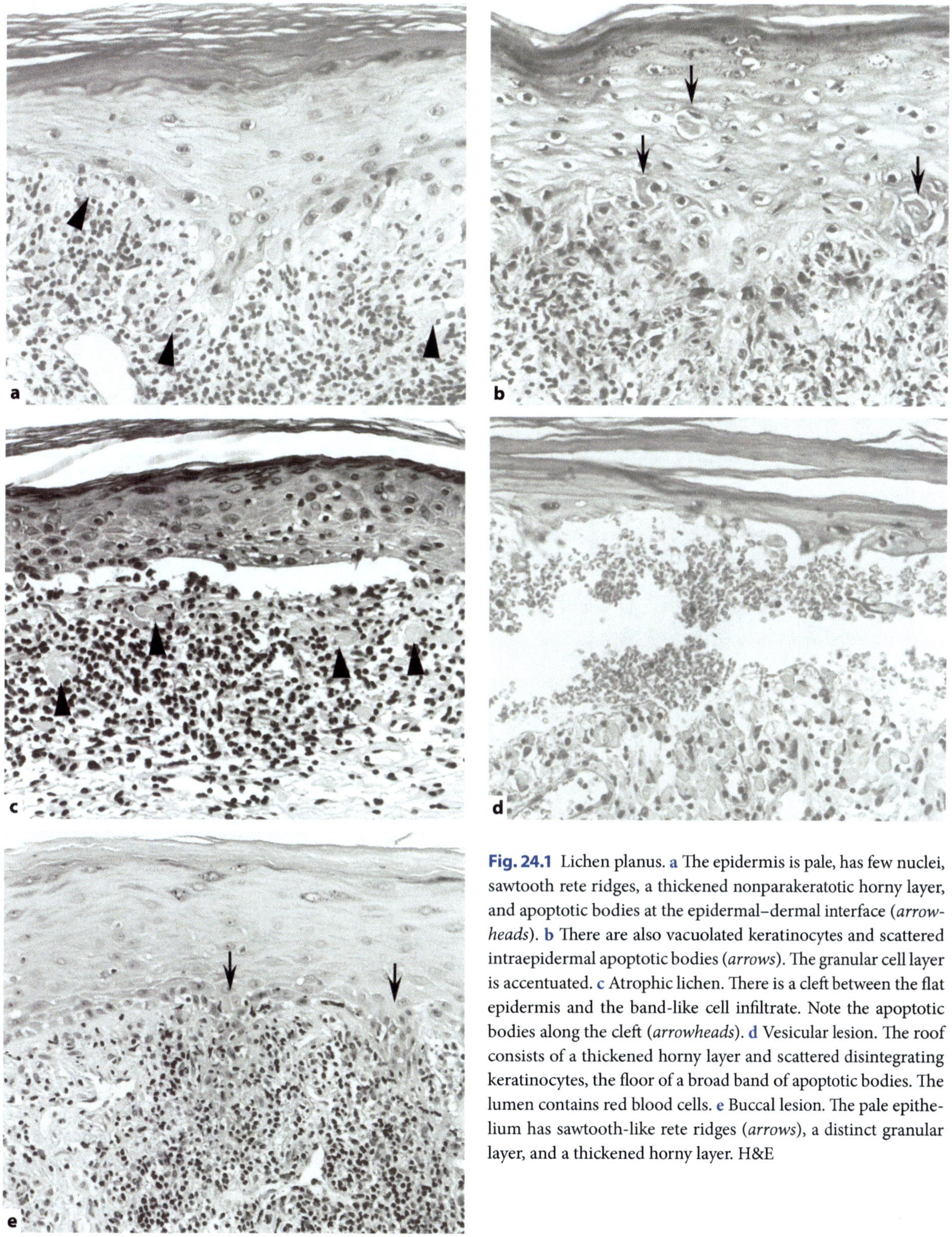

Fig. 24.1 Lichen planus. **a** The epidermis is pale, has few nuclei, sawtooth rete ridges, a thickened nonparakeratotic horny layer, and apoptotic bodies at the epidermal–dermal interface (*arrowheads*). **b** There are also vacuolated keratinocytes and scattered intraepidermal apoptotic bodies (*arrows*). The granular cell layer is accentuated. **c** Atrophic lichen. There is a cleft between the flat epidermis and the band-like cell infiltrate. Note the apoptotic bodies along the cleft (*arrowheads*). **d** Vesicular lesion. The roof consists of a thickened horny layer and scattered disintegrating keratinocytes, the floor of a broad band of apoptotic bodies. The lumen contains red blood cells. **e** Buccal lesion. The pale epithelium has sawtooth-like rete ridges (*arrows*), a distinct granular layer, and a thickened horny layer. H&E

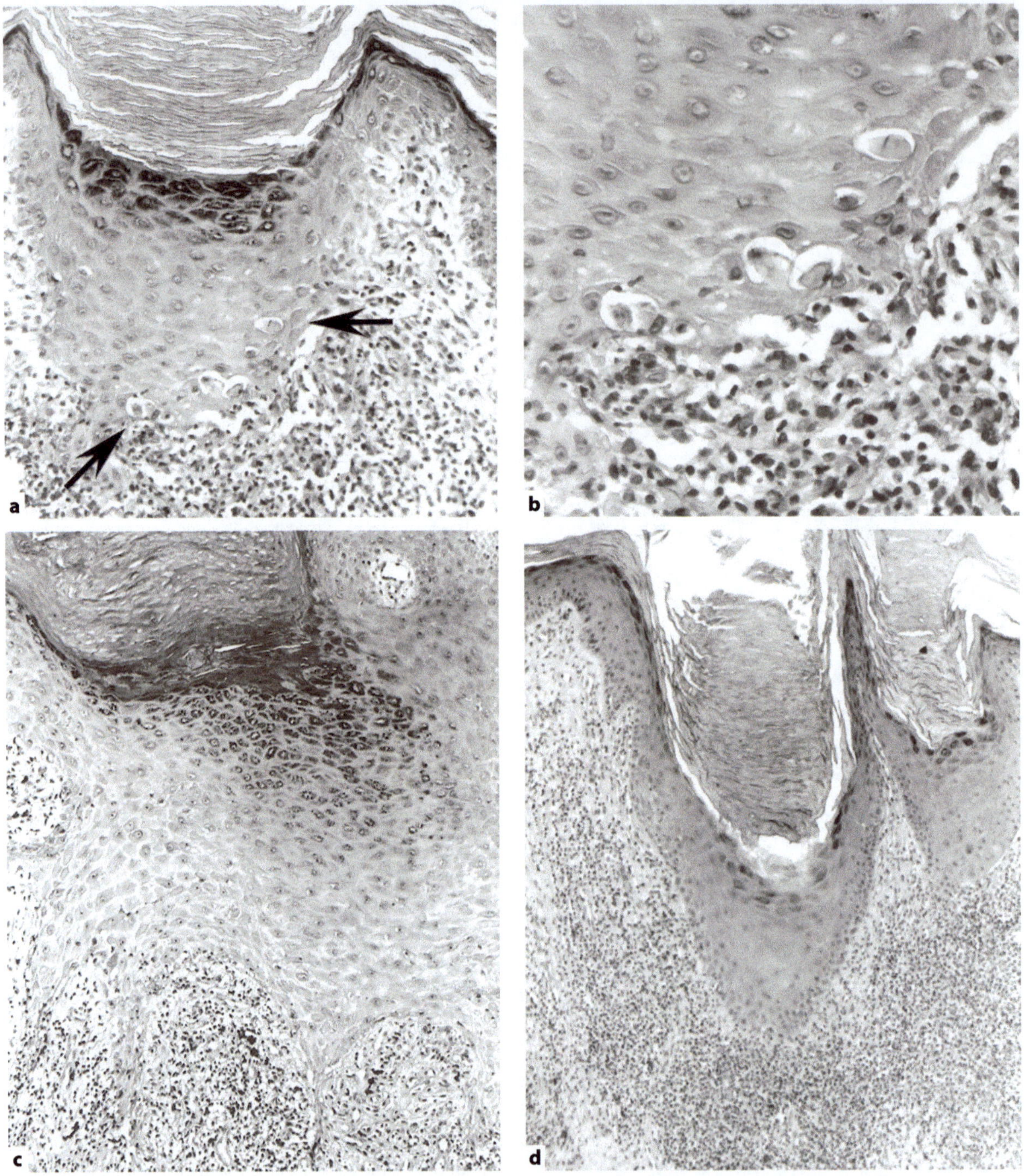

Fig. 24.2 Lichen hypertrophicus and lichen follicularis. **a** The hair follicle is hypertrophic, markedly widened and filled with nonparakeratotic keratin. The stratum granulosum is thickened and the cells are stuffed with large granules. In the area indicated (*arrows*) there are several apoptotic bodies. The dense lymphocytic cell infiltrate appears to gnaw at and is destroying the basic part of the epithelium. **b** Close-up of the area indicated (*arrows*) in **a** shows four large apoptotic bodies just above the interface. **c** In addition to follicular hypertrophy the epidermis is also thickened and shows elongated sawtooth-like rete ridges. **d** The typical band-formed lymphocytic cell infiltrate is confined to the follicles. H&E

In hypertrophic and follicular lichen, both epidermis and follicles or only follicles are hypertrophic (Fig. 24.2). The follicles are enlarged and widened and filled with nonparakeratotic keratin and the granular layer is accentuated. As in common lichen planus, there is a band-like lymphocytic cell infiltrate that appears to gnaw at and destroying the basal part of the follicular epithelium. If only follicles are involved the inflammatory cell infiltrate is more or less confined to the follicular area.

Oral lesions, if not erosive, show the same histopathologic pattern as those of the skin (Fig. 24.1e). Thus there are hyperkeratosis and a granular cell layer, not normally present in the buccal mucosa (compare Fig. 29.6a). Oral erosive (ulcerated) lichen planus is often a difficult histologic diagnosis because the ulceration and dense inflammatory cell infiltrate disguise the typical changes of lichen. In nonulcerated lesions, to establish the typical pattern of lichen demonstrated in Fig. 24.1e is a requirement for the diagnosis.

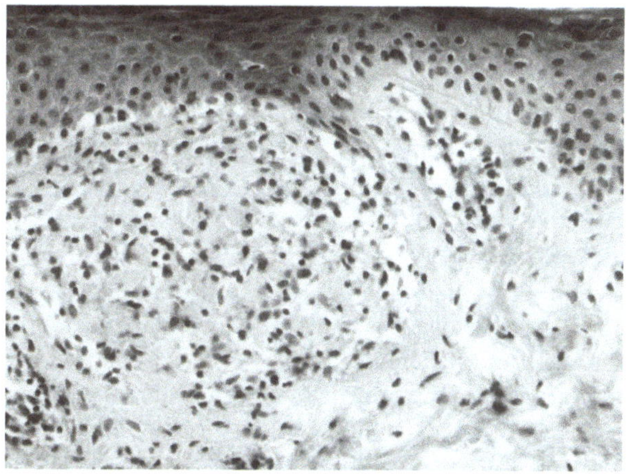

Fig. 24.3 Lichenoid lesion. The epidermis is flattened and has two sawtooth-like rete ridges. Located close to the epidermis there is a large conglomeration of apoptotic bodies, diffusely infiltrated by lymphocytes. H&E (reproduced from Lidén and Brehmer-Andersson 1988, with permission)

24.1.3 Pathogenesis

The cause of lichen planus is not known; however, it is generally thought that the mechanism is an immunologic reaction. Recent investigations have shown that the cell infiltrate in active lichen planus lesions contains a high number of $CD8^+$ (i.e., cytotoxic T cells) and that some $CD8^+$ cells secrete granzyme B granules (see Glossary) and induce apoptosis of the keratinocytes (Akasu et al. 1993: Gadenne et al. 1994; Shimizu et al. 1997). Also the presence of Langerhans cells is increased. These findings indicate that lichen planus may be a type IV hypersensitivity reaction mediated by sensitized $CD8^+$ cells.

24.1.4 Differential Diagnosis

- *Drugs and chemicals* can provoke lichenoid lesions both in the skin and the oral mucosa. The presence of eosinophils in the inflammatory cell infiltrate and/or parakeratosis indicates a drug reaction. Figure 24.3 demonstrates a lichenoid lesion caused by handling the color-developing agent CD-2 (a derivate of *p*-phenylenediamine). In some areas the appearance is lichenoid, in others that of chronic dermatitis. The chemical may be introduced to the body by inhalation, ingestion or absorption through the skin (Lidén and Brehmer-Andersson 1988).
- *Chronic graft-versus-host disease* may be difficult to differentiate histologically from lichen planus. As always it is important to know the case history.
- *Chronic lupus erythematosus* may be similar to lichen atrophicus. Both types of lesion show atrophy of the epidermis and scattered epidermal apoptotic bodies. However, a large number of apoptotic bodies at the epidermal–dermal interface indicates lichen planus.
- *Paraneoplastic pemphigus* may be both clinically and histologically similar to lichen planus (Sect. 25.3).
- *Lichenoid mycosis fungoides* (synonyms, among others, are poikiloderma atrophicans vasculare, and parapsoriasis lichenoides) is a chronic condition which after many years ends up as mycosis fungoides. Earlier stages show a more or less band-like lymphocytic cell infiltrate close to an atrophic epidermis. The cell infiltrate consists mainly of small and normal looking lymphocytes, a fair number of which migrate into the dermis. In contrast to lichen planus there are also a variable number of somewhat larger and more compact cells (atypical lymphocytes). These cells may be found both in the dermal cell infiltrate and in the epidermis, but are most easily seen in the epidermis. There are no apoptotic bodies.
- *Lichen planus pemphigoides* is an autoimmune subepidermal bullous disease. Bullae occur both on lichenoid plaques and on otherwise unaffected skin.

It is provoked by autoantibodies directed against a glycoprotein in the hemidesmosomes (Fig. 25.1) and has nothing to do with lichen planus (Zillikens et al. 1999)

24.2 Lichen Nitidus

Lichen nitidus is much less common than lichen planus. The two diseases have some similarities, both clinically and histologically, and have been observed concurrently in the same patient. It has therefore been seriously discussed as to whether they are variations of one disease or two different dermatoses. The latter view prevails (Daoud and Pittelkow 1999b).

24.2.1 Clinical Appearance

The primary efflorescence is a pinpoint- to pinhead-sized, dome-shaped, flesh-colored, shiny papule. Papules may be closely set, but do not coalesce. Eruptions can be generalized, but are usually confined to one or several areas. Predilection sites are the forearms, penis, abdomen, chest and buttocks. Also the oral mucosa may be affected. Usually eruptions do not itch. The disease is self-limiting.

24.2.2 Histopathologic Appearance

The lesion consists of a small, well-circumscribed granuloma located in a dermal papilla between elongated rete ridges. The epidermis between the elongated rete ridges is flattened and hyperkeratotic, but usually not parakeratotic. Sometimes there is a cleft between the flattened epidermis and the granuloma. The granuloma is composed of histiocytes, a few multinucleated giant cells of Langhans type, and lymphocytes. Apoptotic bodies are not observed.

24.2.3 Pathogenesis

Both the etiology and pathogenesis of lichen nitidus are unknown. An immunophenotypic investigation made on three patients with lichen nitidus showed that the cell infiltrate contained a high number of Langerhans cells, and that the lymphocytes mainly consisted of $CD4^+$ cells (Wright et al. 1990). These findings were then thought to be characteristic also of lichen planus. However, as already mentioned above, recent investigations have shown that most lymphocytes in active lichen planus lesions are $CD8^+$ cells. Furthermore, in lichen nitidus apoptotic bodies are lacking and the cell infiltrate is granulomatous, but mainly lymphocytic in lichen planus. Presumably both diseases are due to a type IV hypersensitivity reaction, but the pathways are different. Thus in lichen nitidus the lesions are initiated by sensitized $CD4^+$ cells and in lichen planus by sensitized cytotoxic $CD8^+$ cells.

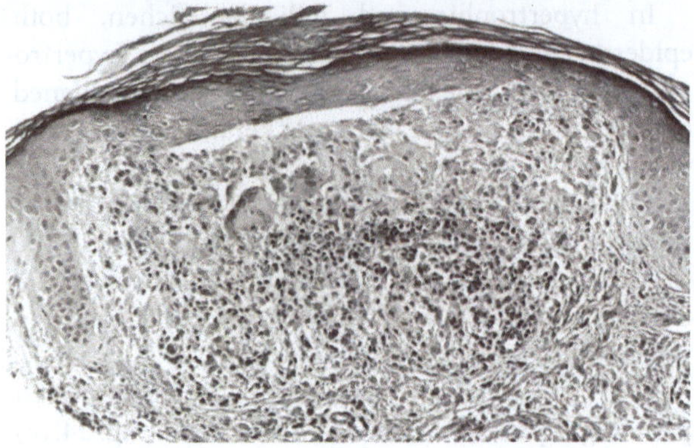

Fig. 24.4 Lichen nitidus. The small and strictly confined lesion is hugged by slightly elongated rete ridges and covered by a flat epidermis with a thickened, nonparakeratotic horny layer. Centrally there is a cleft between the epidermis and the dermal infiltrate, which consists of lymphocytes, histiocytes, and multinucleated giant cells. H&E

24.2.4 Example

Case 1. Lichen Nitidus

A 29-year-old man had observed non-itching papules on the upper extremities and the penile shaft for 6 months. A biopsy specimen taken from the arm showed a typical granuloma described above (Fig. 24.4).

References

1. Abell E, Presbury DGC, Marks R, Ramnarain D (1975) The diagnostic significance of immunoglobulin and fibrin deposition in lichen planus. Br J Dermatol 93:17–24
2. Akasu R, From L, Kahn HJ (1993) Lymphocyte and macrophage subsets in active and inactive lesions of lichen planus. Am J Dermatopathol 15:217–223
3. Boyd AS (1996) Update on the diagnosis of lichenoid dermatitis. Adv Dermatol 11:287–316

4. Daoud MS, Pittelkow MR (1999a) Lichen planus. In: Freedberg IM, Eisen AZ, Wolff K, Austen KF, Goldsmith LA, Katz SI, Fitzpatrick TB (eds) Fitzpatrick's dermatology in general medicine. McGraw-Hill, New York, pp 561–577
5. Daoud MS, Pittelkow MR (1999b) Lichen nitidus. In: Freedberg IM, Eisen AZ, Wolff K, Austen KF, Goldsmith LA, Katz SI, Fitzpatrick TB (eds) Fitzpatrick's dermatology in general medicine. McGraw-Hill, New York, pp 577–581
6. Gadenne A-S, Strucke R, Dunn D, Wagner M, Bleicher P, Bigby M (1994) T-cell lines derived from lesional skin of lichen planus patients contain a distinctive population of T-cell receptor $\gamma\delta$-bearing cells. J Invest Dermatol 103:347–351
7. Lidén C, Brehmer-Andersson E (1988) Occupational dermatoses from colour developing agents. Acta Derm Venereol 68:514–522
8. Mehregan DA, Van Hale HM, Muller SA (1992) Lichen planopilaris: clinical and pathologic study of forty-five patients. J Am Acad Dermatol 27:935–942
9. Shimizu M, Higaki Y, Higaki M, Kawashima M (1997) The role of granzyme B-expressing CD8-positive T cells in apoptosis of keratinocytes in lichen planus. Arch Dermatol Res 289:527–532
10. Wright AL, Mcvittie E, Hunter JAA (1990) An immunophenotypic study of lichen nitidus. Clin Exp Dermatol 15:273–276
11. Zillikens D, Caux F, Mascaro JM Jr, Wesselmann U, Schmidt E, Prost C, Callen JP, Bröcker E-B, Diaz LA, Giudice GJ (1999) Autoantibodies in lichen planus pemphigoides react with a novel epitope within the C-terminal NC16A domain of BP180. J Invest Dermatol 113:117–121

25 Autoimmune Vesicular, Bullous, and Pustular Dermatoses

Autoimmune vesicular, bullous, and pustular dermatoses are caused by autoantibodies directed against different components in *desmosomes*, *hemidesmosomes* or other parts of the epidermal-dermal junction area.

Desmosomes bind keratinocytes together and are composed of two main parts. One of these consists of transmembrane molecules (Fig. 4.2), the other of a plaque located at the inner surface of the cell membrane. The extracellular fraction of the transmembrane part hooks onto the corresponding fraction of the neighboring cells. These two fractions together form the intercellular bridges, which are clearly visible in the spongiotic epidermis (Figs. 5.7c–f and 22.1a). The intracellular fraction of the transmembrane component is via the cytoplasmic plaque connected to *keratin filaments*, which are an integral part of the *cytoskeleton*. This construction stabilizes and strengthens the epithelium. The basal cells differ from other keratinocytes by having both desmosomes and hemidesmosomes. Desmosomes connect basal cells to other keratinocytes and hemidesmosomes connect them to the extracellular component *lamina densa* (Fig. 25.1). At the molecular level, desmosomes and hemidesmosomes are made up of different proteins and glycoproteins, possible to identify by their various molecular weights in kiloDaltons (Anhalt 1999; Woodley and Chen 2001). Relevant components are listed in Table 25.1.

In the electron microscope the epidermal–dermal junction area has four distinct layers (Woodley and Chen 2001):

1. The cell membrane and the hemidesmosomes of the basal keratinocytes.
2. *Lamina lucida*, the transparent layer, which is the only layer that can be visualized under the light microscope as a PAS-positive layer beneath the hemidesmosomes, and here designated the basement membrane. It contains delicate structures called anchoring filaments.
3. *Lamina densa* or the *basal lamina*, the electron-dense layer below the lamina lucida. One of the main components is type IV collagen.
4. The *sublamina densa area*, which contains anchoring fibrils. Collagen type VII is a main component.

Together layers 2–4 form the *basement membrane zone*. Type IV and VII collagens are specific for this region.

25.1 The Pemphigus Group

To this group belong *pemphigus vulgaris* with its variants *pemphigus vegetans of Neumann type* and *pemphigus vegetans of Hallopeau type* and *pemphigus foliaceus* with its variant *pemphigus erythematosus. Pemphigus herpetiformis* is a variant which may end up as either pemphigus foliaceus or pemphigus vulgaris.

Table 25.1 Components of desmosomes and hemidesmosomes

Desmosomal components		Hemidesmosomal components	
Transmembrane glycoproteins	*Cytoplasmic plaque proteins*	*Transmembrane glycoproteins*	*Cytoplasmic plaque proteins*
Desmogleins	Desmoplakin (250 kDa)	BPAg (180 kDa)	BPAg (230 kDa)
Desmocollins	Envoplakin (210 kDa)	Integrins (cell adhesion molecules)	Plectin
	Periplakin (190 kDa)		
	Plakoglobin		

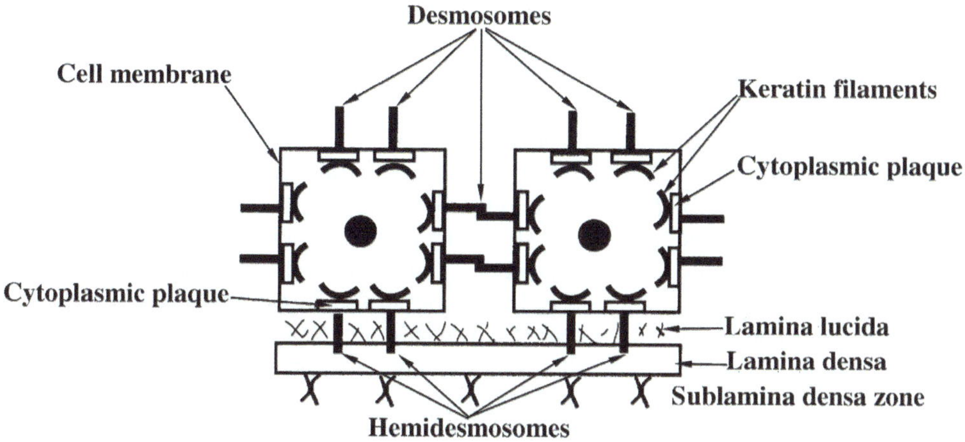

Fig. 25.1 The epidermal–dermal junction area. The drawing shows two basal cells with desmosomes, hemidesmosomes and underlying basement membrane zone. The latter consists of the lamina lucida with anchoring filaments, the lamina densa, and the sublamina densa zone with anchoring fibrils

25.1.1 Pemphigus Vulgaris

Pemphigus vulgaris is a rare disease mostly occurring between the ages of 40 and 60 years. There is a high prevalence among Jewish people. Before the use of corticosteroids the outcome of pemphigus vulgaris was nearly always fatal (Lever 1965). Even with this treatment available it is a serious disease. The incidence is the same in both sexes.

Pemphigus vulgaris in childhood is a very rare disease. Bjarnason and Flosadóttir (1999) reviewed the literature on pemphigus in early life. They found 46 childhood, 9 neonatal, and 3 stillborn cases. In the childhood group, verified by immunofluorescence studies, the mean age of onset was 12 years with only ten patients younger than 11 years. The youngest was 3 years old. At puberty there was an abrupt increase in incidence. The sex ratio was equal. In neonatal patients and stillborns the disease is caused by transplacental transportation of antibodies from mother to fetus. The three stillborn babies had died during the eighth month of gestation. In the nine neonatal cases the prognosis was excellent. In childhood pemphigus most reported cases are not followed for a prolonged time, which is the reason the prognosis is difficult to judge. However, it seems to be better than in adult cases (Wananukul and Pongprasit 1999).

25.1.1.1 Clinical Appearance

Flaccid, rather small vesicles or bullae appear on seemingly normal skin, occasionally on an erythematous base. The blisters are fragile, burst easily, and leave irregular and red denuded areas all over the body. The denuded areas grow in size, coalesce and at the margin show a collar of detached skin. In serious cases the epidermis slides off without preceding vesiculation. Also, in patients with vesicles, a sliding pressure on apparently normal skin made by a finger easily detaches the epidermis. This is called the *Nikolsky* sign. It may also be present in other types of vesicular and bullous diseases such as bullous pemphigoid (Sect. 25.4.1), and toxic epidermal necrolysis (Sect. 28.4). The lesions do not heal, or heal slowly without residue. The oral mucosa is nearly always affected and may be the first and for a long time the only area affected. Often even the lips, perioral area, nostrils, conjunctivae, periorbital area, and genitals are affected.

25.1.1.2 Histopathologic Appearance

The most characteristic histopathologic feature in pemphigus vulgaris and foliaceus as well as in the most relevant differential diseases (i.e., familial benign pemphigus, keratosis follicularis, and transient acantholytic dermatosis) is *primary acantholysis* (Lever 1965). By primary acantholysis is meant dissociation and disintegration of the desmosomes, followed by disintegration of the keratinocytes. This is due either to direct injury to the desmosomes or to some hereditary defect in their construction. In contrast, *secondary acantholysis* is caused by injury to the keratinocytes followed by disintegration of the desmosomes. One example of secondary acantholysis is the dissociation of cells that occurs in herpes simplex and herpes zoster lesions (Fig. 20.1).

In typical pemphigus vulgaris vesicles a suprabasal cleft separates the basal cell layer and the papillary dermis from the rest of the epidermis (Fig. 25.2a). Thus, the floor of the vesicle is made up of papillary dermis covered with basal cells. If the dermal papillae are elongated they protrude into the vesicle. These formations are called *villi* (Fig. 25.2d). The basal cells are attached to the dermis, but are slightly separated from each other. The acantholysis also includes hair follicles (Fig. 25.2c) and sometimes sweat gland ducts (Fig. 25.4b). The roof of the blister consists of the rest of the epidermis; in early vesicles it looks quite normal or contains areas of marked acantholysis (Fig. 25.3b). The lumen of the vesicle contains acantholytic keratinocytes scattered or in sheets (Fig. 25.2d), and also neutrophils and eosinophils, the latter sometimes in abundance. In somewhat older vesicles the roof becomes thin and shrunken (Fig. 25.2a). The roof is sometimes lost during the taking or processing of the specimen, leaving a row of basal cells and some acantholytic cells as the only clue to the diagnosis (Figs. 25.2b and 25.3d). In the early course of the disease the histopathologic pattern is not always clear-cut. It may show that of subacute dermatitis, often with many eosinophils (Figs. 25.2e and 25.4a). Clues to the diagnosis are small areas with a tendency to acantholysis (Fig. 25.4b). In other cases the epithelium looks normal or thickened, but in some areas displays single minute suprabasal clefts (Fig. 25.3c). The papillary epidermis is edematous. The number of inflammatory cells is generally sparse or moderate. Eosinophils are common, but may be lacking. In the oral cavity, older lesions may be difficult to recognize; the roof of the vesicles is often shed and the mucous papillae are heavily infiltrated by inflammatory cells (Fig. 25.3d).

25.1.1.3 Pemphigus Vegetans of Neumann Type

Oral lesions are always present and are often the first to appear. The course is more chronic and more benign than in pemphigus vulgaris. Initially the lesions are identical both clinically and histopathologically. However, in pemphigus vegetans, the blisters soon turn into pustules and later become hypertrophic (vegetative) lesions.

Early hypertrophic lesions show a thickened and acanthotic epidermis, which together with acantholytic clefts contains intraepidermal pustules. The latter are composed of eosinophils and a few acantholytic cells. In older lesions the hypertrophic and acanthotic epithelium remains, but acantholysis and eosinophilic abscesses are absent; the pattern is no longer diagnostic (Lever 1965).

25.1.1.4 Pemphigus Vegetans of Hallopeau Type

Usually the initial lesions are pustules arising on normal-appearing skin. However, affected areas rapidly become hypertrophic, extend peripherally, and coalesce to larger areas. Preferential sites are axilla and groin. The course is chronic and rather benign, but some cases may finish as pemphigus vegetans of Neumann type. Oral lesions are always present.

Histologic investigation of early pustules shows suprabasal acantholysis and eosinophilia. In early hypertrophic lesions the epidermis is hypertrophic and acanthotic and contains intraepidermal abscesses stuffed with eosinophils. Invariably a few acantholytic cells are present. Old lesions show considerable epidermal papillomatosis and acanthosis, but no abscesses or acantholysis (Lever 1965).

25.1.2 Pemphigus Foliaceus

Like pemphigus vulgaris, it is a rare disease, but in comparison has a more favorable prognosis. The majority of patients are middle-aged, but adolescents may also be affected. There is a slight prevalence of Jewish individuals. The incidence is the same for men and women.

25.1.2.1 Clinical Appearance

The disease usually begins slowly with only a few and rather small, flaccid blisters on an erythematous base, which easily break and leave superficial erosions. In some cases only erosions are observed. The first lesions often appear in the center of the face and by spreading give rise to a butterfly-like figure similar to that seen in discoid lupus erythematosus. Sometimes the disease starts abruptly with serpiginous and scaling lesions all over the body. Oral or other mucosal lesions are usually not present. Mostly the course of the disease is chronic, even if not treated, and may disappear without therapy (Lever 1965).

25.1.2.2 Histopathologic Appearance

In pemphigus foliaceus the acantholytic cleft is superficially located. The roof of the cleft consists of the horny layer alone, the horny layer together with a few cells from the stratum granulosum, or the horny layer together with the stratum granulosum and the outermost part of the squamous cell layer (Fig. 25.5a–c). Clefts going down to the deep epidermis and even small suprabasal clefts may be seen, most often at the margins of specimens.

25.1.2.3 Pemphigus Erythematosus

Pemphigus erythematosus is either an abortive form of pemphigus foliaceus or an early manifestation of it (Lever 1965). The lesions consist of circumscribed erythematous scaling or crusted areas on the face, scalp, chest and upper back. Lesions on the face may mimic lupus erythematosus and on the scalp psoriasis or seborrheic dermatitis. Flaccid bullae are seldom seen except on the back. The histopathologic pattern is principally the same as in pemphigus foliaceus. However, hyperkeratosis and acantholysis are more pronounced (Fig. 25.5e,f).

25.1.2.4 Pemphigus Herpetiformis

Pemphigus herpetiformis is considered by some a distinct variant of pemphigus. The eruptions consist of erythematous, vesicular, bullous or papular lesions, which sometimes are similar to those seen in dermatitis herpetiformis, and often associated with severe itching.

The histologic pattern is characterized by spongiosis and intraepidermal vesiculation with infiltration of eosinophils and/or neutrophils. Acantholysis is slight or absent. Oral lesions have been described in some patients. The disease course is benign and the response to treatment is usually good. In spite of this, a fair number of those patients reported eventually developed or had pemphigus foliaceus and occasionally pemphigus vulgaris (Santi et al. 1996).

However, skin lesions showing eosinophilic spongiosis with slight or absent acantholysis have also been considered harbingers of pemphigus foliaceus or vulgaris. Thus Emmerson and Wilson-Jones (1968) described seven such cases, and five of the seven patients developed pemphigus foliaceus and two pemphigus vulgaris. Three of the five patients with pemphigus foliaceus had presented with an atypical initial clinical pattern resembling dermatitis herpetiformis. It might be that lesions interpreted as pemphigus herpetiformis are early manifestations of pemphigus foliaceus or vulgaris.

25.1.3 Pathogenesis

The triggering mechanisms are unknown. However, both pemphigus vulgaris and pemphigus foliaceus and their variants are autoimmune diseases because of the development of autoantibodies against molecular components in desmosomes of the epidermis and oral epithelium (Table 25.1). They are type II hypersensitivity reactions (Sect. 4.3.2).

Since the middle of the 1960s the critical diagnostic finding has been the presence of IgG autoantibodies in the perilesional skin, visualized by means of direct immunofluorescence. Fluorescence is seen on the surface of all cells throughout the epidermis in both pemphigus vulgaris and pemphigus foliaceus, and thus is of no help in differentiating these two types of pemphigus. In addition to the presence of antibodies on the cell surface, in pemphigus erythematosus there are also depositions of IgG and C3 at the basement membrane. In many cases autoantibodies are present also in the patient's serum and may be proved by indirect immunofluorescence on different substrates such as guinea pig or monkey esophagus (Beutner et al. 1965).

In recent years the pemphigus antigens have been characterized at the molecular level by immunologic studies on antibodies present in the serum of patients (Table 25.1). These have revealed that in pemphigus vulgaris with only oral lesions there are antibodies against desmoglein 3. If both the oral mucosa and skin are affected there are antibodies against both desmoglein 3 and desmoglein 1 (Mahoney et al. 1999). This explains why pemphigus vulgaris usually starts in the oral mucosa and for a long time may remain the only affected site, as demonstrated in Case 4 (below). Extension of the disease to the skin is probably due to *epitope spreading* (i.e., when an autoimmune disease evolves, additional antibodies develop against molecules which are either similar in structure or dissimilar but closely located in the affected tissue) (Anhalt 1999). In pemphigus foliaceus the antibodies

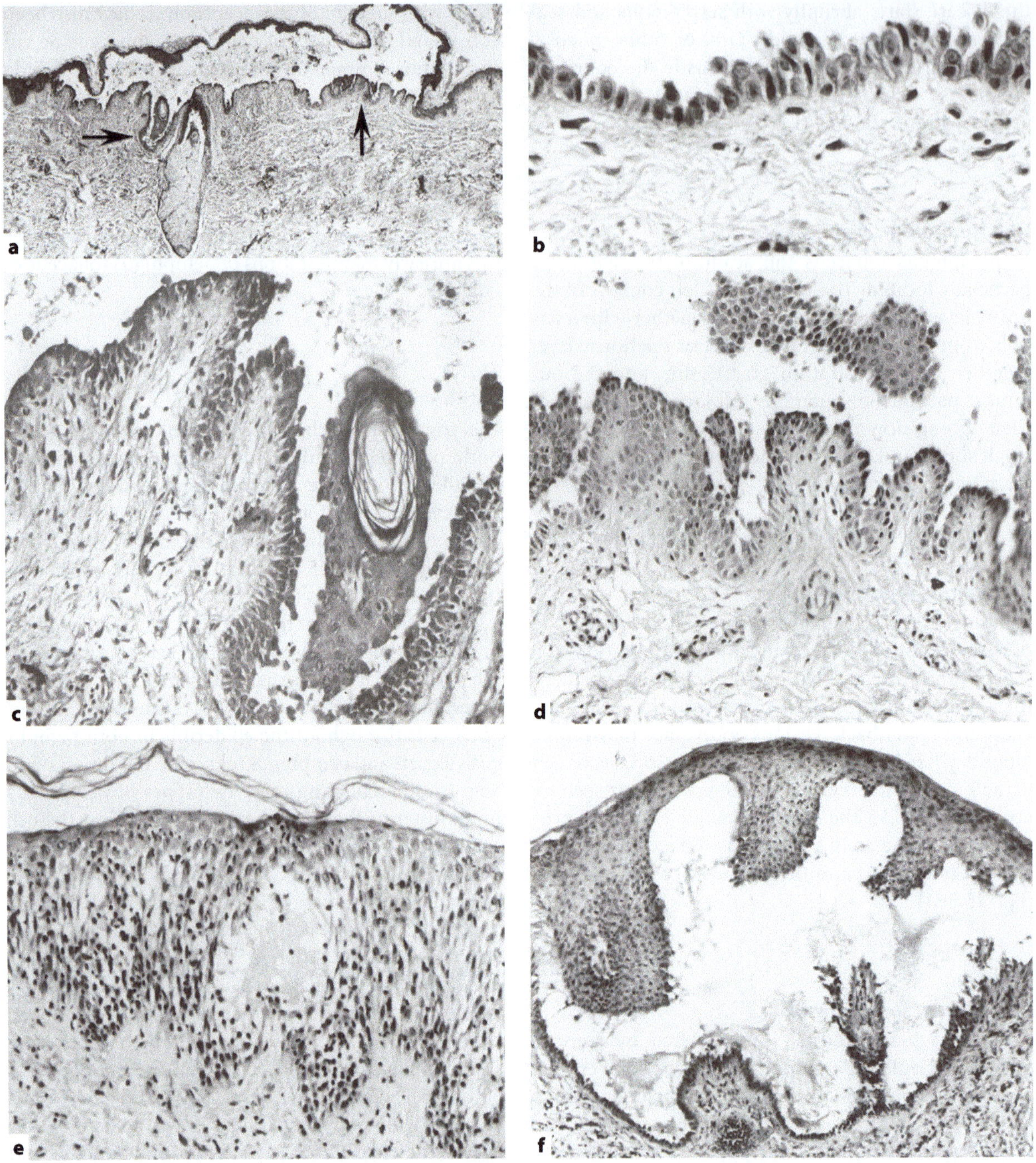

Fig. 25.2 Pemphigus vulgaris. **a** There is a wide acantholytic suprabasal vesicle. A shrunken epidermis makes the roof. The *right arrow* indicates villi covered by basal cells and the *left arrow* an affected hair follicle. **b** The roof may be lost during processing and the only remains of the vesicle will be a row of basal cells and a few more or less detached keratinocytes. **c** Close-up of the hair follicle indicated in **a** shows the conspicuous acantholysis. **d** Close-up of the area indicated by the *right arrow* in **a** shows a sheet of loosely coherent keratinocytes lying free in the lumen above the villi. **e** A lesion from the lower leg shows vesicular dermatitis, but no acantholysis. **f** The anal polyp from the same patient displays a broad acantholytic suprabasal cleft. H&E

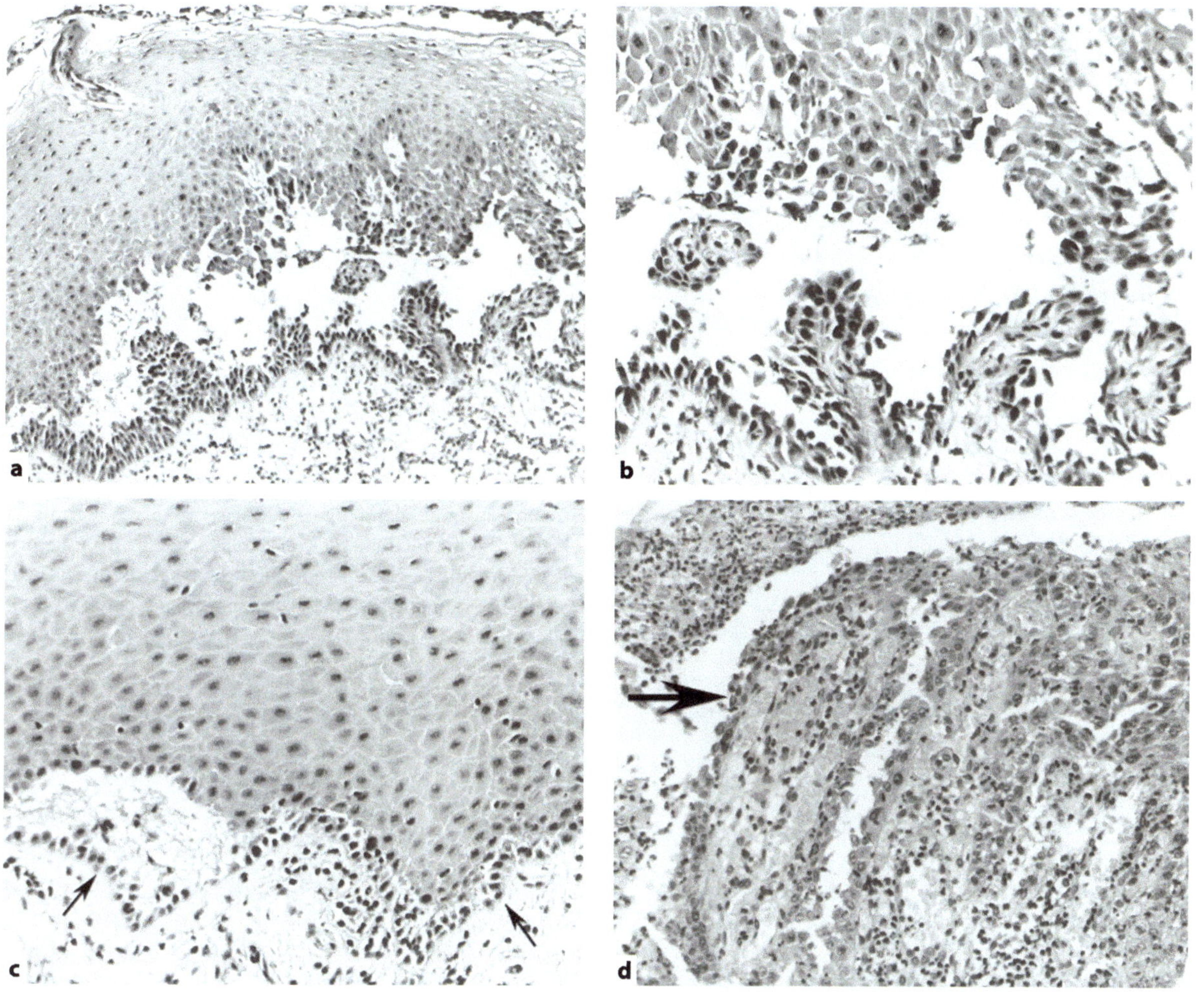

Fig. 25.3 Pemphigus vulgaris: oral lesions. **a** There is a rather wide suprabasal cleft. The roof consists of a thickened epithelium, which partly shows marked acantholysis. **b** Close-up displays the acantholytic part of the roof. The keratinocytes fall apart like pieces of a jigsaw puzzle. Note also the elongated mucosal papillae in the floor. **c** In another area of the same specimen there are only minute gaps between the basal cell layer and the rest of the epithelium (*arrows*). **d** In this case only the floor of the vesicle remains. It consists of elongated mucosal papillae, which are covered with basal cells and massively infiltrated by inflammatory cells. Only the one to the left is clearly discernible (*arrow*). The structure above the arrow is a part of a thick crust composed of inflammatory cells and necrotic tissue. H&E

are directed against desmoglein 1, and are present (expressed) mainly in the superficial parts of the epidermis and mucosal epithelium. Oral lesions are usually absent in pemphigus foliaceus because the expression of desmoglein 3 alone is enough to keep the epithelial cells together in the oral mucosa (Mahoney et al. 1999).

In pemphigus herpetiformis IgG antibodies are found in the skin and in some cases also in the serum. In the majority of cases antibodies develop against desmoglein 1 (Robinson et al. 1999).

25.1.4 Examples

Case 1. Pemphigus Vulgaris

A 48-year-old farmer was admitted to the hospital because of a generalized skin eruption, which had started 3 months previously. He presented with large irregular, bright-red, denuded areas on the trunk and extremities. The lesions were accentuated in the groin and axilla. The oral mucosa, lips, nostrils and the periorbital areas were also affected. In addition, on one lower leg

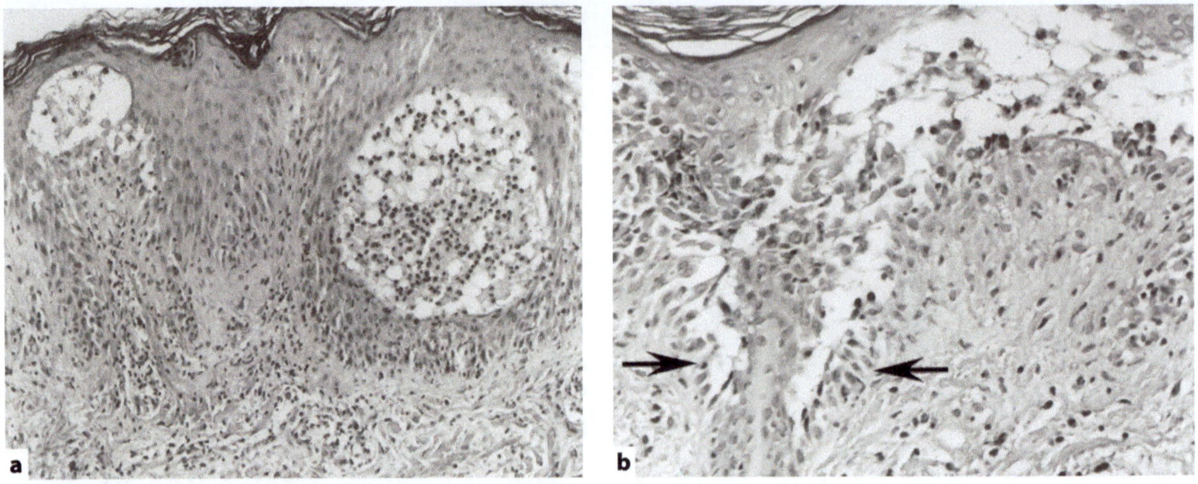

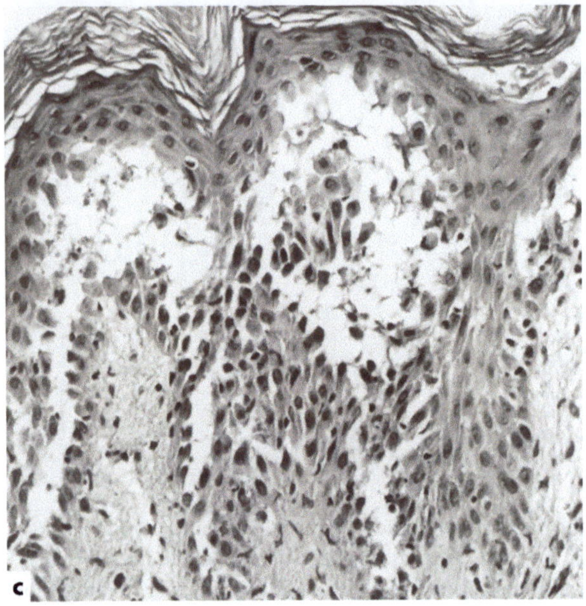

Fig. 25.4 Juvenile pemphigus vulgaris. **a** The epidermis is thickened and contains two vesicles filled with inflammatory cells (eosinophils). There is no acantholysis. **b** Another vesicle is partly acantholytic and includes a sweat gland duct (*arrows*); H&E. **c** In this area there is a suprabasal cleft due to acantholysis. The roof consists of villi; PAS

there was a group of small vesicles on essentially normal skin. One of them was excised whole. The patient died less than 2 years after the onset of the disease in spite of oral treatment with corticosteroids.

Histologic investigation revealed a typical acantholytic vesicle, located above the basal cell layer. Also a hair follicle was acantholytic. The roof was thin and consisted of disintegrating keratinocytes. The lumen contained sheets of keratinocytes, some neutrophils, and eosinophils (Fig. 25.2a,c,d).

Case 2. Pemphigus Vulgaris

A 61-year old woman had had eruptions of scattered different-sized flaccid vesicles on the lower legs for about 6 months. She also had an anal complaint, thought to be due to a hemorrhoidal polyp. This lesion was excised. However, the ailment remained and the operation wound showed a poor tendency to heal. Repeated biopsy specimens and smears were taken from skin lesions. During the course of the disease general onycholysis also occurred. The patient recovered completely after treatment with oral corticosteroids.

Histologic investigation of skin lesions mainly showed the pattern of subacute dermatitis with eosinophils and lymphocytes. In some specimens there was a tendency to acantholysis. Also smears contained many acantholytic cells. The anal operation specimen was reexamined and revealed suprabasal clefts and vesicles typical of pemphigus vulgaris (Fig. 25.2e,f).

Case 3. Oral Pemphigus Vulgaris

A 71-year-old woman presented with large erosions and suspect vesicles on the buccal mucosa.

Histologic investigation disclosed conspicuous acantholysis and wide suprabasal clefts alternating with small discreet suprabasal gaps in an otherwise normal epithelium (Fig. 25.3a–c).

Case 4. Oral Pemphigus Vulgaris

A 55-year-old woman had for 30 years suffered from recurrent spells of edema, vesicles and ulcerations in the mouth and throat, which interfered with eating and drinking. Investigation including virus isolation, and cultures for fungus and bacteria were negative. Later vesicles on the left calf appeared.

The oral biopsy specimen consisted of mucosa and submucosa massively permeated by inflammatory cells. In one area elongated papillae covered only by basal cells were identified. The vesicular skin lesion showed a mixed pattern with eosinophilic vesicular dermatitis in some areas and marked acantholysis in other areas (Fig. 25.3d).

Case 5. Juvenile Pemphigus Vulgaris

A 13-year-old girl presented with rapidly aggravating spells of vesicles and bullae over the trunk and extremities. She also had oral, genital, and periungual erosions. The disease had started insidiously 7 months previously with erythematous and scaling areas on the palms and soles, followed by oral and genital erosions.

A biopsy specimen taken from the arm showed a thickened and acanthotic epidermis which contained one large and several small vesicles. These contained fibrinous exudate and a large number of eosinophils. In addition, there were small acantholytic suprabasal clefts and in one area typical villi. The dermal papillae were edematous. There were small perivascular infiltrates composed of lymphocytes and scattered eosinophils.

Direct and indirect immunofluorescence were positive for IgG antibodies. There was also a diffuse deposition of C3 at the basal membrane. The patient recovered after treatment with oral corticosteroids (Fig. 25.4).

Case 6. Pemphigus Foliaceus

A 52-year-old woman had had spells of flaccid vesicles all over the body for 4 years. They easily ruptured and left an eroded surface.

Histologic investigation showed a thin epidermis with a thickened horny layer without parakeratosis. Due to acantholysis there was a discrete superficial cleft, the roof of which consisted of stratum corneum and scattered keratinocytes. In minute areas slight acantholysis was observed in the outermost cell layer of stratum malpighii (the floor of the vesicle). There were no inflammatory cells in the epidermis and only sparse perivascular infiltrates of lymphocytes in upper dermis (Fig. 25.5a,b).

Case 7. Pemphigus Foliaceus

A 59-year-old man had been treated for 3 months with oral corticosteroids for a vesicular dermatosis when he was referred to the dermatology department. The Nikolsky sign was positive. A biopsy specimen and smears were taken. It was noted that the roof of the vesicle was lost when the biopsy specimen was taken.

The epidermis lacked a horny layer and showed a slight acantholysis in the outermost row of cells. Smears contained large sheets of typical acantholytic cells with a large swollen nucleus, light cytoplasm and a condensed nuclear membrane (Fig. 25.5c,d).

Case 8. Pemphigus Erythematosus

A 71-year-old woman had a scaling lesion on the scalp which she had noticed for a year and which at presentation measured 30 mm in diameter. A biopsy was taken. The clinical suggestions were basal cell carcinoma, psoriasis, or fungal infection. The disease had progressed 3 months later with an outbreak of vesicles on the trunk and on the dorsal aspect of the feet.

In the specimen from the scalp, the epidermis was thickened and had a markedly thickened horny layer. Due to acantholysis there were superficial clefts of the kind seen in pemphigus foliaceus, but also small suprabasal clefts of the kind seen in pemphigus vulgaris. The histopathologic pattern seen in vesicular lesion taken from the trunk and feet was that of pemphigus foliaceus (Fig. 25.5e,f).

25.1.5 Differential Diagnosis

The most important are:

- *Benign pemphigus* (Haily-Haily disease)
- *Keratosis follicularis* (Darier disease)
- *Transient acantholytic dermatosis* (Grover disease)

25.1.5.1 Familial Benign Pemphigus (Haily-Haily Disease)

Familial benign pemphigus is an autosomal, dominant hereditary disease, due to some unknown abnormality in the structure or organization of the desmosomes. The disease usually starts in adolescence or early adult life.

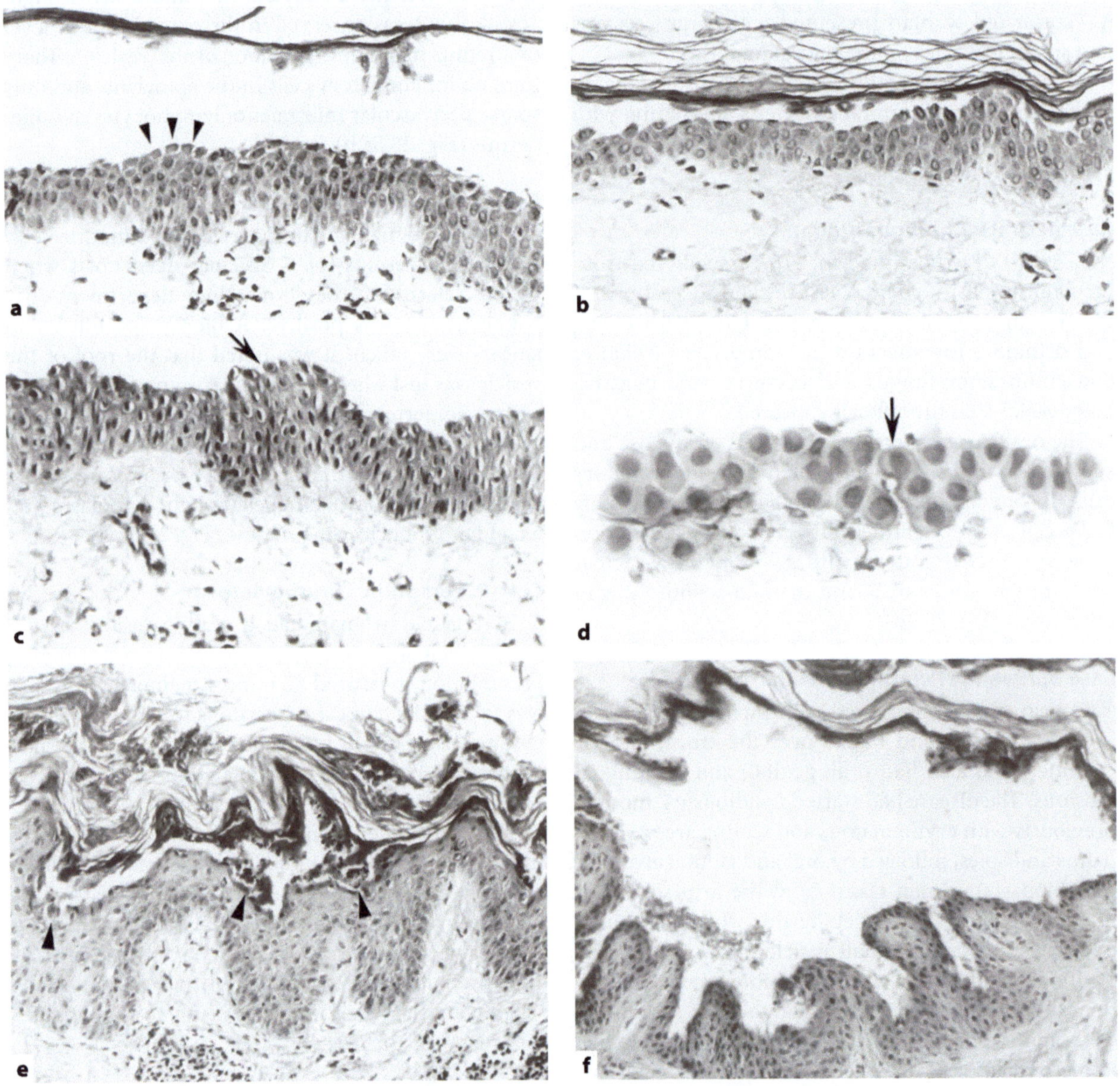

Fig. 25.5 a–d Pemphigus foliaceus; e, f pemphigus erythematosus. a There is a cleft between the horny layer and the rest of the epidermis. The only significant sign of acantholysis is the slightly separated keratinocytes at the surface (*arrowheads*). b In this area the superficial acantholysis is more obvious. c In another case the roof of the superficial vesicle has been lost. Some cells in the outermost cell layer of the floor are slightly dissociated (*arrow*). There are no inflammatory cells in the epidermis and only a few in the upper dermis; H&E. d Smear from the floor shows a sheet of Tzanck cells (*arrow*). The nuclei are swollen and surrounded by a light halo. The cell membranes are accentuated; Mayer stain. e In a biopsy from the scalp there is a wide superficial intraepidermal fissure (*arrowheads*) and a markedly thickened horny layer. f In another area of the same specimen there is a suprabasal vesicle, the floor of which is composed of villi as in pemphigus vulgaris. The roof consists mainly of the horny layer; H&E

Small groups of flaccid blisters arise on normal or reddened skin. Predilection areas are axilla and groin, other intertriginous areas, and the sides and nape of the neck (i.e., sites exposed to pressure). The vesicles break easily, leaving erosions and crusts. Lesions grow peripherally and may form circinate and annular figures. After some time, often months, the lesions heal with pigmentation, but recur in the same areas with little tendency to abate over the course of time. Oral lesions are very rare (Lever 1965).

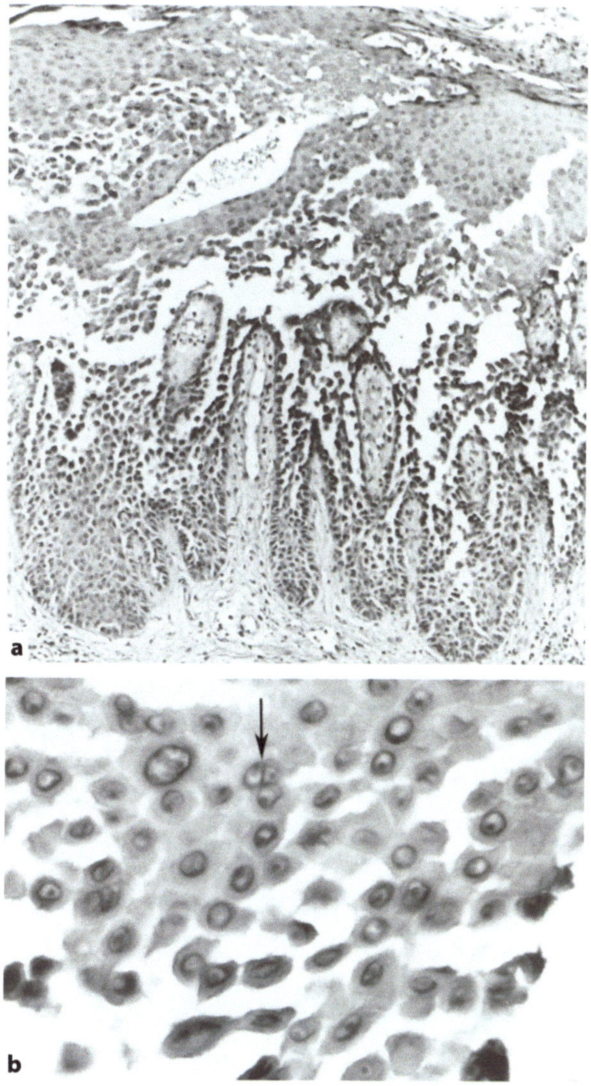

Fig. 25.6 Familial benign pemphigus. **a** The main cleft is suprabasal. The floor consists of acantholytic rete ridges and villi. The roof is thickened and markedly acantholytic. **b** Close-up shows that many cells have a light nucleus, a distinct nucleolus, and condensed nuclear membrane. The *arrow* indicates a cell with two nuclei. To the right of it is a cell with a very large nucleus. H&E

The histopathologic pattern is very much like that of pemphigus vulgaris (Fig. 25.6) and it may be impossible to differentiate the two diseases by means of the histopathologic pattern only (Lever 1965). In benign pemphigus, acantholysis is often more pronounced in the suprabasal part of the vesicle than in pemphigus vulgaris; acanthosis and hyperkeratosis are also more marked. Dyskeratosis with *corps ronds* (see below) may be present.

25.1.5.2 Keratosis Follicularis (Darier Disease)

Keratosis follicularis is an autosomal, dominant hereditary disease, but may occur due to mutation. The primary hereditary abnormality in the structure or organization of the desmosomes is unknown. The disease starts in the first or second decade of life.

Eruptions of persistent, discrete and often follicular papules occur in one or several locations. Predilection sites are the face, forehead, scalp, chest and back. Soles and palms may also be affected. Occasionally the oral mucosa is involved (Lever and Lever-Schaumburg 1990). The primary efflorescences are at first skin colored, but soon become hyperkeratotic, rough and crusted. Papules may coalesce and form hypertrophic plaques, which in intertriginous areas easily become infected. Vesicular and bullous lesions occasionally occur. In association with longstanding keratosis follicularis basal cell carcinoma may develop as in Case 11 (below).

The typical histopathologic changes appear in scattered epidermal foci, including hair follicles and the intraepidermal sweat duct units. The main characteristics are suprabasal clefts due to acantholysis and *acantholytic dyskeratosis*. The base of the clefts either consist of well-developed villi (Fig. 25.7a,d), or of a mainly flat surface from which strings of basal cells grow downwards into the dermis. Typically these strings are composed of only two rows of cells (Fig. 25.7e,f). Above the cleft, the dermis is thickened and occasionally papillomatous (Fig. 25.7a). Dyskeratotic keratinocytes in the form of grains and corps ronds are found in the epidermis, the horny layer and in clefts (Fig. 25.7b–e). By dyskeratosis is meant abnormal and premature keratinization of keratinocytes. Grains are large parakeratotic cells with a longitudinal pyknotic nucleus. They are usually found accumulated in clefts. Typical corps ronds are large round keratinocytes with a central basophilic, large and round nucleus. However, they may vary in size, appearance, and color, presumably according to age. Some of them have a compact and strongly eosinophilic cytoplasm. Between foci of typical changes the epidermis is thickened and hyperkeratotic without parakeratosis. In early lesions the sole and nondiagnostic sign may be small foci of discrete suprabasal acantholysis (Fig. 25.8).

25.1.5.3 Transient Acantholytic Dermatosis (Grover Disease)

Transient acantholytic dermatosis was first described by Grover (1970). Usually elderly persons are affected,

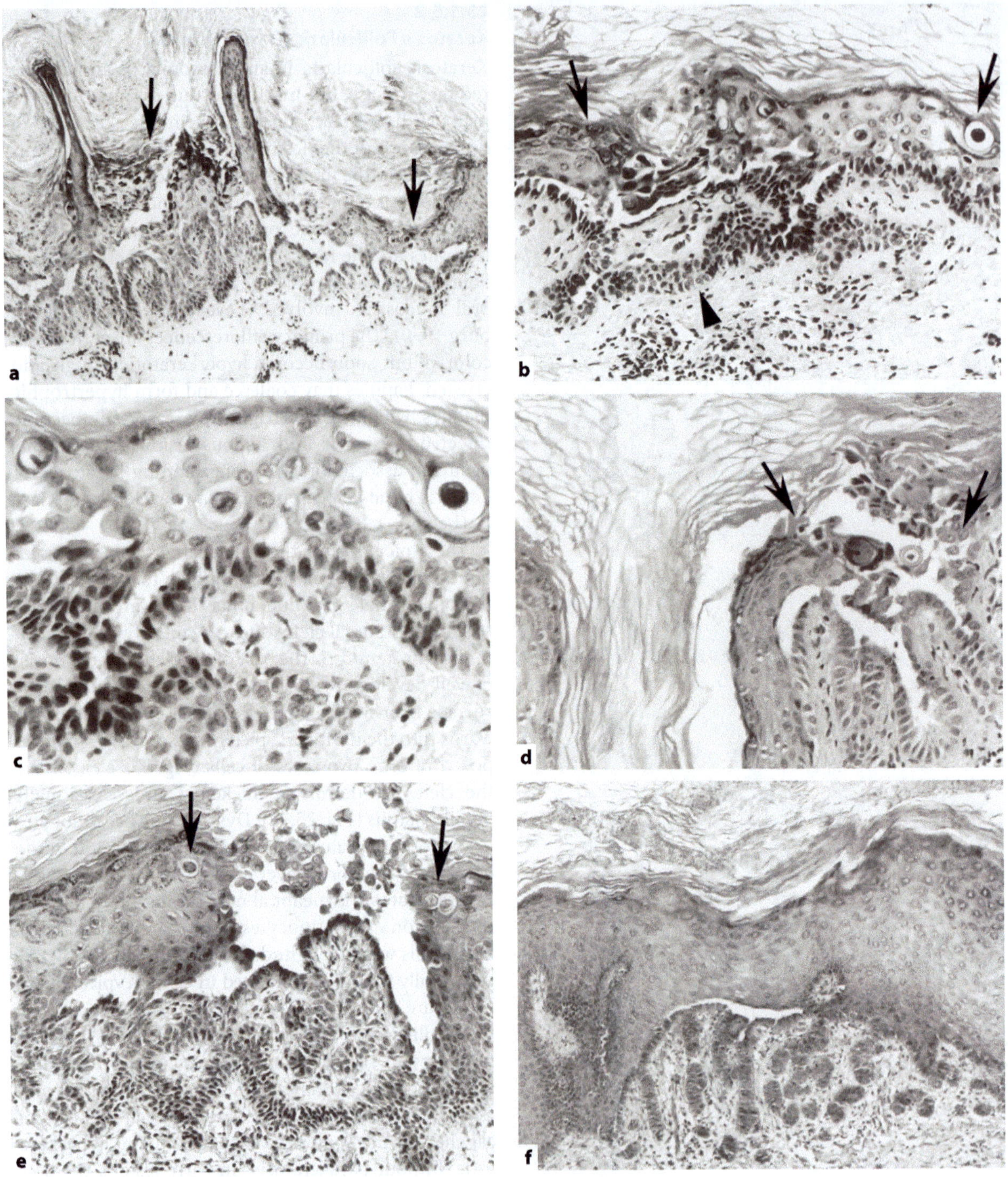

Fig. 25.7 Keratosis follicularis. **a** Papillomatous lesion with marked hyperkeratosis and dyskeratosis (*arrows*) and a suprabasal cleft, the floor of which is composed of villi. **b** Case 10. The dyskeratotic epidermis contains several corps ronds (*arrows*). Bellow the suprabasal fissure there are strands of proliferating basal cells (*arrowhead*). **c** Close-up of the area indicated in **b**. **d** Case 11. A minute lesion close to a hair follicle (*arrows*) contains grains and corps ronds at the top and villi at the base. **e** A cleft in the epidermis comprises dyskeratotic cells (*arrows*) and corps ronds. The papillary dermis is covered with basal cells, which have proliferated as strings in the upper dermis. The longitudinal cleft to the right is probably an affected sweat gland duct. **f** Below a suprabasal gap there are typical strings of proliferating basal cells, composed of two rows of cells. H&E

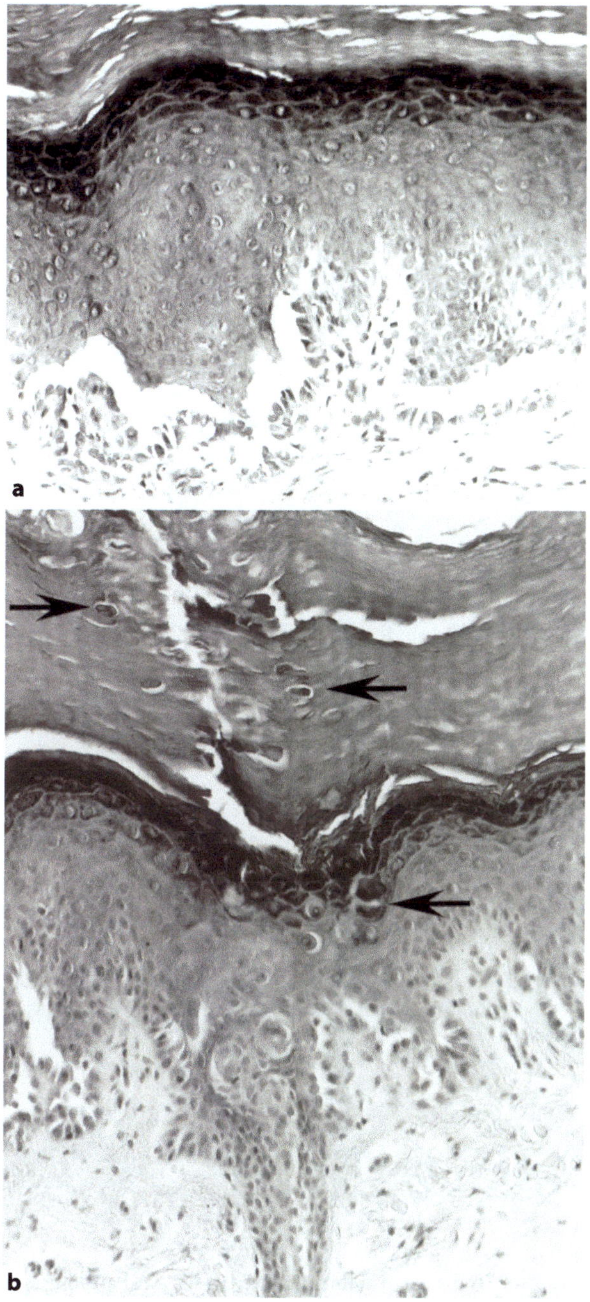

Fig. 25.8 Keratosis follicularis on the palms. **a** There are two small suprabasal clefts not associated with sweat glands and without dyskeratosis. **b** Biopsy specimen taken 1 year later. A sweat gland duct can be followed from the upper dermis through the epidermis to the surface. Along the duct in the granular and horny layers there are scattered dyskeratotic cells (*arrows*). Note also several discrete suprabasal fissures on both sides of the duct. H&E

more often men than women. The cause is unknown, but eruptions have been correlated with intensive sunbathing, sweating and hot baths (Heaphy et al. 1976).

It is clinically characterized by suddenly occurring edematous, and severely itching papules, preferentially located on the chest and back. Lesions usually disappear after some months, but have been reported to remain for more than 2 years (Heaphy et al. 1976).

Histologic investigations have shown that the epidermis contains a few scattered foci, containing clefts or vesicles due to acantholysis. Dyskeratosis may be present or absent. This means that the pattern may mimic small early lesions of pemphigus vulgaris, pemphigus foliaceus, benign familiar pemphigus and keratosis follicularis as well. With such a variable pattern, the case history is decisive of the diagnosis.

Comment

Small foci of acantholytic dyskeratosis, clinically unapparent, are sometimes observed in biopsy specimens from different kinds of lesions, notably tumors such as dermatofibroma, basal cell carcinoma, melanocytic nevus, and malignant melanoma (Ackerman 1972; Schaeppi et al. 2001). In association with a malignant melanoma, localized paraneoplastic pemphigus has been proposed as a label for this phenomenon (Schaeppi et al. 2001). However, systemic involvement and antibodies against desmogleins, present in paraneoplastic pemphigus, are lacking in those cases. This is the reason why the label localized paraneoplastic pemphigus has been firmly rejected by Anhalt (2001).

25.1.5.4 Examples

Case 9. Familial Benign Pemphigus

A 42-year-old man suffered from skin lesions in the axilla and groin. A sister had a similar complaint. The clinical diagnosis was familial benign pemphigus. A biopsy specimen was taken from a plaque in the groin.

The whole epidermis was thickened and hyperkeratotic and showed conspicuous acantholysis. There was a main cleft, the floor of which was made up of villi and elongated, thick rete ridges with marked acantholysis. The upper part of epidermis also displayed large areas of acantholysis and slight dyskeratosis. Many cells had a light nucleus with a distinct nucleolus and a condensed nuclear membrane. Single cells had a very large nucleus. Cells with two nuclei and scattered mitotic figures were also observed (Fig. 25.6).

Case 10. Keratosis Follicularis

A 44-year-old woman presented with widespread follicular hyperkeratotic papules located mainly on the back, at the edge of the scalp, and on the calves. She also had even and confluent hyperkeratosis on the palms and soles. For many years the patient had suffered from a general skin disease with a variable course. The clinical diagnosis was keratosis follicularis. Histologic investigation of a specimen taken from the back disclosed changes typical of keratosis follicularis (Fig. 25.7b,c).

Case 11. Keratosis Follicularis

A 36-year-old woman had had a skin disease from the age of 6 years. Histologic investigation revealed changes typical of keratosis follicularis in close association with an invasive basal cell carcinoma of adenoid type (Fig. 25.7d–f).

Case 12. Keratosis Follicularis

A 15-year-old girl presented with thin, skin-colored papules on the palms and soles. They had been observed for about 6 months and were occasionally pruritic. Histologic investigation of a biopsy specimen from the palm revealed scattered discrete suprabasal clefts (Fig. 25.8a).

The diagnosis was unclear both to the dermatologist and to the present author. The papules continued to occur and a year later a new biopsy was taken. The pattern was regarded by the author as the same as that in the first specimen; thus the diagnosis remained unclear. When several years later old cases with unclear diagnoses were investigated, the referring dermatologist was contacted and provided the information that the patient had gradually developed lesions typical of keratosis follicularis. The slides were reviewed and it was found that in the second specimen the clue to the diagnosis had been overlooked: dyskeratotic cells were present in some epidermal sweat duct units (Fig. 25.8b).

Case 13. Transient Acantholytic Dermatosis

A 73-year-old woman for about 2 months had had pruritic lesions over the sternal area and below the breasts. In these sites closely set erythematous papules and excoriations were observed.

A biopsy specimen revealed a pattern similar to that of keratosis follicularis with two distinct foci, one of which was clearly follicular and showed marked acan-

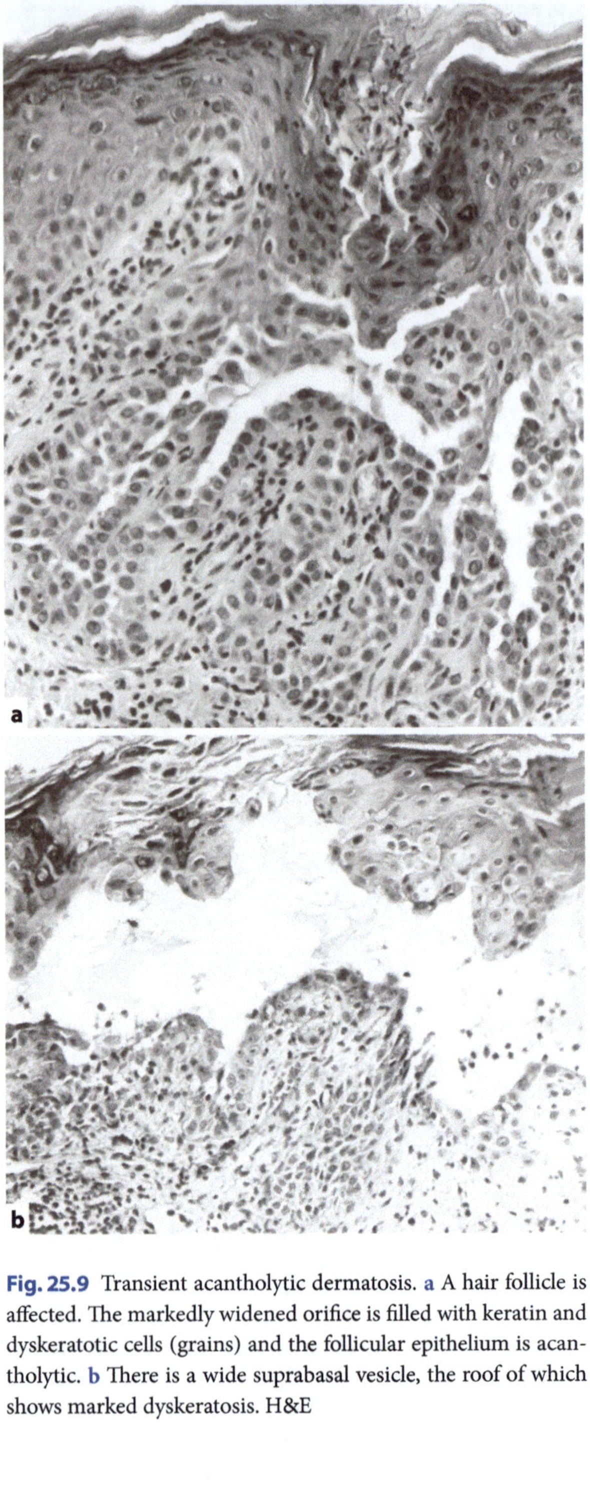

Fig. 25.9 Transient acantholytic dermatosis. **a** A hair follicle is affected. The markedly widened orifice is filled with keratin and dyskeratotic cells (grains) and the follicular epithelium is acantholytic. **b** There is a wide suprabasal vesicle, the roof of which shows marked dyskeratosis. H&E

tholysis. The widened orifice contained grains and a single corps rond (Fig. 25.9a).

Case 14. Transient Acantholytic Dermatosis

A 78-year-old man had suffered for 2 weeks from pruritic papules on the chest and back.

A biopsy specimen showed a central suprabasal vesicle. The floor consisted of villi. The roof was dyskeratotic; some cells resembled corps ronds, others grains. In the papillary dermis there were patchy infiltrates of lymphocytes with scattered eosinophils (Fig. 25.9b).

25.2 Intraepidermal IgA Pustulosis (IgA Pemphigus)

Sneddon and Wilkinson (1956) described a pustular skin disease characterized by outbreaks of sterile neutrophilic pustules strictly located below the stratum corneum; they called it subcorneal pustular dermatosis. This was before the immunofluorescence staining technique was available. However, later direct immunofluorescence revealed intraepidermal deposition of IgA in cases both clinically and histopathologically similar to those described by Sneddon and Wilkinson (Wallach 1992). Also cases with infiltrates of neutrophils in other parts of the epidermis have been reported. These findings initiated a subdivision of the disease into the subcorneal pustular dermatosis type (IgA pemphigus foliaceus) and the intraepidermal neutrophilic type (IgA pemphigus vulgaris).

25.2.1 Clinical Appearance

Characteristically crops of small vesicles on an erythematous base appear on the trunk, the flexor aspect of the extremities, and intertriginous areas. The face

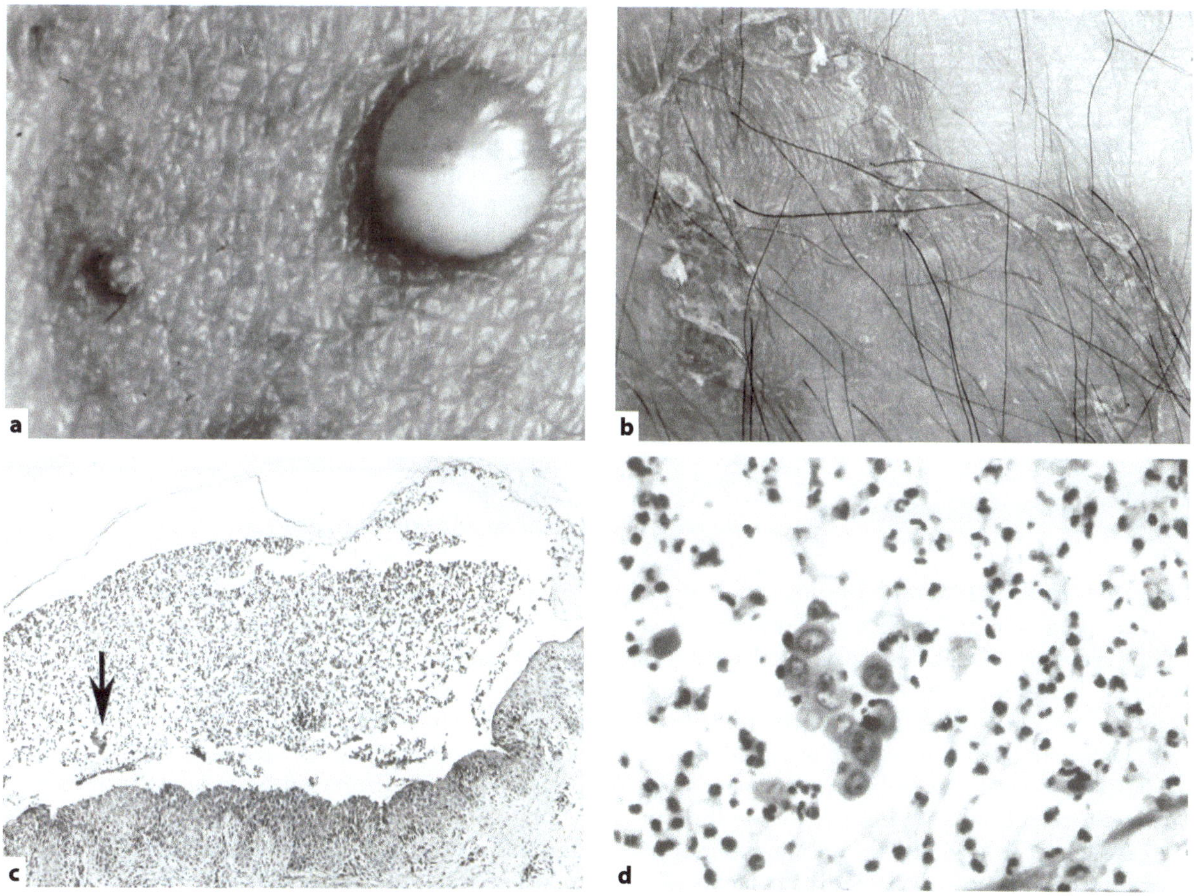

Fig. 25.10 Subcorneal pustular dermatosis. **a** Typical pustule with accumulation of pus in the lower half. **b** Irregular erythematous lesion bordered by large scales. **c** Wide and strictly subcorneal vesicle filled with disintegrating neutrophils and a single small sheet of acantholytic cells (*arrow*). **d** Close-up of the acantholytic cells surrounded by neutrophils. H&E

and scalp are never affected, and palms and soles rarely. The vesicles soon turn into pustules. In a standing position the content of the pustules may form layers, and clear fluid accumulates on the top of a turbid aggregation of neutrophils. The pustules burst after a few days, coalesce and form serpiginous or annular areas with peripheral scales and crusts. New crops wax and wane alternating with periods of remission. The course is benign, but without treatment it may be protracted.

25.2.2 Histopathologic Appearance

The subcorneal pustular dermatosis type is the most common variant. In the intraepidermal neutrophilic type, abscesses may be located in the deep part of the epidermis or the infiltrate may be diffuse. Acantholysis is slight or lacking; spongiosis, if present, is slight. In the upper dermis there are sparse to moderate perivascular infiltrates of neutrophils, lymphocytes and eosinophils.

25.2.3 Pathogenesis

The cause of the disease is not known, nor is the pathogenesis clearly understood. In the subcorneal pustular type IgA is deposited in the upper part of the epidermis, and in the intraepidermal type either in the lower part or in the entire epidermis. In about 50% of patients circulating IgA antibodies against the epithelial cell surface are also present (Robinson et al. 1999).

25.2.4 Example

Case 15. Subcorneal Pustular Dermatosis

A 36-year-old man presented with a widespread and itching eruption which had started 5 weeks previously. Different-sized vesicles and pustules on an erythematous base and large well-circumscribed erythematous areas with peripheral scaling were observed. Some of the pustules showed a layered contents. A biopsy specimen was taken from a vesicular lesion on the trunk. The case was recorded before the immunofluorescence staining technique was available. The contents of the pustules were sterile.

Histologic investigation showed a wide subcorneal pustule. The contents of the pustule consisted of densely packed disintegrating neutrophils and single small sheets of acantholytic keratinocytes. The underlying part of the epidermis was permeated with neutrophils. Spongiosis or acantholysis was not observed. In the upper dermis the perivascular cell infiltrates were composed mainly of lymphocytes (Fig. 25.10).

25.2.5 Differential Diagnosis

- *Bacterial and fungal infections* are excluded by means of culture and PAS staining respectively.
- *Pemphigus foliaceus*. Superficial clefts in pemphigus foliaceus do not contain neutrophils (Fig. 25.5).
- *Psoriasis* has spongiform pustules (Figs. 23.2 and 23.3).

25.2.6 Comment

There is a long list of used or proposed names for this disease (i.e., intraepidermal neutrophilic IgA dermatosis, IgA pemphigus foliaceus, IgA pemphigus vulgaris, atypical neutrophilic dermatosis with subcorneal IgA deposits, intercellular IgA dermatosis, intercellular IgA vesiculopustular dermatosis, IgA herpetiform pemphigus) (Wallach 1992; Robinson et al. 1999). The list mirrors the ambivalence in how to characterize the disease. Is it a pustulosis or is it a kind of pemphigus? Wallach (1992) proposed the TERM *intraepidermal IgA pustulosis*. It seems preferable as long as the pathogenesis is not fully understood. Also acantholysis, the main histologic criterion of pemphigus, is slight or absent in these cases and may be present even in other kinds of pustules such as bullous impetigo.

25.3 Paraneoplastic Pemphigus

Anhalt et al. (1990) described an autoimmune mucocutaneous disease associated with neoplasia observed in five patients. They called the syndrome paraneoplastic pemphigus. Immunofluorescence tests revealed atypical pemphigus-like autoantibodies in perilesional epithelium and in the serum of all five patients. Following this distinctive characterization of the disorder, probably described previously in single case reports as unusual cases of pemphigus vulgaris or erythema multiforme, more than 70 similar patients have been reported (Robinson et al. 1999).

The most common associated neoplasms are in decreasing order of frequency: non-Hodgkin lymphoma, chronic lymphocytic leukemia, and angiofollicular lymph node hyperplasia (Castleman disease); less common are retroperitoneal sarcoma, thymoma (malignant and benign), and Waldenström macroglobulinemia (Anhalt 2001). In approximately two-thirds of the cases the mucocutaneous lesions appear in patients with a known neoplasm. In the remaining one-third a tumor is detected when mucocutaneous symptoms are already present. The prognosis of paraneoplastic pemphigus is poor even if the neoplasm is removed or in complete remission after treatment. Most patients die, either from their autoimmune disease or from complications of treatment (Anhalt 2001). Progressive respiratory failure with clinical features of bronchiolitis obliterans is frequently the cause of death (Nousari et al. 1999).

25.3.1 Clinical Appearance

The constant clinical symptom is severe stomatitis, often associated with conjunctivitis. Skin lesions, if present, are pruritic and polymorphous. In severe cases widespread erythematous maculae or plaques with central vesicles or bullae develop, which break and give rise to large erosions. The condition resembles erythema multiforme or toxic necrolysis and the patient is severely ill with a high fever (Anhalt et al. 1990). In some patients the skin lesions are less acute and consist of widespread lichenoid papules (Ståhle-Bäckdahl et al. 1995).

25.3.2 Histopathologic Appearance

In skin lesions the pattern as a whole may be strikingly lichenoid, as in the two cases demonstrated in Fig. 25.11. Thus in some areas the basic part of the epidermis is destroyed with formation of sawtooth rete ridges, while in the rest of the epidermis keratinocytes are faded and many of them lack a nucleus; scattered intraepidermal apoptotic bodies are also seen. In other areas the epidermis is very thin or necrotic. The granular layer is conspicuous and the horny layer is thickened without parakeratosis. However, subepidermal aggregations of apoptotic bodies typical of lichen planus are lacking (Horn and Anhalt 1992). The most important and discriminating findings are areas of suprabasal vacuolization followed by secondary acantholysis and cleft formation. This phenomenon is emphasized as the hallmark of paraneoplastic pemphigus (Anhalt et al. 1990). However, in contrast to what is the case in pemphigus vulgaris, the floor of the clefts is only partly covered by epithelial cells, and these are more or less disintegrating. In the two demonstrated cases the subepidermal tissue was edematous and contained band-like or patchy cell infiltrates, which mostly were in close contact with the epidermis and consisted of histiocyte-like cells and lymphocytes. Compare Fig. 25.11 with those showing pemphigus vulgaris (Figs. 25.2–25.4) and lichen planus (Figs. 24.1 and 24.2).

25.3.3 Pathogenesis

Direct immunofluorescence shows deposition of IgG in the intercellular spaces of affected skin and mucosal epithelial cells as in pemphigus vulgaris, but in a faint and focal pattern. However, a distinct finding is deposition of complement factor C3 in the epithelial intercellular spaces as well as along the basement membrane (Anhalt 1997). Autoantibodies from the patient's serum also react with monkey esophagus. In contrast to antibodies from pemphigus vulgaris patients, they even react with other kinds of epithelial substrates, most strongly with urinary bladder epithelium, but also with respiratory and intestinal epithelium. The ability of the antibodies to bind to rat urinary bladder has therefore been used as a diagnostic test in suspected cases of paraneoplastic pemphigus (Anhalt et al. 1990).

Immunoprecipitation studies of autoantibodies present in the patient's serum have shown that there are several kinds of antibodies against components of desmosomes and hemidesmosomes (Table 25.1), but not all of them are present in every case. The most common targets are the cytoplasmic plaque proteins envoplakin, periplakin and desmoplakin, and two unidentified antigens, one of 170 kDa and the other of 190 kDa. Antibodies against the transmembrane glycoprotein desmoglein 3 are nearly always found and antibodies against desmoglein 1 occur in two-thirds of cases. However, antibodies against desmogleins are present at a low titer and can only be detected by a special method (Nousari et al. 1999). Sometimes there are also antibodies to the cytoplasmic plaque proteins BPAg (230 kDa) and plectin of the hemidesmosomes (Anhalt 1999).

The release mechanism of the disease is not known. Desmoplakins are present in thymomas and Castleman tumors, and one theory is that autoantibodies directed to desmoplakins in these tumors may cross-react with plakins of the mucocutaneous epithelium. However, the most common neoplasia provoking paraneoplastic pemphigus (non-Hodgkin lymphoma and chronic B-cell leukemia) does not produce desmoplakins (Robinson et al. 1999).

25.3.4 Examples

Case 16. Paraneoplastic Pemphigus

A 55-year-old man was suffering from chronic lymphatic leukemia, diagnosed 2 years previously, when severe stomatitis and conjunctivitis developed. About 6 months later the condition deteriorated. In addition to a high fever and hemorrhagic membranous erosions, widespread skin lesions rapidly developed. The latter consisted of vesicles or bullae on erythematous plaques, which turned into large erosions.

The histopathologic pattern was in accordance of that described above (Fig. 25.11a,b). Direct immunofluorescence showed the presence of IgG throughout the epidermis and complement factor C3 in the basal part of the epidermis as well as at the basal membrane zone. Circulating autoantibodies (titer 1/1280) bound to monkey esophagus with inter- and intracellular fluorescence and to rat bladder transitional epithelium. The serum of the patient immunoprecipitated the antigen complex characteristic of paraneoplastic pemphigus (Ståhle-Bäckdahl et al. 1995).

Case 17. Paraneoplastic Pemphigus

A 71-year old man, previous healthy, presented with erosions on the oral and genital mucosa, conjunctivitis and skin lesions. The latter consisted of areas of densely set lichenoid papules on the trunk and bullae and erosions in intertriginous areas. Investigations revealed that the patient was suffering from B-cell lymphoma.

The histopathologic pattern was in accordance with that described above (Fig. 25.11c–f). Deposition of IgG and C3 were seen in the epidermis and circulating antibodies (titer 1/640) bound to monkey esophagus and to rat bladder epithelium. The serum of the patient immunoprecipitated the antigen complex characteristic of paraneoplastic pemphigus (Ståhle-Bäckdahl et al. 1995).

25.3.5 Comment

The broad spectrum of autoantibodies with predominance for those targeting cytoplasmic proteins of both basal cells and keratinocytes, and the diversity of selection and titer in different patients, may explain the variability in clinical expression and the complex histopathologic pattern of skin lesions in paraneoplastic pemphigus. The latter is distinctly different from that of pemphigus vulgaris, which is due to primary acantholysis caused by autoantibodies against the transmembrane proteins desmogleins 1 and 3. As in lesions of lichen planus, the overwhelming impression is that of primary cell injury, which is in accordance with secondary acantholysis. However, there are also distinct differences between lichen planus and paraneoplastic pemphigus. Scattered apoptotic bodies in the epidermis may be found in both diseases, but aggregations of apoptotic bodies at the epidermal–dermal interface, typical of lichen planus, are not seen in paraneoplastic pemphigus (Horn and Anhalt 1992). Also the suprabasal vesicles present in paraneoplastic pemphigus are not observed in lichen planus or lichen planopilaris.

How then can the similarities in the histopathologic patterns in lichen planus and paraneoplastic pemphigus be explained? In lichen planus, as already mentioned, cytotoxic T cells at the dermal–epidermal junction attack and secrete granzyme B granules and thereby induce apoptosis on basal cells (Shimizu et al. 1997) and progressively cause damage and destruction of keratinocytes from the epidermal–dermal junction towards the surface. The mechanism is a type IV hypersensitivity reaction mediated by sensitized $CD8^+$ cells (Sect. 4.3.4). In paraneoplastic pemphigus the process seems to start in the suprabasal cell layers of the epidermis and progressively causes damage to and destruction of keratinocytes including the basal cells. The presence of autoantibodies against cytoplasmic antigens together with complement justifies considering the process a type II cytotoxic antibody complement-dependent reaction (Sect. 4.3.2). In both lichen

Fig. 25.11 Paraneoplastic pemphigus. **a** Case 16. The pattern is strikingly lichenoid. There are two sawtooth rete ridges (one of them indicated with *small arrows*), and in the basic area vacuolated cells and a single apoptotic body (*large arrow*). The keratinocytes in the rest of the epidermis are faded and many of them lack a nucleus. The stratum granulosum is thickened. There is no parakeratosis. The papillary dermis is edematous and contains a mixed inflammatory cell infiltrate which here is in close contact with the epidermis. **b** Another area shows clefts on both sides of a rete ridge. The floor of the clefts is only partially covered with basal cells (*arrows*). **c** Case 17. Thin, hyperkeratotic epidermal remains with microvesicles in a suprabasal position. **d** Close-up of another area shows severely damaged keratinocytes and small vesicles at the base (*arrow*). Below the left vesicle no keratinocytes can be identified; below the right there is a small chain of flattened keratinocytes. **e** Only thin necrotic epidermal remains are left in close contact with a rather dense inflammatory cell infiltrate (*arrowheads*). **f** Follicular lesion. The pattern is lichenoid, but shows a prominent mainly suprabasal vacuolation and only sparse infiltration of lymphocytes. H&E

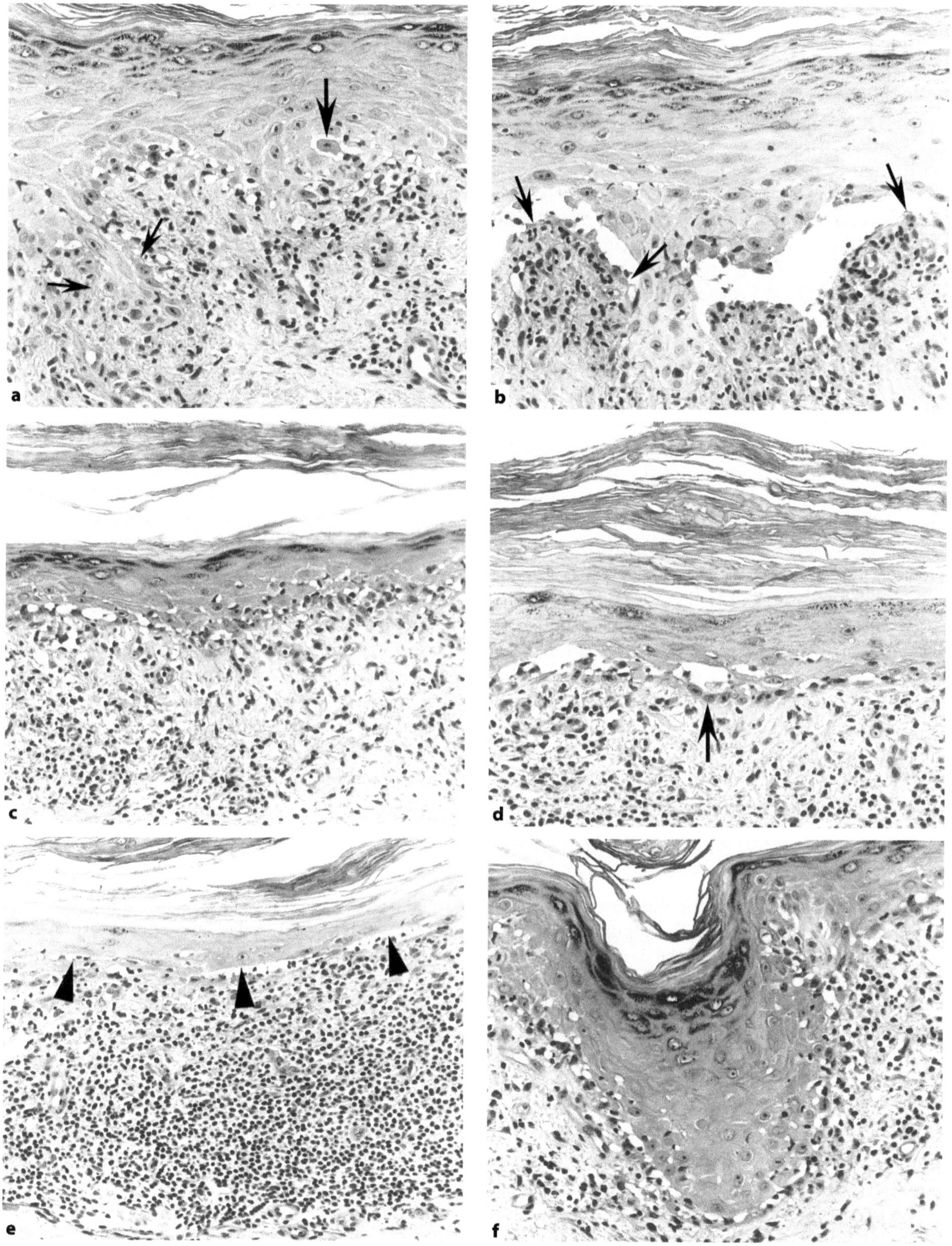
a
b
c
d
e
f

planus and paraneoplastic pemphigus the cell body is primarily attacked, in lichen planus giving rise to many apoptotic bodies and in paraneoplastic pemphigus to secondary acantholysis.

Nousari et al. (1999) investigated two patients, one with Castleman disease and the other with low-grade B-cell non-Hodgkin lymphoma, who developed paraneoplastic pemphigus and died of progressive respiratory failure with clinical features of bronchiolitis obliterans. Endobronchial biopsy specimens showed acantholysis that seemed to be suprabasal. However, respiratory epithelial cells do not express desmogleins or the unidentified 170-kDa antigen, but all plakin antigens recognized by paraneoplastic pemphigus autoantibodies. Also serum from both patients reacted with plakin antigens, which are expressed both by keratinocytes and respiratory epithelial cells. These findings indicate that acantholysis of the respiratory epithelium is a feature of the paraneoplastic syndrome. It is a late complication and may progress after removal or treatment of the underlying neoplasm without evidence of tumor remains. Also mucocutaneous lesions may persist after successful treatment of the tumor. Camisa and Helm (1993) therefore proposed the name neoplasia-induced pemphigus for the syndrome. An even more relevant label might be neoplasia-induced autoimmune mucocutaneous disease (syndrome), which includes the epithelium of the respiratory tract and does not inadequately focus on the pemphigus group.

25.4 Autoimmune Subepidermal Vesicular and Bullous Dermatoses

In autoimmune subepidermal bullous disorders autoantibodies against one or several components are present, which are integral parts of the dermal–epidermal junction area (Fig. 25.1; Table 25.1).

Lever (1965) defined bullous pemphigoid as a subepidermal bullous disorder, clinically and histopathologically different from pemphigus vulgaris. Later bullous pemphigoid and several other kinds of autoimmune subepidermal bullous diseases have been characterized and discriminated by means of immunofluorescence and identification of antigens at the molecular level (Georgi et al. 2001). The value of identifying the exact location of immunoglobulin deposited in the epidermal–dermal junction area has also been focused on. To make this easier salt-split skin technique is used (see Glossary). This preparation splits the skin between the epidermis (layer 1) and lamina lucida (layer 2) and can be used for both direct and indirect immunofluorescence.

25.4.1 Bullous Pemphigoid

Bullous pemphigoid is more common than pemphigus vulgaris and predominantly occurs in old age, but may appear even in young adults and occasionally in small children. Without treatment the course is chronic, but mostly self-healing after months or years. There are periods of remission and exacerbation. The prognosis is good in children and young adults. However, before the use of corticosteroids the mortality was high among older patients (Lever 1965).

25.4.1.1 Clinical Appearance

The disease starts gradually and may in the beginning be localized. Tense bullae, which are often large, appear on seemingly normal skin, or on erythematous areas with serpiginous borders. They may occur all over the body, but predilection sites are the lower abdomen, groin, inner aspect of the thighs and flexor surface of the forearms. Bullae do not break as easily as those in pemphigus vulgaris and denuded areas are small and show a good tendency to heal. About one-third of patients get blisters on the buccal mucosa. As the blisters do not break easily, they are less harmful than oral pemphigus lesions. Usually the lips are not involved.

25.4.1.2 Histopathologic Appearance

Bullous pemphigoid bullae are subepidermal. According to Lever (1965) the process starts with small subepidermal clefts which coalesce and form a bulla (Fig. 25.12a,b). Thus in an early lesion, the floor consists of dermis with the remains of adnexal structures, the roof of the epidermis, which at first is spongiotic or normal, but soon becomes shrunken and finally sheds. As early as after a few days, restoration of the basal part of the epidermis starts at both ends of the bulla (Fig. 27.1f), giving rise at first to an intraepidermal bulla and ultimately to reconstruction of the epidermis. Bullae, which are located on an erythematous base, are filled with eosinophils and the upper dermis is edematous and infiltrated by inflammatory cells, mainly eosinophils. The perilesional parts of the epidermis may be spongiotic and infiltrated by eosinophils. In lesions appearing on seemingly normal skin the inflammatory response is much less conspicuous.

25.4.1.3 Pathogenesis

The triggering cause is usually not known. Occasionally drugs have been suspected. A case control study (Bastuji-Garin et al. 1996) indicated a possible association with neuroleptics and aldosterone-antagonist diuretics. Direct immunofluorescence shows depositions of IgG and C3 along the basement membrane on the epidermal side of salt-split skin. In 80% of patients there are circulating autoantibodies against the 230-kDa BPAg cytoplasmic plaque protein and the 180-kDa BPAg transmembrane glycoprotein of the hemidesmosomes.

25.4.1.4 Differential Diagnosis

- *Anti-P200 pemphigoid*, *anti-P105 pemphigoid*, and *anti-P450 pemphigoid* are variants of bullous pemphigoid (Georgi et al. 2001).
- *Epidermolysis bullosa acquisita* is an autoimmune subepidermal bullous disease induced by trauma and is histologically indistinguishable from bullous pemphigoid. However, deposits of IgG and C3 are located on the dermal side of salt-split skin. Circulating IgG antibodies against collagen VII may be present (Georgi et al. 2001).
- *Acute systemic lupus erythematosus* may give rise to subepidermal vesicles/bullae. Autoantibodies against components in the epidermal–dermal junction area, most often collagen VII, have been found (Georgi et al. 2001).
- *Dermatitis herpetiformis*, *linear IgA dermatosis*, *cicatricial pemphigoid* and *acquired porphyria cutanea tarda* (sporadic or type I) are other dermatoses that histopathologically may be difficult to differentiate from bullous pemphigoid. See below.

25.4.2 Dermatitis Herpetiformis

Dermatitis herpetiformis is a chronic, lifelong disease that may affect both children and adults, but usually starts in the second to fourth decades of life.

25.4.2.1 Clinical Appearance

Typical lesions consist of eruptions of severely itching groups of erythematous papules and papulovesicles symmetrically distributed on elbows, knees, buttocks, shoulders, and the sacral area. However, widespread non-grouped lesions may also appear, and occasionally there are large bullae. Mucosal lesions and eruptions on palms and soles are rare; in the latter two locations, lesions may be hemorrhagic. Eruptions wax and wane. Old papulovesicles become crusted and resolve leaving pigmentation.

25.4.2.2 Histopathologic Appearance

In early lesions small pustules composed of neutrophils, located on the top of dermal papillae, are highly characteristic (Piérard and Whimster 1961; MacVicar et al. 1963). These small pustules coalesce and form a large subepidermal vesicle or bulla filled mainly with neutrophils; the latter is in contrast to bullous pemphigoid where most cells are eosinophils. Sometimes suprapapillary pustules may be seen besides large vesicles (Fig. 25.12c,d)

25.4.2.3 Pathogenesis

Immunofluorescence shows deposition of granular IgA mostly in the dermal papillae and sometimes along the basement membrane. The target antigen is not known. HLA typing has shown that a high number of patients with dermatitis herpetiformis have the human histocompatibility antigen HLA-B8. The disease is nearly always associated with gluten-sensitive enteropathy.

25.4.3 Linear IgA Dermatosis

Linear IgA dermatosis is a rare autoimmune disease. It was previously regarded as a variant of dermatitis herpetiformis, but is now thought to be a separate disease with several patterns of clinical expression. Clinically it may be similar to dermatitis herpetiformis, epidermolysis bullosa acquisita, bullous pemphigoid or cicatricial pemphigus. Most commonly it mimics dermatitis herpetiformis and is often associated with severe itch. Oral lesions are common, and sometimes there are also conjunctival lesions mimicking cicatricial pemphigoid (Hall 1999).

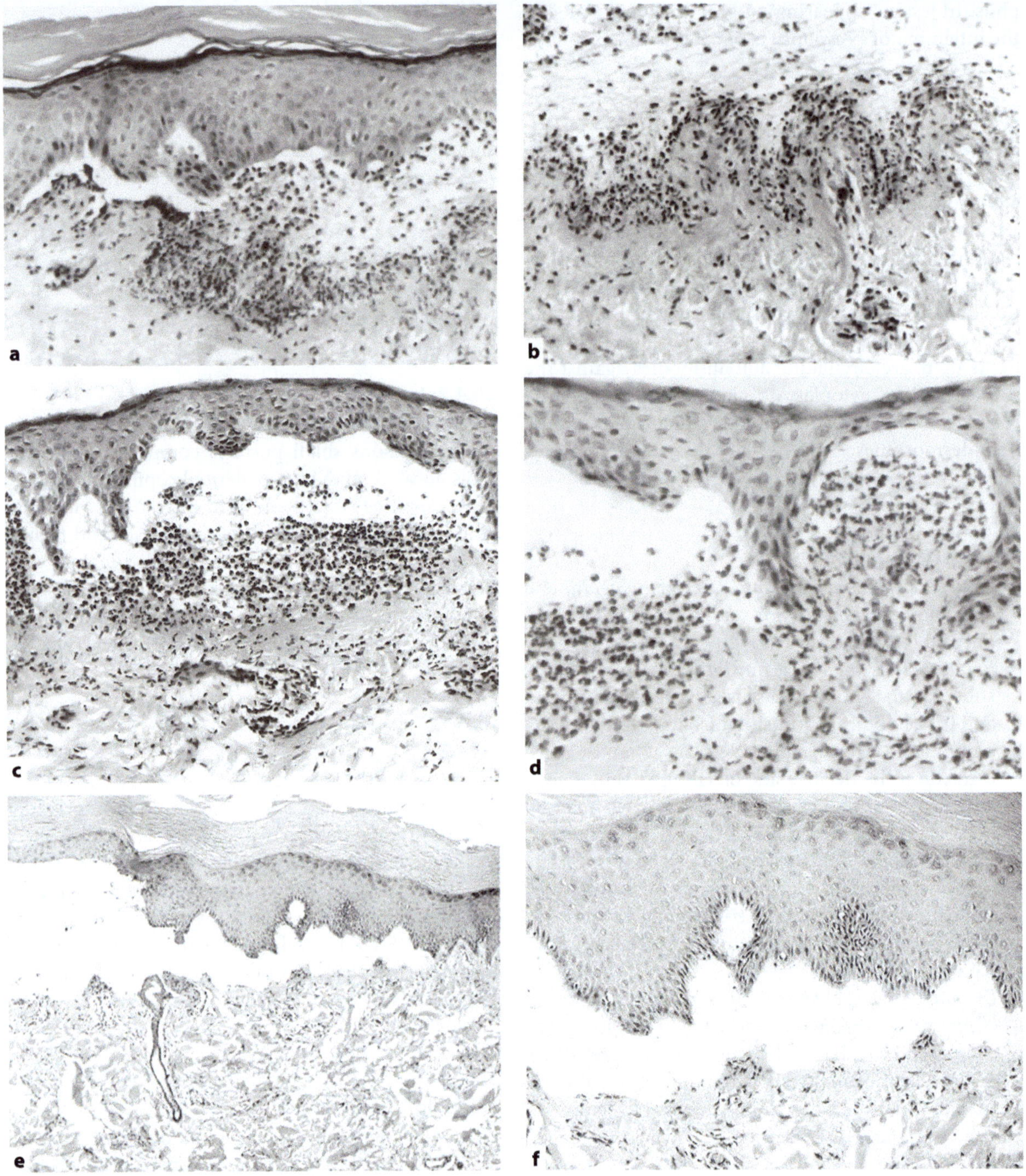

Fig. 25.12 Autoimmune subepidermal bullous diseases: **a, b** bullous pemphigoid; **c, d** dermatitis herpetiformis; **e, f** porphyria cutanea tarda. **a** A fresh subepidermal bulla contains a dense inflammatory cell infiltrate. **b** Close-up of the floor shows elongated dermal papillae, densely infiltrated by inflammatory cells (eosinophils). **c** There is a large subepidermal vesicle containing many neutrophils. **d** Close-up of the area to the right of the large vesicle shows a typical suprapapillary abscess composed of neutrophils. **e** A part of a subepidermal bulla. The cleft cuts through a sweat duct. The epidermis is well preserved at the end; in the center shrunken. **f** Close-up of well-preserved epidermis and dermal papillae. The inflammatory cell infiltrate is sparse. H&E

Histologically there are subepidermal vesicles filled mainly with neutrophils. In contrast to dermatitis herpetiformis, it shows linear deposition of IgA along the basement membrane. There are indications of more than one target antigen, and electron microscopy has shown that a blister forms either within the lamina lucida or in the sublamina densa layer.

Linear IgA dermatitis may be triggered by drugs and is sometimes associated with neoplasm. The disease has no association with enteropathy. *Chronic bullous disease of childhood* is a variant of linear IgA dermatosis.

25.4.4 Cicatricial Pemphigoid

Cicatricial pemphigoid is an uncommon chronic autoimmune disease with many previous labels, the most common of which is *benign mucous membrane pemphigoid*. It affects elderly individuals, women more often than men.

Clinically there are vesicles and erosions with predilection for the oral mucosa and conjunctiva. However, other mucosal membranes as well as the skin may be affected. At least some lesions heal with scarring. The vesicles are subepidermal. Immunofluorescence and autoantigen studies have indicated that cicatricial pemphigoid is not a single disease (Yancey 1999).

25.4.5 Acquired Porphyria Cutanea Tarda (Sporadic or Type I)

Acquired porphyria cutanea tarda usually starts in the third or fourth decade of life. Exposure to sunlight and minor trauma result in vesicles on the dorsal aspect of the hands and feet and sometimes on the face. The lesions heal with slight scarring. In affected areas the skin may become thickened and sclerotic. On the face hypertrichosis is common.

The blisters are subepidermal. The dermal papillae are well preserved and protrude into the bulla. The inflammatory response is slight (Fig. 25.12e,f). Immunofluorescence shows deposition of granular C3 and IgG along the dermal–epidermal junction and sometimes also in and around vessel walls (Bickers et al. 1999).

Liver damage provoked by, for example, alcohol abuse or treatment with drugs such as estrogenic hormones may disturb the synthesis of the heme part of hemoglobin. The disturbed production of hemoglobin results in high levels of porphyrins both in the urine and the skin. In the skin, the porphyrins provoke the development of fragile blisters when activated by ultraviolet light.

Blisters with the same histopathologic pattern as that seen in porphyria cutanea tarda also occur in phototoxic drug eruptions (Sect. 28.6).

References

1. Ackerman AB (1972) Focal acantholytic dyskeratosis. Arch Dermatol 106:702–706
2. Anhalt GJ (1997) Paraneoplastic pemphigus. Adv Dermatol 12:77–96
3. Anhalt GJ (1999) Making sense of antigens and antibodies in pemphigus. J Am Acad Dermatol 40:763–766
4. Anhalt GJ (2001) Paraneoplastic pemphigus. The role of tumors and drugs. Br J Dermatol 144:1101–1104
5. Anhalt GJ, Kim S, Stanley JR, Korman NJ, Jabs DA, Kory M, Izumi H, Ratrie H, Mutasim D, Ariss-Abdo L, Labib RS (1990) Paraneoplastic pemphigus. An autoimmune mucocutaneous disease associated with neoplasia. N Engl J Med 323:1729–1735
6. Bastuji-Garin S, Joly P, Picard-Dahan C, Bernard P, Vaillant L, Pauwels C, Salagnac V, Lok C, Roujeau J-C (1996) Drugs associated with bullous pemphigoid. A case control study. Arch Dermatol 132:272–276
7. Beutner EH, Lever WF, Witebsky E, Jordon R, Chertock B (1965) Autoantibodies in pemphigus vulgaris. Response to an intercellular substance of epidermis. JAMA 192:682–688
8. Bickers DR, Pathak MA, Lim HW (1999) The porphyrias. In: Freedberg IM, Eisen AZ, Wolff K, Austen KF, Goldsmith LA, Katz SI, Fitzpatrick TB (eds) Fitzpatrick's dermatology in general medicine. McGraw-Hill, New York, pp 1766–1803
9. Bjarnason B, Flosadóttir E (1999) Childhood, neonatal, and stillborn pemphigus vulgaris. Int J Dermatol 38:680–688
10. Camisa C, Helm TN (1993) Paraneoplastic pemphigus is a distinct neoplasia-induced autoimmune disease. Arch Dermatol 129:883–886
11. Emmerson RW, Wilson-Jones E (1968) Eosinophilic spongiosis in pemphigus. A report of an unusual histological change in pemphigus. Arch Dermatol 97:252–257
12. Georgi M, Jainta S, Bröcker EB, Zillikens D (2001) Autoantigens of subepidermal bullous autoimmune dermatoses (in German). Hautarzt 52:1079–1089
13. Grover RW (1970) Transient acantholytic dermatosis. Arch Dermatol 101:426–434
14. Hall RP (1999) Linear IgA dermatosis and chronic bullous disease of childhood. In: Freedberg IM, Eisen AZ, Wolff K, Austen KF, Goldsmith LA, Katz SI, Fitzpatrick TB (eds) Fitzpatrick's dermatology in general medicine. McGraw-Hill, New York, pp 680–685

15. Heaphy MR, Tucker SB, Winkelmann RK (1976) Benign papular acantholytic dermatosis. Arch Dermatol 112:814–821
16. Horn TD, Anhalt GJ (1992) Histologic features of paraneoplastic pemphigus. Arch Dermatol 128:1091–1095
17. Lever WF (1965) Pemphigus and pemphigoid. Charles C. Thomas, Springfield
18. Lever W, Schaumburg-Lever G (1990) Histopathology of the skin. J.B. Lippincott, Philadelphia
19. MacVicar DN, Graham JH, Burgoon CF (1963) Dermatitis herpetiformis, erythema multiforme and bullous pemphigoid. A comparative histopathologic and histochemical study. J Invest Dermatol 41:289–300
20. Mahoney MG, Wang Z, Rothenberger K, Koch PJ, Amagai M, Stanley JR (1999) Explanations for the clinical and microscopic localization of lesions in pemphigus foliaceus and vulgaris. J Clin Invest 103:461–468
21. Nousari HC, Deterding R, Wojtczack H, Aho S, Uitto J, Hashimoto T, Anhalt GJ (1999) The mechanism of respiratory failure in paraneoplastic pemphigus. N Engl J Med 340:1406–1410
22. Piérard J, Whimster I (1961) The histological diagnosis of dermatitis herpetiformis, bullous pemphigoid and erythema multiforme. Br J Dermatol 73:253–266
23. Robinson ND, Hashimoto T, Amagai M, Chan LS (1999) The new pemphigus variants. J Am Acad Dermatol 40:649–671
24. Santi CG, Maruta CW, Aoki V, Sotto MN, Rivitti EA, Diaz LA (1996) Pemphigus herpetiformis is a rare clinical expression of nonendemic pemphigus foliaceus, fogo selvagem, and pemphigus vulgaris. J Am Acad Dermatol 34:40–46
25. Schaeppi H, Bauer JW, Hametner R, Metze D, Ortiz-Urda S, Salmhofer W, Rappersberger K, Hintner H (2001) A localized variant of paraneoplastic pemphigus. Acantholysis associated with malignant melanoma. Br J Dermatol 144:1249–1254
26. Shimizu M, Higaki Y, Higaki M, Kawashima M (1997) The role of granzyme B-expressing CD8-positive T cells in apoptosis of keratinocytes in lichen planus. Arch Dermatol Res 289:527–532
27. Sneddon IB, Wilkinson DS (1956) Subcorneal pustular dermatosis. Br J Dermatol 68:385–394
28. Ståhle-Bäckdahl M, Hedblad M-A, Skoglund C, Fagerholm P, Anhalt GJ (1995) Paraneoplastic pemphigus: a report of two patients responding to cyclosporin. Eur J Dermatol 5:671–675
29. Wallach D (1992) Intraepidermal IgA pustulosis. J Am Acad Dermatol 27:993–1000
30. Wananukul S, Pongprasit P (1999) Childhood pemphigus. Int J Dermatol 38:29–35
31. Woodley DT, Chen M (2001) The basement membrane zone. In: Freinkel RK, Woodley DT (eds) The biology of the skin. Parthenon, New York, pp 133–152
32. Yancey KB (1999) Cicatricial pemphigoid. In: Freedberg IM, Eisen AZ, Wolff K, Austen KF, Goldsmith LA, Katz SI, Fitzpatrick TB (eds) Fitzpatrick's dermatology in general medicine. McGraw-Hill, New York, pp 674–679

Chapter 26

Recurrent Vesicular Eruptions 26

Erythema multiforme (EM), *eosinophilic cellulitis*, and *pityriasis lichenoides et varioliformis acuta* are three different vesicular conditions with some common traits: they appear suddenly, are self-healing and often recur at intervals over several years, sometimes decades.

26.1 Erythema Multiforme

The nomenclature concerning EM is confusing. The clinical pattern of a group of similar diseases was first described by Hebra in 1866 and by him called erythema exudativum multiforme (Fritsch and Ruiz-Maldonado 1999). The less-severe variant in this group was called *erythema multiforme minor*. The reason was to differentiate it from Stevens-Johnson disease, considered to be a more serious variant of EM and therefore also called *erythema multiforme major*. However, today Stevens-Johnson disease is considered a less-severe variant of *toxic epidermal necrolysis* (Sect. 28.4).

26.1.1 Clinical Appearance

EM is characterized by a sudden eruption of erythematous, rounded, urticaria-like efflorescences, which vary in size from a few to 20–30 mm in diameter. They have a symmetrical, acral position and are mainly located on the hands, forearms and face. Some of these lesions develop into so-called target lesions, the clinical hallmark of EM. A typical target lesion is less than 3 cm in diameter, has a well-defined border and is composed of at least three concentric rings of different colors: a dark center is surrounded by a light rim, which in turn is encircled by a peripheral erythematous area (Bastuji-Garin et al. 1993). Sometimes the center becomes vesicular and may give rise to denuded areas. The first eruption is sometimes followed by one or a few new eruptions at short intervals. In some patients the oral mucosa is slightly or moderately affected. General symptoms are slight or absent. The disease is self-healing in a few weeks, but recurrences are frequent. The disease predominantly affects adolescents and young adults.

26.1.2 Histopathologic Appearance

Histopathologically two variants of EM are described: *dermal type* and *epidermal type*.

EM of dermal type is characterized by a conspicuous subepidermal edema in which an essentially normal epidermis is detached giving rise to a vesicle in the center of the lesion (Fig. 26.1a,b). In the underlying dermis there are dense, perivascular or diffuse cell infiltrates composed of mononuclear cells. Occasionally there is an admixture of eosinophils. There may be extravasation of erythrocytes, but no vasculitis (Lever and Schaumburg-Lever 1990).

EM of epidermal type starts as an interface dermatitis. Inflammatory cells invade the basal epidermis which shows intercellular edema, focal cell necrosis and subepithelial vesiculation. In a fully developed lesion there is a subepidermal vesicle showing necrosis and/or reticular degeneration of the epidermis (Fig. 26.1c–f). In the upper dermis there are infiltrates of lymphocytes and histiocytes and often extravasation of erythrocytes, but no vasculitis.

The two types of EM have become a matter of controversy. Some authors maintain that there is only one type, the epidermal (Ackerman et al. 1971; Ackerman and Ragaz 1985), others that both variants exist (Bedi and Pinkus 1976; Lever 1985; Reed 1985).

Orfanos et al. (1974) investigated biopsy specimens from 24 patients with EM by means of light and electron microscopy. Electron microscopy showed that in bullae caused by subepidermal edema the roof included the basal lamina, while in the other kind, the basal lamina, if identified, was located at the floor. There was a clear difference between dermal and epidermal vesicles; a mixed pattern was not observed.

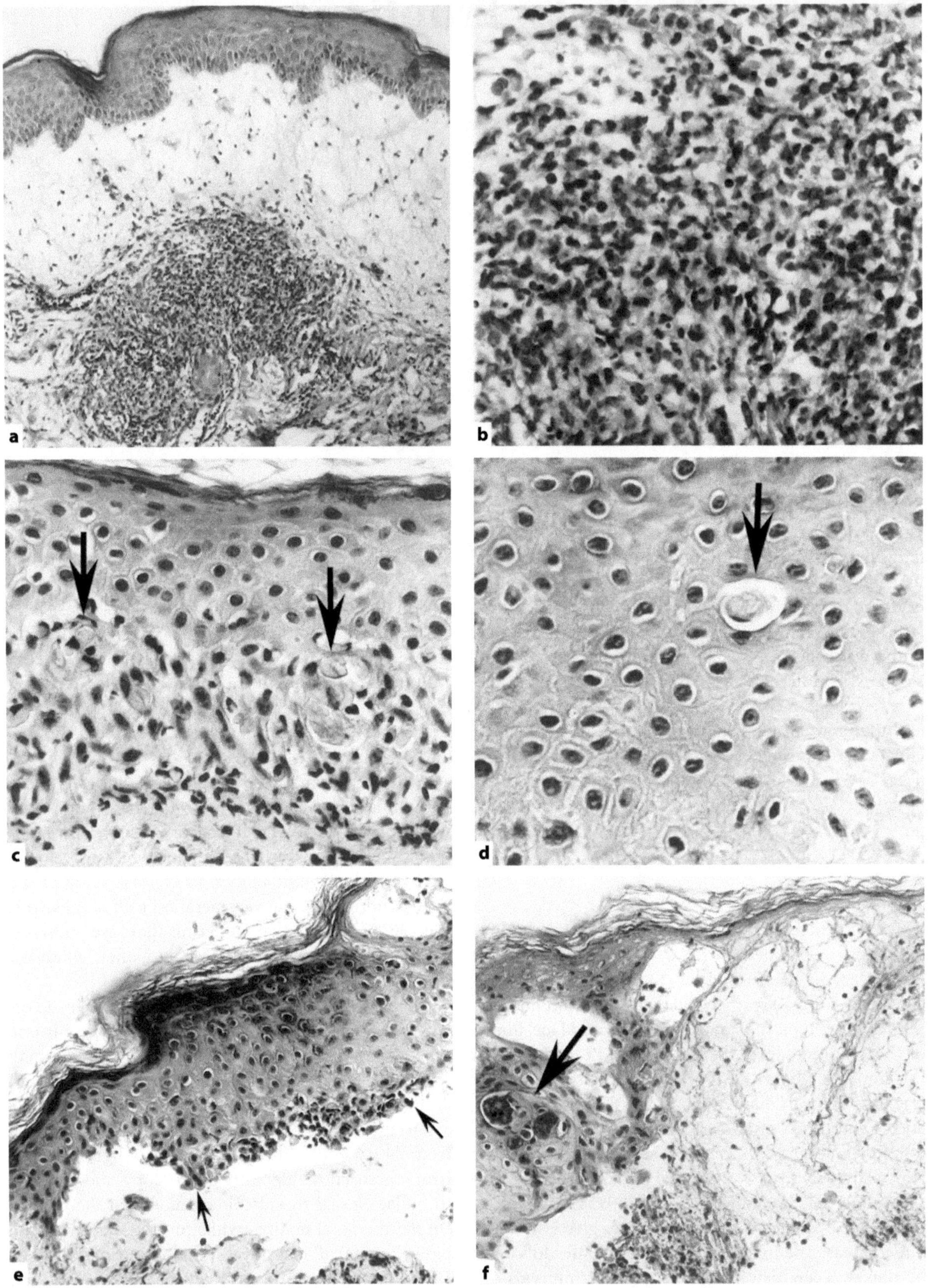
a
b
c
d
e
f

26.1.3 Pathogenesis

EM has been associated with infections and drugs. In some patients, but not in all, recurrent spells of herpes simplex are after a while (a few days to 2 weeks) followed by an outbreak of EM. A close relationship between the two diseases has for a long time been suspected, but the presence of HSV in lesions of EM has not been possible to prove by means of culture or in situ hybridization. However, in recent years, investigations by the more sensitive PCR technique (see Glossary) have shown that during a spell of EM, fragments of herpes simplex DNA are present both in blood cells and in keratinocytes of lesional skin. In healed skin the fragments remain for about 1 to 5 months (Brice et al. 1994; Imafuku et al. 1997; Aurelian et al. 2004). The inflammatory cells in EM lesions are primarily HSV-specific $CD4^{+}$-1 cells, which produce IFN-γ. The latter may then upregulate different kinds of cytokines including TGF-β (Sect. 4.1.5). The inflammation is amplified and may, by recruitment of cytotoxic lymphocytes ($CD8^{+}$ cells and NK cells), give rise to epidermal damage. The mechanism is not fully understood. However, it is thought that during a spell of herpes simplex, virus DNA is picked up and fragmented by macrophages or by precursors of Langerhans cells, present in the circulation, and then deposited in the skin. According to Aurelian et al. (2004) the presence of primarily HSV-specific $CD4^{+}$-1 cells, IFN-γ and TGF-β, but not TNF-α, is typical of EM caused by HSV.

EM without signs of infection with HSV has been associated with infections caused by VZV, CMV, or *Mycoplasma pneumoniae*, and with drugs (Aurelian et al. 2004).

Fig. 26.1 Erythema multiforme. **a** Dermal type. The epidermis is detached from the dermis by a conspicuous subepidermal edema. In the upper dermis there is a dense patchy cell infiltrate. **b** The infiltrate consists mainly of mononuclear cells, but contains even nuclear fragments. **c** Epidermal type. Inflammatory cells invade the dermal–epidermal interface. In the lower part of the epidermis there are groups of apoptotic bodies (*arrows*). **d** Close-up of another area of the epidermis shows a single apoptotic body (*arrow*). **e** Epidermal type. In this case one end of the bulla consists of a subepidermal cleft. The overlying epidermis is well preserved, but is basically invaded by inflammatory cells (*arrows*). **f** The rest of the lesion consists of a sub- and intraepidermal bulla with marked reticular degeneration and superficial thin and necrotic remains of the epidermis. The *arrow* indicates eosinophilic necrosis and apoptotic bodies in the better-preserved part of the epidermis. H&E

26.1.4 Examples

Case 1. Erythema Multiforme of Epidermal Type

A 20-year-old woman had had a spell of herpes simplex on the left buttock 5 months previously. Nine days after a recurrence at the same location she presented with EM lesions on the hands and forearms. She also had vesicles in the mouth and vulva. A biopsy specimen was taken from the forearm.

Histologic investigation showed a wide area of marked interface dermatitis with invading inflammatory cells and aggregates of apoptotic bodies. This area passed into a large subepidermal vesicle with a thin and eosinophilic roof. Between slender rete ridges there were the remains of reticular degeneration and aggregates of large and highly degenerated epithelial cells. The pattern was very like that seen in an advanced herpes vesicle with reticular degeneration (Fig. 20.2a–c), but no giant cells or inclusion bodies were identified. In the upper dermis there were small perivascular infiltrates of lymphocytes (Fig. 26.1c,d).

Case 2. Erythema Multiforme of Epidermal Type

A 32-year-old man presented with classical EM lesions on the trunk and extremities. The consulting form did not note possible HSV infection.

Histologic investigation revealed a subepidermal bulla, the roof of which showed conspicuous reticular degeneration, areas of eosinophilic necrosis, and small groups of apoptotic bodies (Fig. 26.1e,f). The pattern was very much similar to that seen in Case 1, and thus like an advanced herpes vesicle without inclusion bodies or giant cells.

26.1.5 Comment

It is evident that lesions considered clinically to be EM may show one or the other histopathologic pattern. However, the author has seen the dermal variant in specimens from lesions which were associated with drug administration, but clinically did not resemble EM. The two cases described above emphasize the association between HSV infection and EM. It is tempting to think that the epidermal variant exclusively appears in HSV-induced cases and the dermal variant exclusively in EM of other causes. Maybe this is not the case. The only way to resolve this issue would be to investigate biopsy specimens from patients with clinically well-documented EM for the presence or absence of HSV and with respect to the histopathologic as well as the molecular pattern.

26.1.6 Differential Diagnosis

- *Bullous pemphigoid* may be mistaken for EM of dermal type. However, the bullae in bullous pemphigoid, due to antibodies against components of the epidermal–dermal junction area, have abrupt and rather distinct ends, while the bullae in dermal EM, due to a marked edema in the uppermost dermis, gradually tail off. Also bullae in pemphigoid usually contain many eosinophils, while bullae of dermal EM contain a sparse or moderate number of lymphocytes.
- A lesion from recurrent EM of epidermal type associated with HSV may be difficult to differentiate from an old herpes vesicle. In the latter, identification of virus giant cells is crucial (Chapter 20).

26.2 Eosinophilic Cellulitis

Wells and Smith (1979) described a series of patients, who presented with suddenly appearing skin lesions that showed a striking histopathologic pattern and followed a characteristic course. The disease was first called granulomatous dermatitis with eosinophilia and later eosinophilic cellulitis. It is also known as Wells syndrome.

26.2.1 Clinical Appearance

Eosinophilic cellulitis is a rare disease that may affect persons of all ages, even small children (Anderson et al. 1995). Recurrences at short or long intervals, sometimes of a year or more, are common. In typical cases the patient suddenly experiences a spell of edema and erythema in one or several locations. The lesions often cover large areas and some of them show vesicles or bullae in the central part. New lesions appear, while others subside. The eruption may be associated with severe itch, a burning sensation, or pain. If not treated, the acute edema and redness subside and affected areas become indurated and take on a bluish color. The induration and discoloration successively abate and the lesions heal after a few or several weeks without residue (Wells and Smith 1979). Blood eosinophilia is common. Fever may occur, but other general symptoms are absent.

26.2.2 Histopathologic Appearance

Both the dermis and subcutaneous tissue may be affected and show conspicuous edema and massive infiltration of inflammatory cells in addition to so-called *flame figures* (Fig. 26.2). In H&E-stained sections, the flame figure is bright red and composed of a collagen bundle, to which aggregates of eosinophilic granules are attached. In an early flame figure the aggregates of granules are rather small and the surrounding edematous tissue contains eosinophils, disintegrating eosinophils, extruded eosinophilic granules, and basophilic nuclear fragments (Fig. 26.2b). The core of older lesions consists of dense aggregates of eosinophilic granules around a normal-looking piece of collagen and is encircled by a more or less well-developed granuloma. The granuloma is composed of histiocytes and lymphocytes, and sometimes a few multinucleated giant cells (Fig. 26.2c,d). There may be only a single flame figure or many, some of which may be located in the subcutis (Fig. 26.2a,c). The collagen making up the core of the flame figure stains normally with H&E and vG. Intracellular eosinophilic granules, extruded granules and aggregates of granules adherent to collagen bundles are stained bright red with H&E and dusky yellow with vG.

The formation of vesicles and bullae may be due to subepidermal edema, intraepidermal vesiculation or a combination of both. Sometimes there is central ulceration. The inflammatory cell infiltrate in the dermis and subcutis is both diffuse and patchy with aggregates of lymphocytes and eosinophils. There are also histiocytes and a few mast cells. Neutrophils are usually sparse. There are many dilated thin-walled vessels (venules and lymphatics), but no vasculitis or necrosis.

26.2.3 Pathogenesis

The triggering factor in eosinophilic cellulitis is in most cases unknown. Arthropod bite, infections and drugs have been suggested or proved in some cases (Wells and Smith 1979; Schorr et al. 1984; Brehmer-Andersson et al. 1986). The mechanism of the disease is not known. Human eosinophilic granules contain, among other proteins, major basic protein (MBP), which makes up >50% of the granular protein, eosinophilic cationic protein and eosinophil-derived neurotoxin (Peters et al. 1986). All three proteins have cytotoxic properties. A possible cytotoxic effect of eosinophilic granules is the reason for considering the flame figure to be degenerated collagen and the granuloma formation around them secondary to necrosis (Wells and Smith 1979; Spigel and Winkelmann 1979).

However, by using an indirect immunofluorescence technique, Peters et al. (1983) were able to localize the MBP in lesions of eosinophilic cellulitis. Areas of fluo-

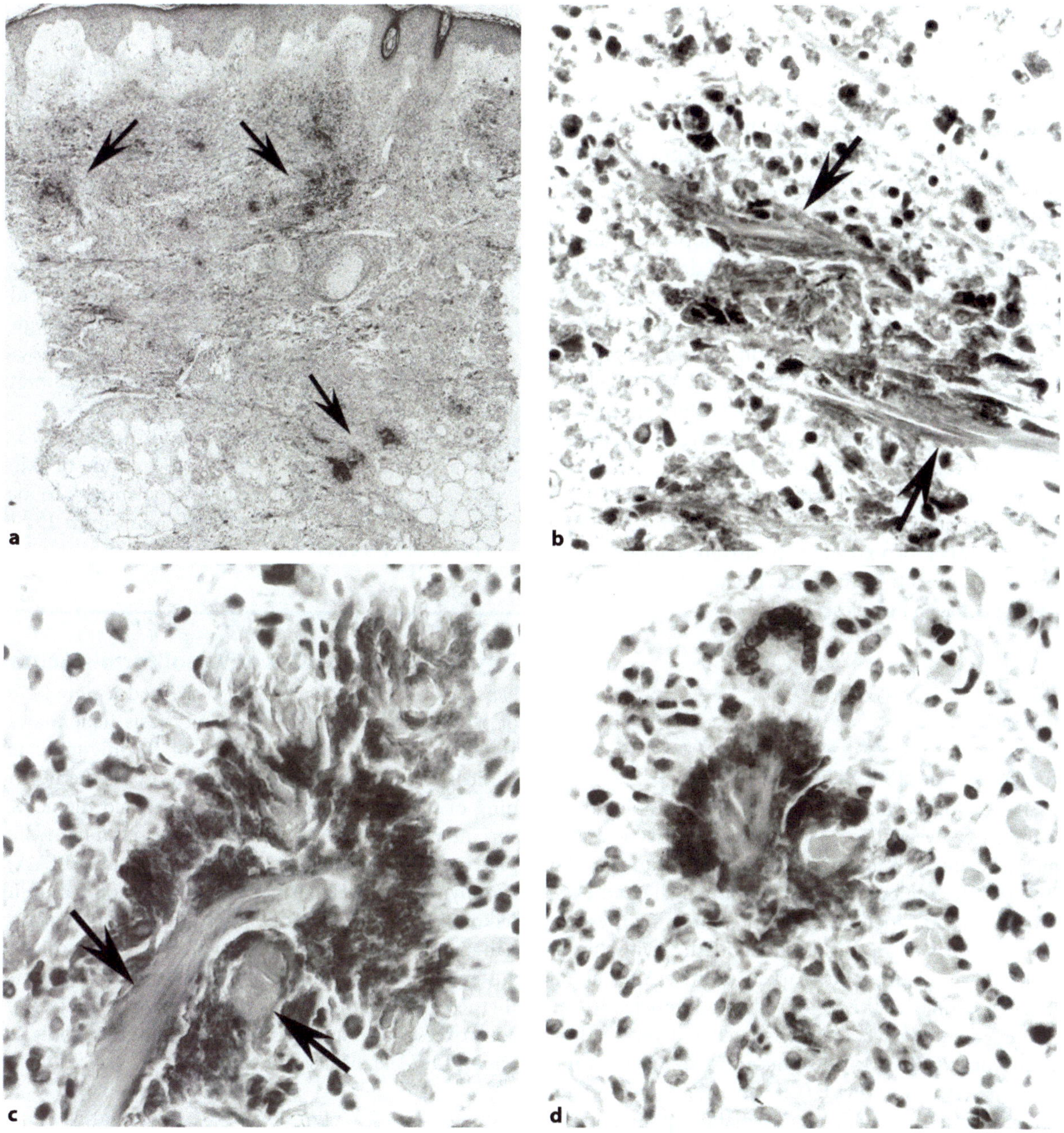

Fig. 26.2 Eosinophilic cellulitis. **a** There is a subepidermal edema with a vesicle in the making. The dermis and subcutis are edematous and densely infiltrated by inflammatory cells. The *arrows* indicate groups of flame figures. **b** Detail from the upper dermis. Two fragments of collagen bundles (*arrows*) are in close contact with, or partly covered by, aggregates of extruded eosinophilic granules. The surrounding edematous tissue contains eosinophils expelling granules, disintegrating inflammatory cells, nuclear fragments, and lymphocytes. **c** Close-up of one of the flame figures in the subcutis. Collagen bundles (*arrows*) are coated by thick and dense layers of eosinophilic granules and surrounded by inflammatory cells. **d** A flame figure encircled by a well-developed granuloma containing histiocytes and a giant cell of Langhans type. H&E (**b**, **d** reproduced from Brehmer-Andersson et al. 1986, with permission)

rescence exactly mirrored the flame figures, indicating that they consist of MBP. The collagen in the center of the flame figures was not reactive. Furthermore, investigations of flame figures by electron microscopy have shown that free eosinophilic granules cover otherwise normal collagen bundles. Eosinophilic granules have also been observed in histiocytes (macrophages) surrounding the flame figures (Stern et al. 1984; Ferrier et al. 1988). The core structure of eosinophilic granules is poorly soluble and thus difficult to destroy (Zucker-Franklin 1978), a prerequisite for foreign body granuloma formation (Sect. 5.3.2). Together all these findings and the staining qualities in routinely prepared and stained specimens tell against necrosis (necrobiosis) as the cause of flame figures (Peters et al. 1983; Stern et al. 1984; Ferrier et al. 1988; Brehmer-Andersson et al. 1986). According to Majno and Joris (1996) collagen has a negatively charged surface, and this has led to the question: are flame figures formed when a large number of extruded, positively charged MBP molecules are attracted by the negatively charged surface of collagen bundles?

26.2.4 Example

Case 3. Eosinophilic Cellulitis

A 56-year-old woman had had chronic lymphatic leukemia for 7 years. For 2 years she had been treated periodically with chlorambucil. Every summer for 3 years after the treatment was stopped she had experienced several spells of severely itching skin lesions. The episodes always started suddenly with shooting pain, erythema and marked edema. After about 24 hours some of the lesions showed vesicles in the center. One or several lesions occurred on the face, trunk or extremities. They varied in size from a few centimeters to very large (i.e., covering large parts of the extremities). Usually they vanished spontaneously after 2–3 weeks. No triggering factor was known. Except for moderate blood eosinophilia, her laboratory status was normal. Biopsy specimens were taken from an erythematous and edematous lesion a few hours old and from a lesion 24 hours old with a crust in the center.

Histologic investigation of the early lesion showed only edema. In the 24-hour-old lesion there was a conspicuous subepidermal edema and in the whole dermis and the subcutaneous tissue dense infiltrates of eosinophils with a large number of flame figures in different stages. In a biopsy of a new 24-hour-old eruption, dense infiltrates of eosinophils, but no flame figures were observed (Fig. 23.2).

26.2.5 Differential Diagnosis

- The diagnosis of eosinophilic cellulitis also requires, in addition to a typical clinical appearance and course, the presence of flame figures, the histopathologic hallmark of the disease. This is crucial, because flame figures may be missing in a given biopsy specimen and possibly also in a given eruption of the disease (Brehmer-Andersson et al. 1986). In these cases acute dermatitis (eczema) and drug reactions with eosinophilia, and autoimmune bullous diseases with uncharacteristic histopathologic pattern will be important differential diagnoses. Several biopsies from lesions of different ages may be necessary.
- Flame figures are sometimes found incidentally in biopsy specimens taken from other kinds of skin diseases or from localized lesions known to be caused by arthropod bites (Wells and Smith 1979; Schorr et al. 1984).

26.3 Pityriasis Lichenoides et Varioliformis Acuta

Neisser and Jadassohn (1894) described a new kind of skin eruption and named it pityriasis lichenoides. The concept included a spectrum of chronic to acute clinical and histopathologic conditions. At the beginning of the 20th century, Mucha described the acute variant as a distinct disease and Habermann named it pityriasis lichenoides et varioliformis acuta (PLEVA), synonym Mucha-Habermann disease (Daoud and Pittelkow 1999). The chronic variant was called pityriasis lichenoides chronica (PLC), synonym parapsoriasis guttata. If PLEVA and PLC are variants of the same theme or two different diseases is still the subject of controversy. The author favors the latter hypothesis. Only PLEVA is discussed here.

26.3.1 Clinical Appearance

PLEVA may affect all ages, but preferentially children and young adults. Intermittent episodes occur, sometimes over several years. Crops of discrete papular lesions from a few to about 10 mm in diameter appear, usually on the extremities and trunk. However, eruptions may be generalized and sometimes even mucous membranes are involved. The lesions develop and disappear over a period of weeks. Fresh papules are pink and edematous, and sometimes hemorrhagic. Later they increase somewhat in size, become darker, vesicular, crusted, or necrotic. The lesions finally heal with hypo- or hyperpigmentation or a small scar. The eruptions may occasionally be associated with itch and general malaise.

26.3.2 Histopathologic Appearance

Histologically there is a dense mainly lymphocytic subepidermal cell infiltrate that invades the lower part of the epidermis and more or less obscures the epidermal–dermal junction. The epidermis is edematous, and may be vesicular or necrotic; typically it contains many erythrocytes. The horny layer may be thickened and parakeratotic and occasionally contains neutrophils. The dermis is edematous and contains patchy or confluent infiltrates of lymphocytes and histiocytes and many extravasated erythrocytes. Venules are dilated and filled with erythrocytes. In some cases a single thrombotic venule with fibrinoid wall necrosis surrounded by a lymphocytic cell infiltrate is observed. Atypical lymphocytes may be present in the epidermis and/or in the dermis (Black and Jones 1972). This is discussed further in Sect. 26.3.5.

26.3.3 Pathogenesis

The triggering factors in PLEVA are not known. The pathogenesis is also unknown, but an immunologic reaction is suspected. The infiltrating cells are T cells, the majority of which are $CD8^+$ (Jang et al. 2001).

26.3.4 Examples

Case 4. Pityriasis Lichenoides et Varioliformis Acuta

A 16-year-old boy had suffered from a non-itching eruption on the trunk and extremities for 3 weeks. A biopsy was taken from the forearm. Pityriasis lichenoides et varioliformis acuta was suggested.

In the central part of the lesion the epidermis was necrotic and in the whole specimen the epidermal–dermal junction was obscured by a dense cell infiltrate consisting of a mixture of lymphocytes, nuclear dust and neutrophils. There were a high number of extravasated erythrocytes and capillaries and venules were dilated and filled with erythrocytes. Also a single small venule contained a fibrin thrombus. In the whole dermis, with accentuation in the upper and middle parts, there were perivascular and interstitial infiltrates composed of small lymphocytes and histiocytes with an admixture of neutrophils. No atypical cells were observed (Fig. 26.3a).

Case 5. Pityriasis Lichenoides et Varioliformis Acuta with Stimulated Lymphocytes

A 25-year-old woman had had discrete eruptions on the trunk and extremities for 1 month. The non-itching lesions occurred in crops and started as small red, infiltrated papules, some of which were hemorrhagic. The papules increased in size, became scaling and sometimes vesicular, gradually took on a brown or bluish color, became crusted, and finally disappeared leaving pigmentation. The clinical appearance was considered perfectly in agreement with pityriasis lichenoides et varioliformis acuta. Lymph nodes were not involved and a bone marrow biopsy specimen was normal. However, the histologic investigation showed an admixture of atypical lymphocytes. Seven years after the first spell of the disease, the patient reported that she now and then still had isolated efflorescences of the same type. These healed without treatment and she felt well.

During a 7-year follow up three more skin biopsy specimens were taken. All showed in principle the same histopathologic pattern of subacute to acute dermatitis with a dense lymphocytic cell infiltrate containing many rather small atypical lymphocytes and mitotic figures at the dermal–epidermal junction. There were also scattered small aggregations of atypical cells high up in the epidermis resembling Pautrier abscesses (see Glossary). In the upper dermis there were perivascular infiltrates of small lymphocytes. Fresh hemorrhages were seen in intradermal vesicles and in the papillae. In one of the specimens a totally necrotic venule surrounded by a dense infiltrate of small lymphocytes was observed in the upper dermis.

Cytologic smears obtained by means of tape-stripping showed aggregations of different-sized lymphoid cells containing an irregular nucleus with a large nucleolus and course chromatin (Fig. 26.3b–d).

Case 6. Pityriasis Lichenoides et Varioliformis Acuta with Stimulated Lymphocytes

A 28-year-old woman had suffered from suddenly occurring papules up to 1 cm on the trunk and extremities from the age of 13 years. The lesions healed with scarring. She was followed for 4 years. Several investigations showed only scattered papules, some of them hemorrhagic or crusted, and many small, shallow scars. Clinically the diagnosis pityriasis lichenoides et varioliformis acuta was settled. A fresh 4 mm hemorrhagic papule on the forearm was taken for histologic investigation.

In the upper dermis there was a dense perifollicular and perivascular cell infiltrate, which slightly involved the overlying epidermis. The infiltrate consisted mainly of atypical lymphoid cells with one or several

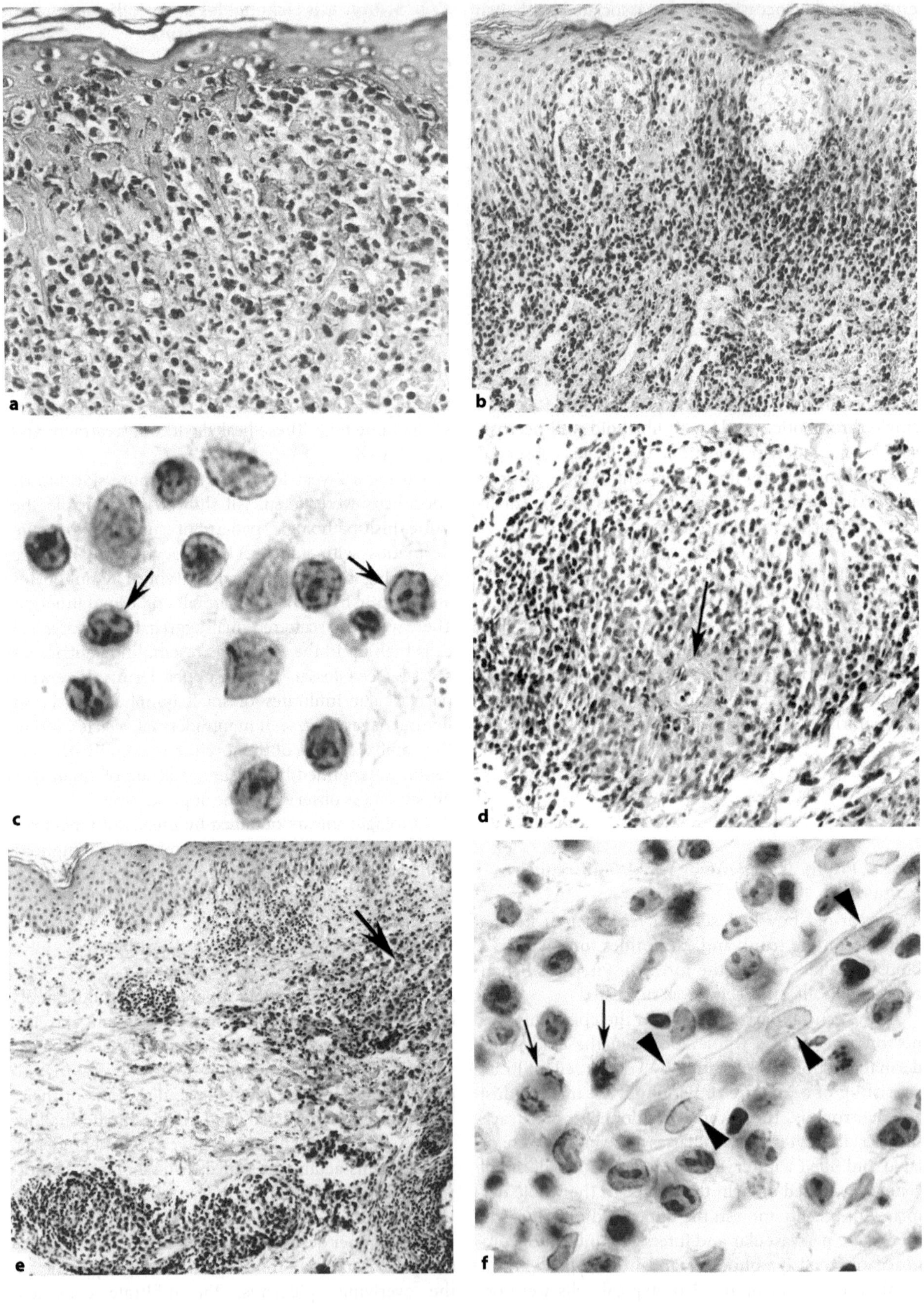
a
b
c
d
e
f

large nucleoli. Several mitotic figures were observed. There were also many extravasated erythrocytes, but no obvious vasculitis (Fig. 26.3e,f).

26.3.5 Comment

Case 5 has been described previously and discussed in detail (Brehmer-Andersson 1976; Brehmer-Andersson 1981). With respect to the histopathologic pattern, a malignant lymphoma, most probably mycosis fungoides was initially suspected. Between 1956 and 1976, there were several case reports and two larger reported series of otherwise healthy patients who had lesions clinically typical of PLEVA, but showed a histologic pattern suggestive of malignant lymphoma. Macaulay (1968) described one such patient and coined the concept *lymphomatoid papulosis*. Analysis of 25 reported cases distinguished two different groups of patients with respect to the morphology of the atypical cells. In one group the degree of atypia and number of atypical cells were prominent, and in the other the degree of atypia and number of atypical cells were moderate (Brehmer-Andersson 1976). The case of Macaulay belonged to the first group and Case 5 to the second.

In the EORTC classification for primary cutaneous lymphomas of 1997 (Willemze et al. 1997) lymphomatoid papulosis is defined as a chronic, recurrent, self-healing papulonodular skin eruption with histologic features (suggestive) of a cutaneous T-cell lymphoma, which runs a chronic mostly benign course. With respect to the morphology, infiltrates of lymphomatoid papulosis may be divided into types A, B and C as follows:

- *Type A* is characterized by extensive infiltrates of inflammatory cells. These are composed of histiocytes, small lymphocytes, neutrophils, and/or eosinophils, scattered or small clusters of large atypical and sometimes multinucleated or Reed-Sternberg-like cells. Initially the infiltrate is nonepidermotropic.
- *Type B* has perivascular or band-like epidermotropic infiltrates with predominance of small to medium-sized atypical lymphoid cells with cerebriform nuclei. The pattern is similar to that of plaque-stage mycosis fungoides.
- *Type C* has features suggestive of a large T-cell lymphoma and is composed of large clusters of the same large atypical cells as those seen in type A, but contains relatively few inflammatory cells.

The immunophenotypes of atypical cells in the different types are as follows:

Types A and C: $CD30^+$ (large atypical cells), $CD2^{-/+}$, $CD3^+$; $CD4^{+/-}$, $CD5^{-/+}$; $CD8^-$, $CD30^+$, $CD15^-$, EMA^-

Type B: Atypical cerebriform cells $CD3^+$, $CD4^+$, $CD8^-$, $CD30^-$

Clonally rearranged TCR genes (see Glossary) have been detected in approximately 60% of lesions of lymphomatoid papulosis.

In cases 5 and 6 described above, the immunophenotype and genetic features of the lymphocytes were not investigated, but the clinical features as well as histopathologic pattern and course were well in accordance with type B lymphomatoid papulosis of EORTC.

Recently two investigations have been performed on PLEVA with respect to the immunophenotype of cells and the presence of a dominant T-cell clone (Dereure et al. 2000; Weinberg et al. 2002). Dereure et al. investigated 20 cases with clinical and histopathologic typical PLEVA. The cell infiltrate consisted mainly of lymphocytes with phenotype $CD2^+$, $CD3^+$, $CD8^+$ and little or no $CD30^+$. They found a dominant clone in 13 of the 20 cases. With respect to their results, the authors favored the hypothesis that PLEVA is a clonal T-cell cutaneous lymphoproliferative disorder, but leave open the possibility that the dominant T-cell clone in PLEVA may be a clonal immunologic response to an unknown antigen or infectious agent. Weinberg et al. (2002) investigated the presence of T-cell clonality in lesions from 14 patients with PLEVA and from 13 patients with PLC diagnosed with respect to clinical and histopathologic characteristics. Monoclonal T-cell receptor gene rearrangement was found in eight PLEVA lesions and in one PLC lesion. The authors concluded that PLEVA is a benign clonal T-cell disorder and considered the T-cell clonality as the result of varying host immune responses to different pathogenic factors.

Fig. 26.3 Pityriasis lichenoides et varioliformis acuta. **a** The epidermal–dermal junction is obscured by a dense cell infiltrate consisting of lymphocytes, neutrophils and erythrocytes. The epidermis is edematous and partly necrotic. **b** The epidermal–dermal interface is obscured by a dense infiltrate of lymphocytes and the epidermis contains vesicles filled with erythrocytes and lymphocytes. **c** Smear obtained after tape stripping of the epidermis. It shows atypical lymphocytes with irregular nuclei, course chromatin and a distinct nucleolus (*arrows*). **d** A single necrotic venule in the upper dermis is densely surrounded by small lymphocytes (*arrow*). **e** Case 6. There are dense infiltrates of lymphoid cells mainly arranged around a hair follicle (not included) and around perifollicular venules. **f** Close-up of the area indicated (*arrow*) in **e** displays a thin-walled vessel (*arrowheads*) which is surrounded by atypical lymphocytes with one or several distinct nucleoli and several mitotic figures. The *arrows* indicate two distinct mitotic figures. H&E

As already demonstrated, atypical lymphocytes are now and then observed in skin lesions of known causes such as herpes virus infections and drugs (Figs. 22.5c and 7.5). Also well known are skin lesions with a lymphomatoid pattern due to anticonvulsive and antihistaminic drugs (Ploysangam et al. 1998; Magro and Crowson 1995). In all probability the atypical cells in these cases have undergone blast transformation and proliferated at the local site, a phenomenon parallel to the development of lymphocytomas with B cells as the main actors (Sect. 4.1.4). Consequently, from a histopathologic point of view the lesions demonstrated in Case 5 and Case 6 may represent either an immune response to a pathogenic factor or lymphomatoid papulosis. The number of atypical cells is not decisive. It may differ according to the age and severity of the lesion, and in routinely processed slides may be difficult to evaluate and even discover. Identification of different immunophenotypes of T cells present in clonal immunologic response to antigens and T cells present in lymphomatoid papulosis may be a way to distinguish the two conditions. More sophisticated investigation techniques focus on chromosomal abnormalities (Kadin 2002).

26.3.6 Differential Diagnosis

- *Subacute dermatitis* and vesicular PLEVA may be mixed up. An obscured epidermal–dermal interface and many erythrocytes in the epidermis are typical of PLEVA.
- *Lymphomatoid papulosis* and *mycosis fungoides* have to be considered if there is an admixture of atypical lymphocytes.

References

1. Ackerman AB, Ragaz A (1985) Erythema multiforme. Am J Dermatopathol 7:133–139
2. Ackerman AB, Penneys NS, Clark WH (1971) Erythema multiforme exudativum: distinctive pathological process. Br J Dermatol 84:554–566
3. Anderson CR, Jenkins D, Tron V, Prendiville JS (1995) Wells' syndrome in childhood. Case report and review of the literature. J Am Acad Dermatol 33:857–864
4. Aurelian L, Ono F, Burnett J (2004) Herpes simplex virus (HSV)-associated erythema multiforme (HAEM). A viral disease with an autoimmune component. Dermatol Online J 9:1–27
5. Bastuji-Garin S, Rzany B, Stern RS, Shear NH, Naldi L, Roujeau J-C (1993) Clinical classification of cases of toxic epidermal necrolysis, Stevens-Johnson syndrome, and erythema multiforme. Arch Dermatol 129:92–96
6. Bedi TR, Pinkus H (1976) Histopathologic spectrum of erythema multiforme. Br J Dermatol 95:243–250
7. Black MM, Jones EW (1972) "Lymphomatoid" pityriasis lichenoides. A variant with histological features simulating lymphoma. A clinical and histopathological study of 15 cases with details of long term follow up. Br J Dermatol 86:329–347
8. Brehmer-Andersson E (1976) Mycosis fungoides and its relation to Sézary's syndrome, lymphomatoid papulosis and primary cutaneous Hodgkin's disease. A clinical, histopathologic and cytologic study of fourteen cases and a critical review of the literature. Acta Derm Venereol Suppl (Stockh) 56:3–142
9. Brehmer-Andersson E (1981) Lymphomatoid papulosis. A concept which encompasses more than one disease process. Am J Dermatopathol 3:169–174
10. Brehmer-Andersson E, Kaaman T, Skog E, Frithz A (1986) The histopathogenesis of flame figures in Wells' syndrome based on five cases. Acta Derm Venereol 66:213–219
11. Brice SL, Leahy MA, Ong L, Krecji S, Stockert SS, Huff JC, Weston, WL (1994) Examination of non-involved skin, previously involved skin, and peripheral blood for herpes simplex virus DNA in patients with recurrent herpes-associated erythema multiforme. J Cutan Pathol 21:408–412
12. Daoud MS, Pittelkow MR (1999) Pityriasis lichenoides. In: Freedberg I, Eisen A, Wolff K, Austen KF, Goldsmith LA, Katz SI (eds) Fitzpatrick's dermatology in gerneral medicine. McGraw-Hill, New York, pp 553–560
13. Dereure O, Levi E, Kadin ME (2000) T-cell clonality in pityriasis lichenoides et varioliformis acuta. Arch Dermatol 136:1483–1486
14. Ferrier MC, Janin-Mercier A, Souteyrand P, Bourges M, Hermier C (1988) Eosinophilic cellulitis (Wells' syndrome). Ultrastructural study of a case with circulating immune complexes. Dermatologica 176:299–304
15. Fritsch PO, Ruiz-Maldonado R (1999) Erythema multiforme. In: Freedberg IM, Eisen AZ, Wolff K, Austen KF, Goldsmith LA, Katz SI, Fitzpatrick TB (eds). Fitzpatrick's Dermatology in general medicine. McGraw-Hill, New York, pp 636–644
16. Imafuku S, Kokuba H, Aurelian L, Burnett J (1997) Expression of herpes simplex virus DNA fragments located in epidermal keratinocytes and germinative cells is associated with the development of erythema multiforme lesions. J Invest Dermatol 109:550–556
17. Jang K-A, Choi J-C, Choi J-H (2001) Expression of cutaneous lymphocyte-associated antigen and TIA-1 by lymphocytes in pityriasis lichenoides et varioliformis acuta and lymphomatoid papulosis. Immunohistochemical study. J Cutan Pathol 28:453–459

18. Kadin ME (2002) T-cell clonality in pityriasis lichenoides. Evidence for a premalignant or reactive immune disorder? Arch Dermatol 138:1089–1090
19. Lever WF (1985) My concept of erythema multiforme. Am J Dermatopathol 7:141–142
20. Lever W, Schaumburg-Lever G (1990) Histopathology of the skin. J.B. Lippincott, Philadelphia
21. Macaulay WL (1968) Lymphomatoid papulosis. A continuing, self-healing eruption, clinically benign—histologically malignant. Arch Dermatol 97:23–30
22. Magro CM, Crowson AN (1995) Drugs with antihistaminic properties as a cause of atypical cutaneous lymphoid hyperplasia. J Am Acad Dermatol 32:419–428
23. Majno G, Joris I (1996) Cells, tissues and disease. Principles of general pathology. Blackwell Science, Cambridge, Massachusetts, USA
24. Orfanos CE, Schaumburg-Lever G, Lever WF (1974) Dermal and epidermal types of erythema multiforme. Arch Dermatol 109:682–688
25. Peters MS, Schroeter AL, Gleich GJ (1983) Immunofluorescence identification of eosinophil granule major basic protein in the flame figures of Wells' syndrome. Br J Dermatol 109:141–148
26. Peters MS, Rodriguez M, Gleich GJ (1986) Localization of human eosinophil granule major basic protein, eosinophil cationic protein, and eosinophil-derived neurotoxin by immunoelectron microscopy. Lab Invest 54:656–662
27. Ploysangam T, Breneman DL, Mutasim DF (1998) Cutaneous pseudolymphomas. J Am Acad Dermatol 38:877–905
28. Reed RJ (1985) Erythema multiforme. A clinical syndrome and a histologic complex. Am J Dermatopathol 7:143–152
29. Schorr WF, Tauscheck AL, Dickson KB, Melski JW (1984) Eosinophilic cellulitis (Wells' syndrome). Histologic and clinical features in arthropod bite reactions. J Am Acad Dermatol 11:1043–1049
30. Spigel GT, Winkelmann RK (1979) Wells' syndrome. Recurrent granulomatous dermatitis with eosinophilia. Arch Dermatol 115:611–613
31. Stern JB, Sobel HJ, Rotchford JP (1984) Wells' syndrome. Is there collagen damage in the flame figures? J Cutan Pathol 11:501–505
32. Weinberg JM, Kristal L, Chooback L, Honig PJ, Kramer EM, Lessin SR (2002) The clonal nature of pityriasis lichenoides. Arch Dermatol 138:1063–1067
33. Wells GC, Smith NP (1979) Eosinophilic cellulitis. Br J Dermatol 100:101–109
34. Willemze R, Kerl H, Sterry W, Berti E, Cerroni L, Chimenti S, Diaz-Peréz JL, Geerts ML, Goos M, Knobler R, Ralfkiaer E, Santucci M, Smith N, Wechsler J, van Vloten WA, Meijer CJLM (1997) EORTC classification for primary cutaneous lymphomas. A proposal from the Cutaneous Lymphoma Study Group of the European Organization for Research and Treatment of Cancer. Blood 90:354–371
35. Zucker-Franklin D (1978) Eosinophil function related to cutaneous disorders. J Invest Dermatol 71:100–105

27 Profiles of the Epidermal/Dermal Area in some Vesicular/Bullous Dermatoses

The profile of the epidermal/dermal area is sometimes helpful in the differential diagnosis.

27.1 Vesicular/Bullous Dermatitis (Eczema)

In subacute and acute dermatitis (eczema) vesicles and bullae are located in the epidermis (Chapter 22). The basement membrane is not destroyed. When the causing agent is removed or becomes weaker the epithelium is repaired. This is probably a rather fast process, which starts in the preserved surrounding epithelium. A shedding horny layer, containing exudate, may then be the only sign indicating the possibility of acute/subacute dermatitis (Figs. 22.1d and 27.1a).

27.2 Necrolytic Migratory Erythema

Necrolytic migratory erythema is a rare kind of eruption, which in most cases is due to a *glucagonoma*, a pancreatic tumor which secretes the polypeptide hormone glucagon, normally produced by cells in the pancreatic islets. The condition is called the *glucagonoma syndrome* which, in addition to the skin eruption and high serum levels of glucagon, includes other symptoms such as mild diabetes mellitus, weight loss, anemia, and stomatitis. Glucagonoma is a slowly growing tumor which may be benign or malignant. The skin eruption appears often before the underlying tumor becomes evident. Occasionally necrolytic migratory erythema appears without the presence of a glucagonoma. In these cases the underlying disease may be another kind of tumor, liver disease, inflammatory bowel disease, or malabsorption disorders (Tierney and Badger 2004).

The eruption consists of erythematous areas which become infiltrated and then vesicular and crusted. They may be widespread, but are most common on the trunk and extremities and in periorificial areas. The lesions spread outwards and heal in the center, giving rise to annular or circinate figures. They wax and wane over periods of 7–14 days (Mallinson et al. 1974).

The characteristic histopathologic findings are multiple small areas of necrosis in different stages of development and repair, which are located above a preserved and sometimes hyperplastic basal cell layer (Fig. 27.1b). Above the epidermis one to three generations of shed necrotic epithelium may be observed. This is in contrast to toxic epidermal necrolysis, in which the whole epidermis becomes necrotic and sheds (Fig. 28.5d). In the dermis there are edema and infiltrates of inflammatory cells, mainly composed of lymphocytes (Mallinson et al. 1974; Pujol et al. 2004).

Fig. 27.1 Profiles of the epidermal/dermal area. **a** Epidermal vesicular lesion during healing. The shed horny layer contains exudate and inflammatory cells. The underlying part of the epidermis is slightly hyperkeratotic and acanthotic and sparsely infiltrated by lymphocytes; H&E. **b** Necrolytic migratory erythema. The thin epidermis contains focal necroses of different ages. The *small arrows* indicate a fresh necrotic area above the basal cells and the *large arrow* an area of repair. A large necrotic flake covers the whole lesion; H&E. **c** Vesicular SLE. To the right there is a widened follicle with a keratin plug and to the left a subepidermal vesicle containing fibrinous exudate. Both the epidermis and the follicular epithelium are reduced to a few rows of cells. The upper dermis is edematous, but contains only a few inflammatory cells; vG. **d** Vesicular dermatomyositis. The pattern is very much the same as that demonstrated in **c**; H&E. **e** Lichen sclerosus et atrophicus. The epidermis is very thin, but the horny layer is conspicuously thickened. To the right a small part of a plugged follicle is visible. Below a subepidermal cleft there is a hyaline zone. A part of the underlying band-formed infiltrate of lymphocytes is exposed in the left lower corner; H&E. **f** Bullous pemphigoid. There is a subepidermal bulla. The *arrow* indicates the beginning of restoration of the basement membrane. Note also the degenerated roof of the bulla. H&E

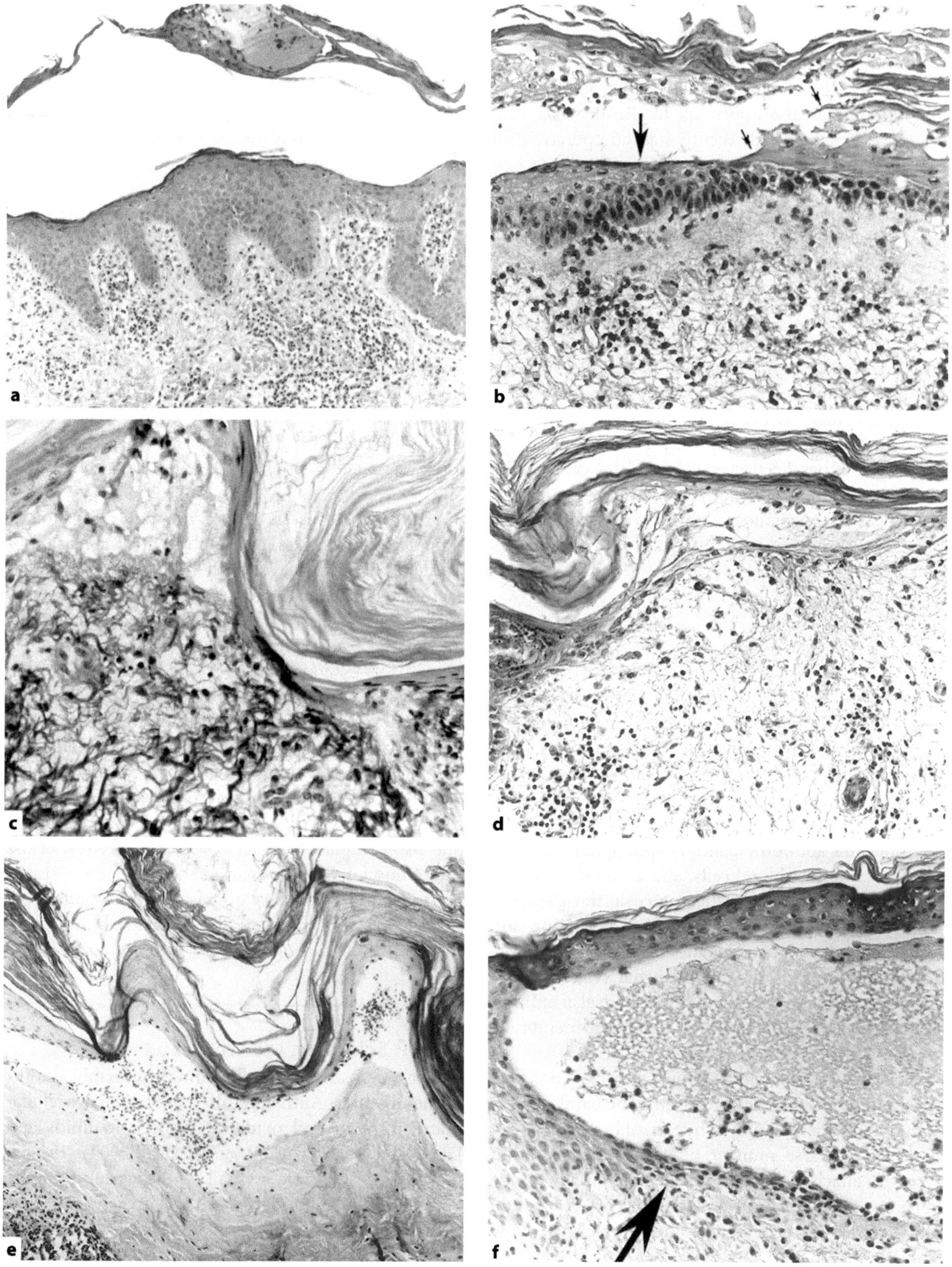
a
b
c
d
e
f

27.2.1 Example

Case 1. Necrolytic Migratory Erythema[1]

An 80-year old woman presented with coalescent annular lesions on the upper lip, forehead, trunk and thighs. The patient had recently had an operation for carcinoma of the breast and was thought also to be suffering from Sjögren syndrome (see Glossary). The lesions, which had progressed for some time, were considered an expression of lupus erythematosus. However, an increased level of plasmachromogranin A was the reason, and even the possibility of a neuroendocrine tumor was discussed. The patient died before further investigations could be done and autopsy was not performed, and thus the character of the underlying disease remained unclear.

The histologic investigation showed a thin epidermis, which contained multiple areas of necrosis above the preserved basal cell layer. One to three generations of shed necrotic epithelium covered the epidermis. There was a conspicuous subepidermal edema and rather dense perivascular infiltrates of lymphocytes (Fig. 27.1b).

27.3 Vesicular/Bullous Eruption in Systemic Lupus Erythematosus and Dermatomyositis

Systemic lupus erythematosus (SLE) is an autoimmune disease which may involve several organs or tissues, differing with respect to numbers and combinations. A characteristic trait is the presence of a wide variety of circulating autoantibodies such as antinuclear and anticytoplasmic antibodies, antiphospholipid antibodies, antibodies against blood cells, and antibodies against various tissues such as gastric mucosa, muscle sarcolemma and neurons (Bos and de Rie 2005). The skin lesions may be acute, subacute, or chronic. In acute erythematous eruptions subepidermal vesicles/bullae sometimes occur. In these cases there are also antibodies against a component in the basement membrane zone, mostly collagen IV (Georgi et al. 2001).

Histologic investigation shows a conspicuous destruction of the epidermis including the basal cells. In some places there is only a hypertrophic horny layer, to which a sparse number of degenerated keratinocytes are attached, above a vesicle or bulla filled with fibrinous exudate. However, inflammatory cells are remarkably few. Widened hair follicles and sweat gland orifices plugged with keratin are also typical.

Dermatomyositis is an autoimmune disease in which groups of striated muscles and the skin are affected. The mechanism of the disease is unclear. However, especially in elderly women, there is an association with malignant disease of internal organs. Vesicular/bullous lesions appear occasionally. The histopathologic pattern is the same as that seen in vesicular/bullous lesions of SLE (McCollough and Cockerell 1998). Consequently, it is not possible to differentiate between the two diseases only by means of the histopathologic pattern of the vesicular/bullous lesions.

27.3.1 Examples

Case 2. SLE with Acute Vesicular Eruption

A 19-year-old man suffering from SLE had had a widespread and intensely erythematous skin eruption for 4 months. The disease course was short and fatal. Autopsy revealed glomerulonephritis characteristic of SLE.

Histologic investigation of lesional skin showed subepidermal vesicles, the roof of which consisted of a thickened horny layer with the minor remains of regressively changed epidermis and the roof of markedly edematous tissue. Hair follicles were widened and filled with keratin (Fig. 27.1c).

Case 3. Dermatomyositis with Vesicles

A 65-year old woman had had slowly progressing and itching skin lesions for 4 months. The lesions had started on the face and spread to the trunk and extremities. Investigation showed circinate, erythematous areas with peripheral scaling and central healing. She also complained of weakness and soreness of the thigh muscles. Six years earlier she had been operated on for pulmonary carcinoma. The histopathologic pattern was very much similar to that seen in Case 2 (Fig. 27.1d).

27.4 Lichen Sclerosus et Atrophicus

Lichen sclerosus is a chronic and presumably autoimmune disease. Autoantibodies against extracellular matrix protein and oxidative damage to lipids and DNA have been proved (Sander et al. 2004). The primary efflorescence is a small whitish, round papule. Papules coalesce into larger whitish areas with prominent widened hair follicles and sweat gland orifices filled with yellow or brown keratin plugs. Occasionally vesicles or bullae appear. Details are best studied on the upper trunk, but are most common and most severe in the anogenital area in women, and on the prepuce in men.

1 Courtesy of Dr. Ismini Vassilaki, Danderyd Hospital, Stockholm, Sweden

The histopathologic pattern is typical. As in lupus erythematosus and dermatomyositis, there is successive destruction of the epidermis from the basal cell layer outwards, massive hyperkeratosis, and follicular plugging. Also in some areas the havoc in the epidermis leaves the horny layer with only a few keratinocytes attached that in combination with subepidermal edema gives rise to a vesicle or bulla. However, in contrast to vesicles/bullae in SLE and dermatomyositis, the floor consists of a band of hyaline collagen tissue, beneath which there is a band-formed infiltrate of lymphocytes, sometimes with an admixture of plasma cells.

27.4.1 Example

Case 4. Lichen Sclerosus et Atrophicus

A 66-year-old woman had had non-itching lesions on the upper back for several years, which clinically as well as histologically were typical of lichen sclerosus et atrophicus (Fig. 27.1e).

27.5 Bullous Pemphigoid

In bullous pemphigoid, as mentioned above, circulating autoantibodies directed against the hemidesmosomes give rise to subepidermal bullae, the roof of which consists of epidermis and the floor of the papillary dermis (Sect. 25.4.1.2). Restoration of a new epidermis starts as early as after a few days (Lever 1965). A change in morphology and function of the keratinocytes in the perilesional epidermis (edges of the bulla and adnexal remnants) allow them to migrate over the denuded dermal area and at the same time reconstruct the basement membrane. When the whole dermal surface is covered by basal cells and a new basement membrane is formed the migration stops and the basal cells proliferate and differentiate normally (Falabella and Falanga 2001). The process takes some time and when completed no shed remains of the roof are left.

27.5.1 Example

Case 5. Bullous Pemphigoid

An 80-year-old woman had had bullae on the extremities, partly developed on a nonerythematous base, for about 1 month.

The subepidermal bulla contained fibrinous exudate and many eosinophils. In the dermis there were diffusely spread neutrophils and small perivascular infiltrates of lymphocytes. At both ends of the bulla the beginning of the restoration of a new basal cell layer was evident (Fig. 27.1f).

27.6 Comment

When the injury is located in the epidermis and the basement membrane is intact, the restoration time is short and shed epidermal remains, significant for the diagnosis, may be observed in the biopsy specimen (Figs. 22.1d and 27.1a,b; see also biting lesions on the buccal mucosa and tongue, Fig. 29.6c,d). If the basement membrane or deeper parts of the basement membrane zone are injured, the restoration (if it occurs) takes more time, and thus shed remains are not found in a biopsy specimen from an active lesion.

In Case 1 the possible diagnosis was the subject of much discussion. The two diagnoses proposed were Sjögren syndrome associated with lupus erythematosus and necrolytic migratory erythema. In both diseases skin lesions and stomatitis may occur. However, the histopathologic pattern with focal areas of epithelial necrosis and shed flakes of necrotic epithelium excludes lupus erythematosus and strongly supports the diagnosis necrolytic migratory erythema.

References

1. Bos JD, de Rie MA (2005) Lupus erythematosus. In: Bos JD (ed) Skin immune system. Cutaneous immunology and clinical immunodermatology. CRC Press, London, pp 545–552
2. Falabella AF, Falanga V (2001) Wound healing. In: Freinkel RK, Woodley DT (eds) The biology of the skin. Parthenon, New York, pp 281–297
3. Georgi M, Jainta S, Bröcker E-B, Zillikens D (2001) Autoantigens of subepidermal bullous autoimmune dermatoses (in German). Hautarzt 52:1079–1089
4. Lever WF (1965) Pemphigus and pemphigoid. Charles C. Thomas, Springfield
5. Mallinson CN, Bloom SR, Warin AP, Salmon PR, Cox B (1974) A glucagonoma syndrome. Lancet 2:1–5
6. McCollough ML, Cockerell CJ (1998) Vesiculo-bullous dermatomyositis. Am J Dermatopathol 20:170–174
7. Pujol RM, Wang C-YE, el-Azhary RA, Su WPD, Gibson LE, Schroeter AL (2004) Necrolytic migratory erythema. Clinicopathologic study of 13 cases. Int J Dermatol 43:12–18
8. Sander CS, Ali I, Dean D, Thiele JJ, Wojnarowska F (2004) Oxidative stress is implicated in the pathogenesis of lichen sclerosus. Br J Dermatol 151:627–635
9. Tierney EP, Badger J (2004) Etiology and pathogenesis of necrolytic migratory erythema. Review of the literature. Med Gen Med 6:1–8

28 Skin Lesions Due to Drugs

Due to a constantly increasing number and use of drugs, reactions provoked by drugs or their metabolites are very common and may affect internal organs as well as the skin. However, it is important to realize that food additives, such as preservatives, colorings and quinine (used in tonic water), and chemicals, inhaled or absorbed through the skin, may also cause adverse skin reactions.

Adverse reactions to drugs are usually not serious if they are recognized and the drug withdrawn, but occasionally become critical, and even fatal. Skin eruptions are probably the most prevalent and include a wide spectrum of clinical and histopathologic patterns. A particular drug, or a metabolite of it, may give rise to several kinds of eruptions, but usually one kind prevails. Stubb et al. (1994) reported on 1997 consecutive patients with drug-related eruptions seen during a period of 35 years at the Department of Dermatology of the University Central Hospital, Helsinki, Finland. Most of the patients were hospitalized and in nearly all cases the causative drug was verified by oral provocation. Maculopapular exanthemata, urticaria, and fixed eruptions were the most common kinds of lesions. Antibiotics, antipyretic/antiinflammatory analgesics, and drugs acting on the central nervous system were the most common causative drugs. In another large study, Hunziker et al. (1997) analyzed the records of 1317 hospitalized patients with definite or probable drug-induced skin reactions, observed during a 20-year period in the divisions of general internal medicine in Berne and St. Gallen in Switzerland. The incidence was 2.7%. The reactions comprised maculopapular exanthema (91.2%), urticaria (5.9%), and vasculitis (1.4%). Only six cases (0.5%) of fixed eruption were observed and none of toxic epidermal necrolysis.

In the previous chapters a number of skin lesions that may be provoked by drugs are exemplified and/or discussed:

- Neutrophilic venular vasculitis (Sect. 7.1)
- Lymphocytic venular vasculitis (Sect. 7.2)
- Livedo reticularis (Sect. 7.5.4)
- Thrombocytopenia (Sect. 8.3)
- Thrombotic-thrombocytopenic purpura (Sect. 8.3)
- Hypercoagulability (Sect. 8.4)
- Warfarin skin necrosis (Sect. 8.5)
- Contact dermatitis (Sect. 4.5)
- Erythroderma (Sect. 22.5)
- Lichenoid lesions (Sect. 24.1.4)
- Erythema multiforme (Sect. 26.1.3)
- Eosinophilic cellulitis (Sect. 26.2.3)
- Lymphomatoid drug reactions (Sect. 26.3.5)

Skin eruptions caused by drugs can be divided roughly into two groups: those due to an immunologic (allergic) reaction and those that are nonallergic. Allergic skin reactions may be categorized as belonging to one of the hypersensitivity reactions types I–IV. Best elucidated are the mechanisms of those related to type I (urticaria, angioedema), type II (such as drug-induced thrombocytopenia), and type III (leukocytoclastic vasculitis) (described in Sect. 4.3), and the mechanism of delayed hypersensitivity reaction type IV in contact dermatitis (described in Sect. 4.5). However, the pathways of drug reactions thought to belong to delayed hypersensitivity reaction type IV are much more complicated and variable. Naisbitt et al. (2001) and Pichler et al. (2002) have summarized the possible occurrences.

Most drugs are proteins with a low molecular weight (haptens) and are not antigenic until they have bound covalently (strongly) to a larger protein, a carrier molecule (Sect. 4.1). To be able to bind covalently to the carrier protein, the drug or metabolite must become chemically reactive. It is believed that most adverse drug reactions that give rise to delayed-type immune-mediated reaction are caused by chemically reactive metabolites, generated by the normal process of drug metabolism. This is called drug bioactivation and usually takes place in hepatocytes, but may also take place in other kinds of cells such as professional antigen presenting cells (i.e., macrophages, dendritic cells, B cells), and even in epidermal keratinocytes.

T cells recognize small peptide fragments of the original antigen, presented on a MHC molecule by antigen-presenting cells. The process of presenting antigen peptides can take place inside or outside the antigen-presenting cell. Endogenous antigens are presented on MHC class I molecules to $CD8^+$ cells, whereas exogenous antigens are presented on MHC class II molecules to $CD4^+$ cells.

The following are examples of these processes:

- Reactive drug metabolites generated in the liver and bound to some intracellular protein are processed to peptides inside the liver cells. The process is endogenic and the antigen is consequently presented to cytotoxic $CD8^+$ T cells by MHC class I molecules.
- A drug protein bound to a carrier molecule may escape endogenous processing to antigenic peptides in the liver and enter the peripheral circulation. This exogenous antigen may instead be processed in professional antigen-presenting cells and presented to $CD4^+$ T cells on MHC class II molecules. However, it is not known whether drug metabolites formed in the liver are stable enough to circulate in the periphery.
- A circulating drug (stable or reactive hepatic metabolite) may accumulate inside a specific type of cell, e.g. macrophages. Processing may occur in the cell giving rise to endogenous antigen presented on MHC class I molecules to $CD8^+$ T cells or outside the cell as a cell-surface reaction with antigen presentation on MHC class II molecules to $CD4^+$ cells.
- Some chemically nonreactive drugs (metabolites) may also bind directly and noncovalently to MHC molecules and may be able to provoke adverse immunologic reactions without going through bioactivation. The binding is MHC-restricted, but less stable.

The diversity of the pathways of T-cell recognition of drug antigens explains why drugs may activate both $CD8^+$ and $CD4^+$ T cells. Also the kind of stimulated T cell is of importance:

- $CD4^+$-1 cells secrete IFN-γ, which gives rise to the $CD8^+$ response, and IL-2 secrefion.
- $CD4^+$-2 cells secrete IL-4 and IL-5. These attract eosinophils.
- $CD4^+$-3 cells secrete transforming growth factor β (TGF-β) and IL-10.

TGF-β and IL-10 counteract cytokines secreted by $CD4^+$-1 and $CD4^+$-2 cells and the cellular immune response does not appear. This is referred to as the *silent immune response* and may explain why most individuals do not develop adverse reactions.

Furthermore, investigations have revealed that, as compared to maculopapular lesions, vesicular and bullous lesions contain a higher number of infiltrating $CD8^+$ cells and a higher level of IL-5 secretion. The latter, together with the chemokine eotaxin (present in T cells, endothelial cells, and keratinocytes), is probably responsible for the conspicuous eosinophilia often seen in vesicular and bullous lesions (Pichler 2002).

It has also been proved that some types of T cells may attract a large number of neutrophils and even that drugs may give rise to drug-specific T cell lines and clones (Britschgi and Pichler 2002).

The final activation of the cellular immune response is thought to occur via two signals between the antigen-presenting cell and the lymphocyte. The binding (receptor–ligand interaction) between the MHC-restricted antigen and the TCR is the first signal. The second signal occurs through further receptor–ligand interactions, called *costimulatory interactions*. However, there is probably a third signal, the *danger signal*, represented by the cytokine IL-1 in the case of $CD4^+$ cells and of IL-12 in the case of $CD8^+$ cells. Cells that are under oxidative stress (see Glossary), cells infected with virus, necrotic cells, and cells undergoing apoptosis release the third signal.

From the above and previous discussion it is evident that the scenarios of drug eruptions are legion. A few are discussed in detail here.

28.1 Acute Allergic Urticaria/Angioedema

Acute allergic urticaria with or without angioedema is the second most common skin reaction caused by drugs. The condition appears at any age, but is most common in young adults.

28.1.1 Clinical Appearance

Acute allergic urticaria is characterized by a sudden and more or less widespread eruption of swellings (wheals) with a white center surrounded by an erythematous area and usually associated with severe itch. The size and form vary from small papules to large lesions, which may be rounded, irregular, annular, or serpiginous. The rash is transient and individual efflorescences usually disappear within 24 hours. When angioedema occurs, the face is the most common location.

28.1.2 Histopathologic Appearance

A typical urticaria wheal below an essentially normal epidermis shows subepidermal edema and small cell infiltrates consisting mainly of lymphocytes with an admixture of both neutrophils and eosinophils. Thin-walled vessels (lymphatics and venules) are dilated and some venules are filled with erythrocytes. There is no vasculitis. In angioedema the edema includes the deep dermis and subcutaneous tissue.

28.1.3 Pathogenesis

Allergic urticaria is due to a hypersensitivity type I reaction, in which $CD4^{+}$-2 T cells are activated. These cells secrete IL-4 and IL-5, which is followed by production of IgE antibodies, release of histamine from mast cells, and activation of eosinophils. The reaction may be provoked by, for example, drugs, food and food additives.

Urticaria vasculitis, a type III reaction, is better considered as a variant of neutrophilic venular vasculitis (leukocytoclastic vasculitis) which is described in Section 7.1. Drugs may also cause non-allergic urticaria by direct release of histamine from mast cells (pharmacologic reaction).

28.1.4 Examples

Case 1. Urticaria Caused by Penicillin

A 51-year-old woman showed an urticarial reaction after treatment with penicillin. A palm-sized area had remained for more than 24 hours; thus urticaria vasculitis was suggested.

Histologic investigation showed marked subepidermal edema and in the upper half of the dermis sparse to moderate dense perivascular and interstitial cell infiltrates composed of lymphocytes, neutrophils, nuclear fragment, and eosinophils. Vasculitis was not observed (Fig. 28.1a).

Case 2. Urticaria Caused by Methimazole

A 40-year-old woman was given methimazole for hyperthyroidism. Three days later severe itching occurred all over the body and she presented with erythematous papules in the axilla. A biopsy specimen was taken from a papule.

Below a subepidermal edema there were sparse perivascular and interstitial cell infiltrates composed of lymphocytes, neutrophils and eosinophils. Vasculitis was not observed (Fig. 28.1b).

28.2 Maculopapular Eruptions

This group of reactions, also called exanthemata, is the most common drug eruption.

28.2.1 Clinical Appearance

Eruptions may be morbilliform, scarlatiniform or rubelliform. They are usually discrete and subside when the causative drug is withdrawn. However, occasion-

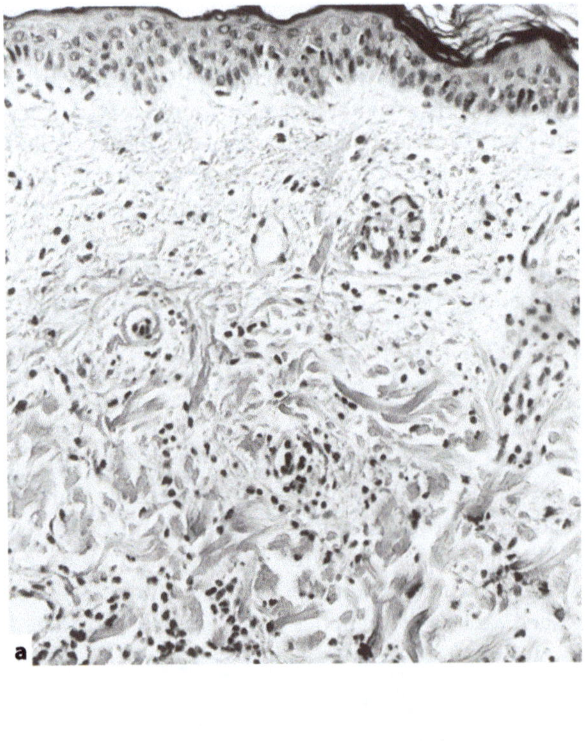

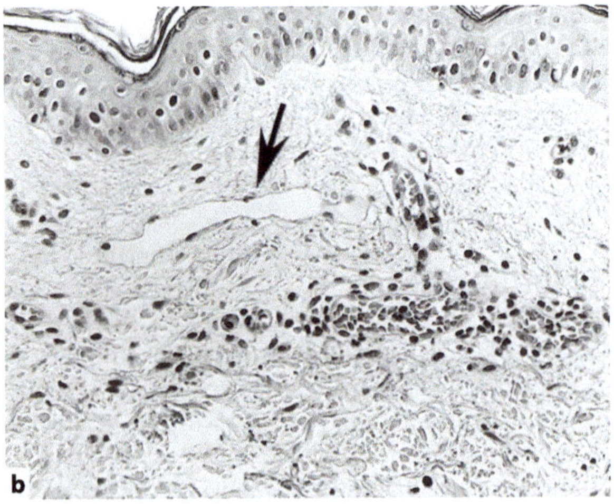

Fig. 28.1 Urticaria. **a, b** In the upper dermis there are marked edema and sparse diffuse infiltrates of lymphocytes with a slight admixture of neutrophils and eosinophils. Lymphatics are dilated (*arrow*) and venules are filled with erythrocytes. H&E

ally they become widespread and may represent either the initial phase of erythroderma or toxic necrolysis.

28.2.2 Histopathologic Appearance

The pattern is nonspecific. In the upper dermis there are sparse to moderate perivascular infiltrates of lymphocytes, histiocyte-like cells, and occasionally eosinophils. In the epidermis there are intercellular edema, some lymphocytes, and scattered necrotic keratinocytes in the basal part (Yawalkar and Pichler 2001).

28.2.3 Pathogenesis

Maculopapular eruptions are hypersensitivity type IV reactions. The cell infiltrate in the dermis consists of $CD4^+$ cells and in the dermal–epidermal junction of equal numbers of $CD4^+$ and $CD8^+$ cells secreting IFN-γ and IL-5. Both the $CD4^+$ cells and the $CD8^+$ cells contain perforin and granzyme B granules (see Glossary), which are cytotoxic. Histiocyte-like cells are either $CD1a^+$ dendritic cells or $CD68^+$ macrophages (Yawalkar and Pichler 2001).

28.2.4 Differential Diagnosis

The differential diagnosis includes eruption caused by infectious agents such as morbilli, scarlatina and rubella.

28.3 Fixed Drug Eruptions

By a fixed drug reaction is meant a sharply demarcated skin lesion which disappears when the drug is withdrawn and reappears at the same location when the drug is given anew.

28.3.1 Clinical Appearance

An active lesion usually consists of a rounded, erythematous, and edematous area up to about 50 mm in diameter. Some lesions may be vesicular or bullous. Fixed eruptions may also mimic other dermatoses such as lichen planus, erythema multiforme, and psoriasis. In inactive periods, the area may show a slight hyperpigmentation. There may be more than one lesion, and the eruption is rarely generalized. Preferential sites are the face and genitalia (Mahboob and Haroon 1998).

28.3.2 Histopathologic Appearance

The pattern is variable, but mostly resembles either the dermal or the epidermal pattern of erythema multiforme. In inactive hyperpigmented lesions only macrophages containing melanin pigment are observed in the upper dermis, indicating a previous injury to the basic epidermis.

28.3.3 Pathogenesis

A large number of drugs, of which sulfonamides and tetracyclines are the most common, may provoke a fixed drug eruption (Mahboob and Haroon 1998). The pathogenesis is not clearly understood. However, investigations have indicated that the phenomenon may be due to a localized disturbance of the regulation of the activity of memory $CD8^+$ T cells, normally homing in the epidermis (Shiohara et al. 2002).

28.3.4 Examples

Case 3. Fixed Drug Eruption of Unknown Cause

A 34-year-old man had had a frequently recurrent itching skin lesion for 2 years, always located at the bend of the left arm. He presented with an erythematous plaque that measured 30×15 mm. He returned 2 months later with a new lesion, 10 mm in diameter, at the same location. The patient denied using drugs. Biopsy specimens were taken from both lesions.

Both specimens showed the same histologic pattern. The epidermis was slightly acanthotic, but otherwise normal. In addition to marked subepidermal edema, dense perivascular cell infiltrates composed of lymphocytes were observed throughout the dermis. Some vessels were dilated and filled with erythrocytes. Also extravasated erythrocytes were seen, but no vasculitis. (Fig. 28.2)

Case 4. Fixed Drug Eruption Caused by Pindolol

A 66-year-old man for 4 months had experienced several recurrences of a distinct erythematous lesion with a large central vesicle, always located on the same area of the scrotum. He had been given, together with several other drugs, the β-receptor blocking agent pindolol. This was suspected to be the culprit. After withdrawal of the drug no recurrences appeared.

Histologic investigations showed both intraepidermal and subepidermal vesicles. The latter were stuffed with eosinophils. Between the vesicles, the dermal epidermal interface was totally obscured by densely

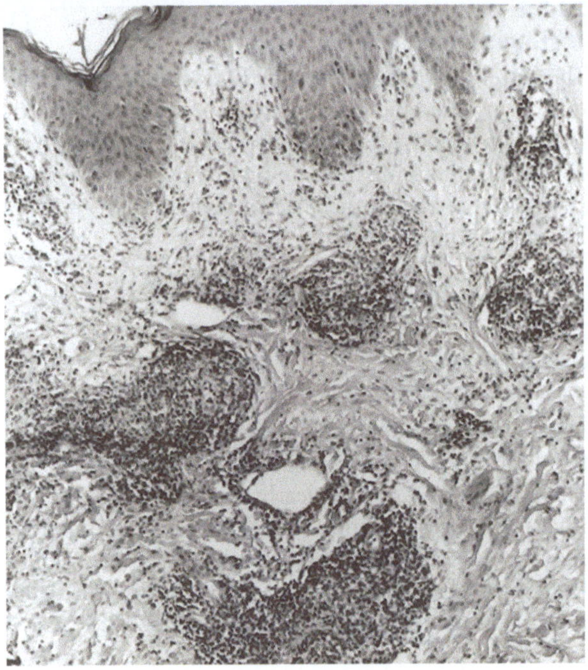

Fig. 28.2 Fixed drug eruption. The epidermis is thickened and acanthotic. There are marked edema and moderate infiltrates of lymphocytes in the papillary dermis. In the rest of the dermis there are dense well-circumscribed infiltrates of lymphocytes. H&E

packed eosinophils. In the dermis there was a rather dense diffuse cell infiltrate consisting of eosinophils and lymphocytes. Veins were dilated and had prominent endothelial cells. Vasculitis was not observed (Fig. 28.3).

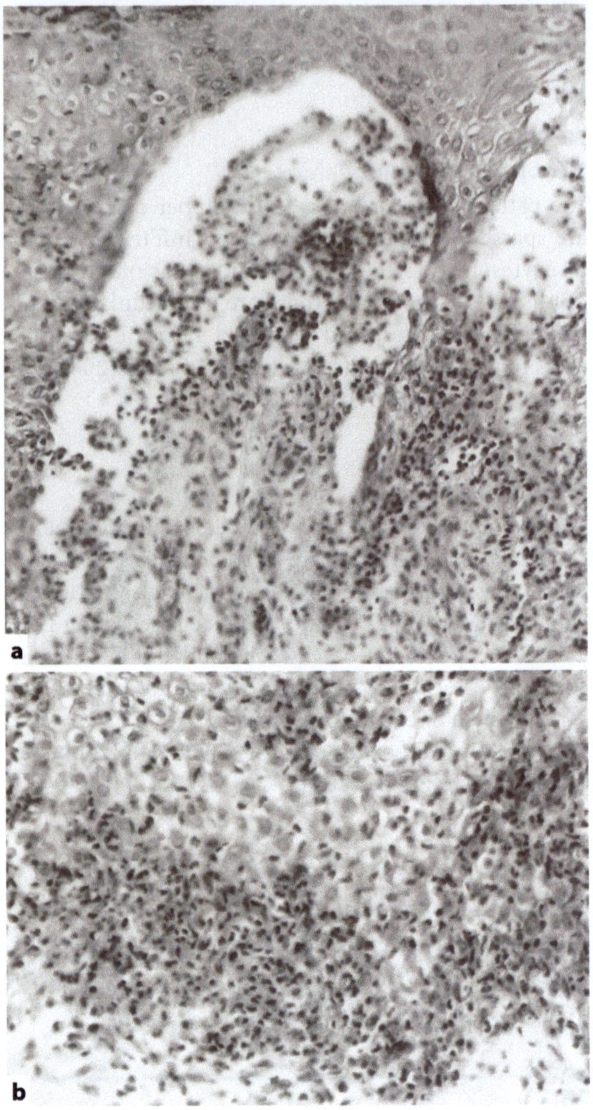

Fig. 28.3 Fixed drug eruption provoked by pindolol. **a** A cleft between the dermis and epidermis contains a large number of eosinophils. **b** A broad band of densely packed eosinophils obscures the dermal–epidermal interface. H&E

28.4 Toxic Epidermal Necrolysis and Stevens-Johnson Syndrome

Toxic epidermal necrolysis (TEN) is the most serious form of drug reaction and Stevens-Johnson syndrome (SJS) is considered to be a somewhat less severe variant of TEN. Lyell (1956) reported on four adult patients with extensive areas of epidermal necrolysis and called the condition toxic epidermal necrolysis. He regarded it as closely related to a disease described previously in children by Stevens and Johnson. Both variants are rare. The estimated incidence ranges from 0.4 to 6 per million persons per year. Conditions in which the immunologic status is disturbed, such as lupus erythematosus and HIV infection, increase the risk of reacting with TEN (Roujeau and Stern 1994).

28.4.1 Clinical Appearance

Both variants usually start with poorly defined erythematous maculae with purpuric centers symmetrically located on the face and upper trunk. Within a few days the lesions spread all over the body, coalesce and turn into flaccid bullae due to epidermal necrosis. The necrotic epidermis desquamates in sheets and leaves large denuded areas. In most patients, the mucous membranes and conjunctivae are also affected, and occasionally even the epithelium of the trachea, bronchi and gastrointestinal tract. The condition is as-

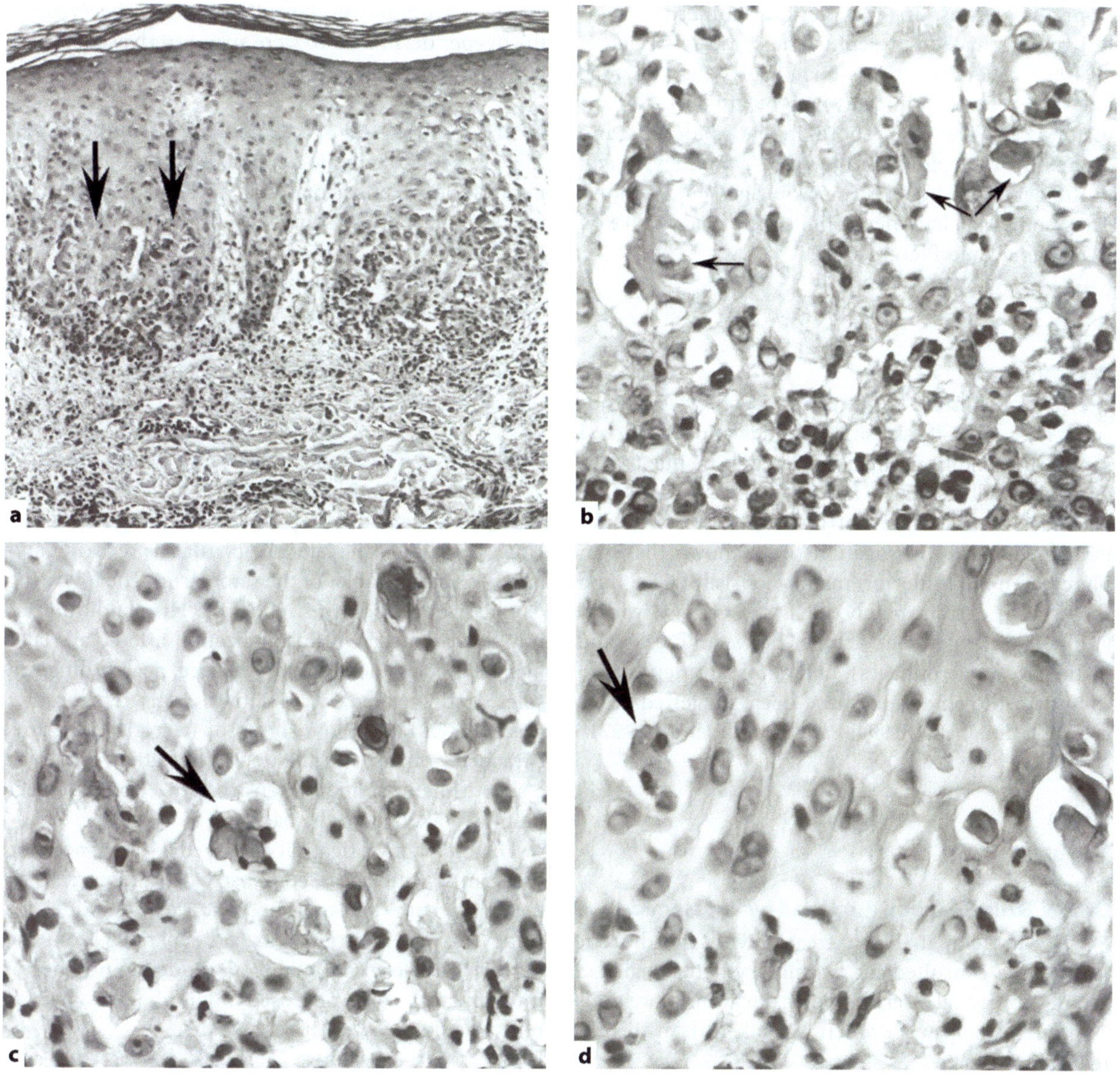

Fig. 28.4 Drug reaction provoked by furosemide. a The epidermis is thickened with elongated and broad rete ridges, which in the lower half are disintegrating and contain aggregates of apoptotic bodies (*arrows*) and lymphocytes. In the papillae and upper dermis there are rather sparse infiltrates of lymphocytes. b Close-up of the area indicated (*arrows*) in a. c, d Other areas of epidermis with aggregates of apoptotic bodies, in to two of which lymphocytes are attached (*arrows*). H&E

sociated with a high fever and general illness (Roujeau and Stern 1994).

The two disorders merge into each other. A patient in whom the detached area is less than 10% is considered to have SJS and a patient with more than 30% of detachment to have TEN. In borderline cases detachment is between 10% and 30%. In SJS atypical target lesions (i.e., lesions similar to those described as target lesions in erythema multiforme) may be observed (Bastuji-Garin et al. 1993). Both SJS and TEN are life-threatening. If the patient survives, the lesions heal without remnants within 3 weeks. However, some lesions may heal with scars and ocular sequelae are common (Roujeau and Stern 1994).

28.4.2 Histopathologic Appearance

In full-blown cases of TEN the epidermis becomes necrotic. The necrotic epidermis consists of faded shadow cells alternating with areas of necrotic eosinophilic keratinocytes, and is in large areas separated from the dermis. In early lesions numerous apoptotic bodies may be present in the epidermis (Paul et al. 1996). They sometimes form aggregates to which one or several lymphocytes may be attached. Inflammatory cells are sparse both in the epidermis and dermis. In the epidermis there are lymphocytes and in the dermis histiocytes (macrophages) and lymphocytes; somewhat later neutrophils are added (Paul et al. 1996; Paquet and Piérard 1997).

28.4.3 Pathogenesis

The most common causative drugs reported to provoke TEN and SJS are sulfonamides and anticonvulsants. The conditions are considered to be due to one or several cell-mediated immunologic reactions, the pathways of which are not fully understood. Immunohistochemical investigations have shown that lymphocytes in the epidermis mainly consist of $CD8^+$ and those in the dermis mainly of $CD4^+$ T cells (Miyauchi et al. 1991). Synergistic activity between T cells and histiocytes (macrophages), and abundant deposits of TNF-α in the epidermis, have been suggested to be critical (Paquet et al. 1994; Paquet and Piérard 1997).

28.4.4 Examples

Case 5. Drug Reaction Provoked by Furosemide

A 57-year-old man being treated with the diuretic furosemide consulted for itching erythema that had rapidly spread all over the body during the previous 24 hours. A biopsy specimen was taken from the gluteal area.

Investigation showed a thickened and acanthotic epidermis, the lower half of which was edematous and contained numerous apoptotic bodies. Some apoptotic bodies formed aggregates to which scattered lymphocytes were attached (Fig. 28.4).

Case 6. Drug Reaction Provoked by Phenytoin

A 63-year-old man was given the antiepileptic drug phenytoin after a brain tumor operation and suffered a widespread and itching maculopapular exanthema associated with a high fever. A biopsy specimen was taken the day after the eruption started. Within a few days TEN developed.

The epidermis contained aggregates of apoptotic bodies. The surrounding keratinocytes were faded and disintegrating. At the dermal–epidermal interface, edema and sparse infiltrates of lymphocytes with scattered neutrophils and eosinophils were observed. In the deeper dermis there were sparse perivascular infiltrates of lymphocytes (Fig. 28.5a,b).

Case 7. Drug Reaction Provoked by Carbamazepine

A 37-year-old alcoholic woman, who was also suffering from lupus erythematosus, developed generalized flaccid bullae after treatment with the anticonvulsant carbamazepine.

Histologic investigation revealed a subepidermal bulla caused by detachment of a totally necrotic epidermis. The dermis was edematous and contained dilated thin-walled vessels and sparse lymphocytes (Fig. 28.5c,d).

Case 8. Drug Reaction Provoked by Sulfonamide

A 28-year-old man had received a sulfonamide on a previous occasion for prostatitis with good effect. However, some time later the prostatitis recurred and he took a single tablet of the same drug. The following day his whole body was reddened. His condition rapidly deteriorated. On hospitalization a few days later he had vesicles and bullae on the face, neck, palms and soles, and purulent conjunctivitis. His temperature was 40.7°C. Later large sheets of necrotic epidermis detached from all over the body. The patient died after a short time in spite of intensive care. A biopsy specimen was taken from the back.

Histologic investigation displayed a totally necrotic epidermis, which was composed of shadow cells alternating with areas of necrotic eosinophilic keratinocytes, and in large areas was separated from the dermis. The dermis contained a moderate number of inflammatory cells composed of lymphocytes, neutrophils, and histiocytes (Fig. 28.6).

28.4.4.1 Comment

In Case 5 as well as in Case 6 biopsy specimens were taken on the second day of the eruption. In Case 5 the condition promptly ameliorated and healed after withdrawal of the drug, whereas in Case 6 typical TEN developed. Thus the presence of numerous apoptotic bodies in a more or less preserved epidermis may appear early in SJS as well as in TEN.

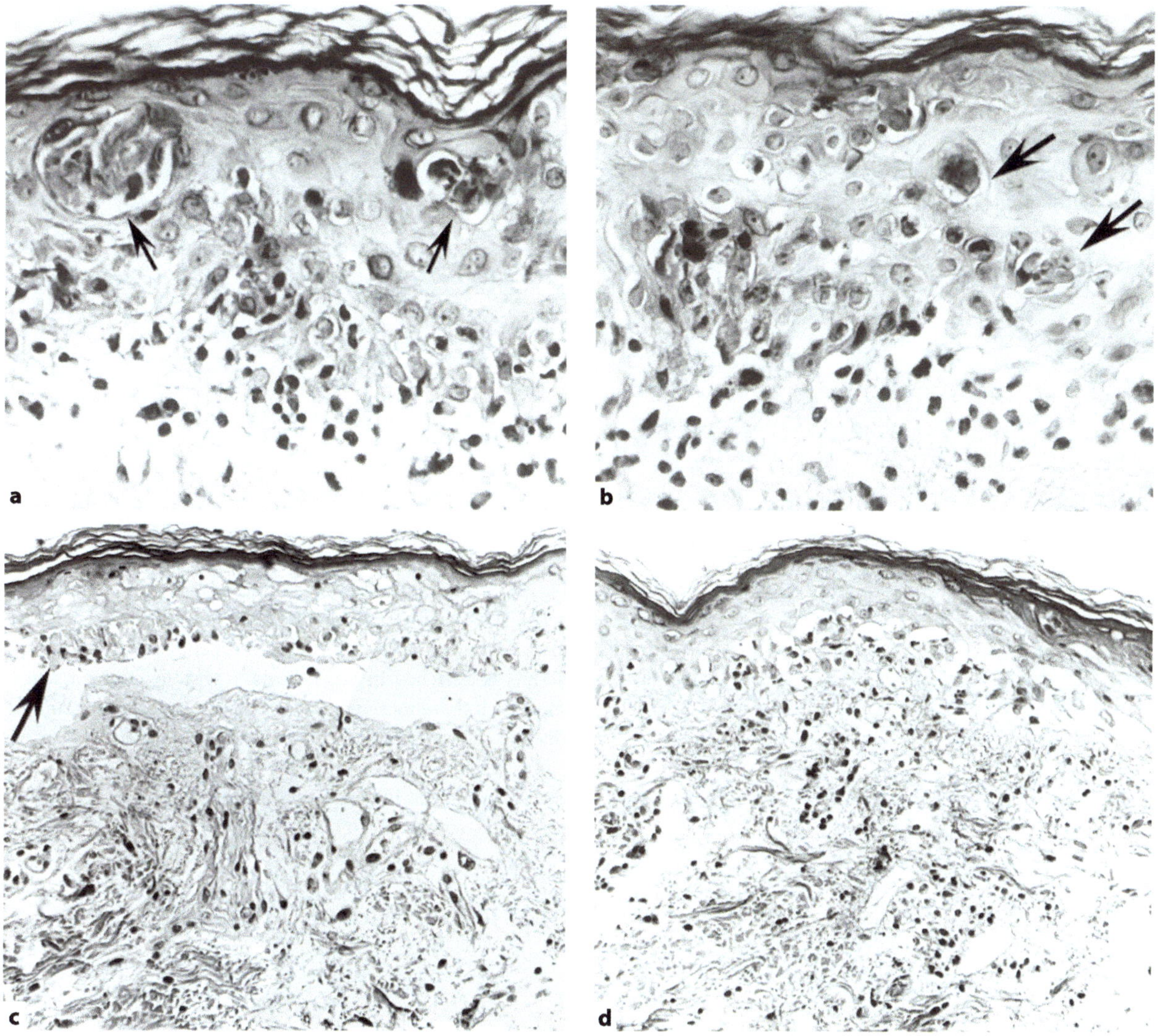

Fig. 28.5 Toxic epidermal necrolysis. **a** Provoked by phenytoin. The epidermis contains aggregates of apoptotic bodies (*arrows*). The surrounding keratinocytes are faded or disintegrated. **b** There is marked subepidermal edema and a moderate number of lymphocytes (*arrows*). **c** Provoked by carbamazepine. In the center of the lesion the epidermis is necrotic and detached from the dermis. In the left corner there are the remains of apoptotic bodies (*arrow*). **d** The margin of the lesion shows interface dermatitis with a sparse number of lymphocytes. The dermis is edematous and contains thin-walled dilated vessels and a few lymphocytes. H&E

28.4.5 Differential Diagnosis

- *Herpes simplex, herpes zoster* in advanced stage (Sect. 20).
- The *staphylococcal scalded-skin syndrome* (Sect. 12.5).
- *Acute graft-versus-host disease* may be impossible to differentiate from toxic necrolysis.
- *Phytophotodermatitis* also has to be considered (Sect. 29.4.3).

28.5 Acute Generalized Exanthematous Pustulosis

Acute generalized exanthematous pustulosis (AGEP) was previously considered as pustular psoriasis. It was differentiated from pustular psoriasis by Baker and Ryan (1968) and since then has had different names such as exanthematous pustular psoriasis, toxic pustuloderma, and pustular drug rash (Sidoroff et al. 2001).

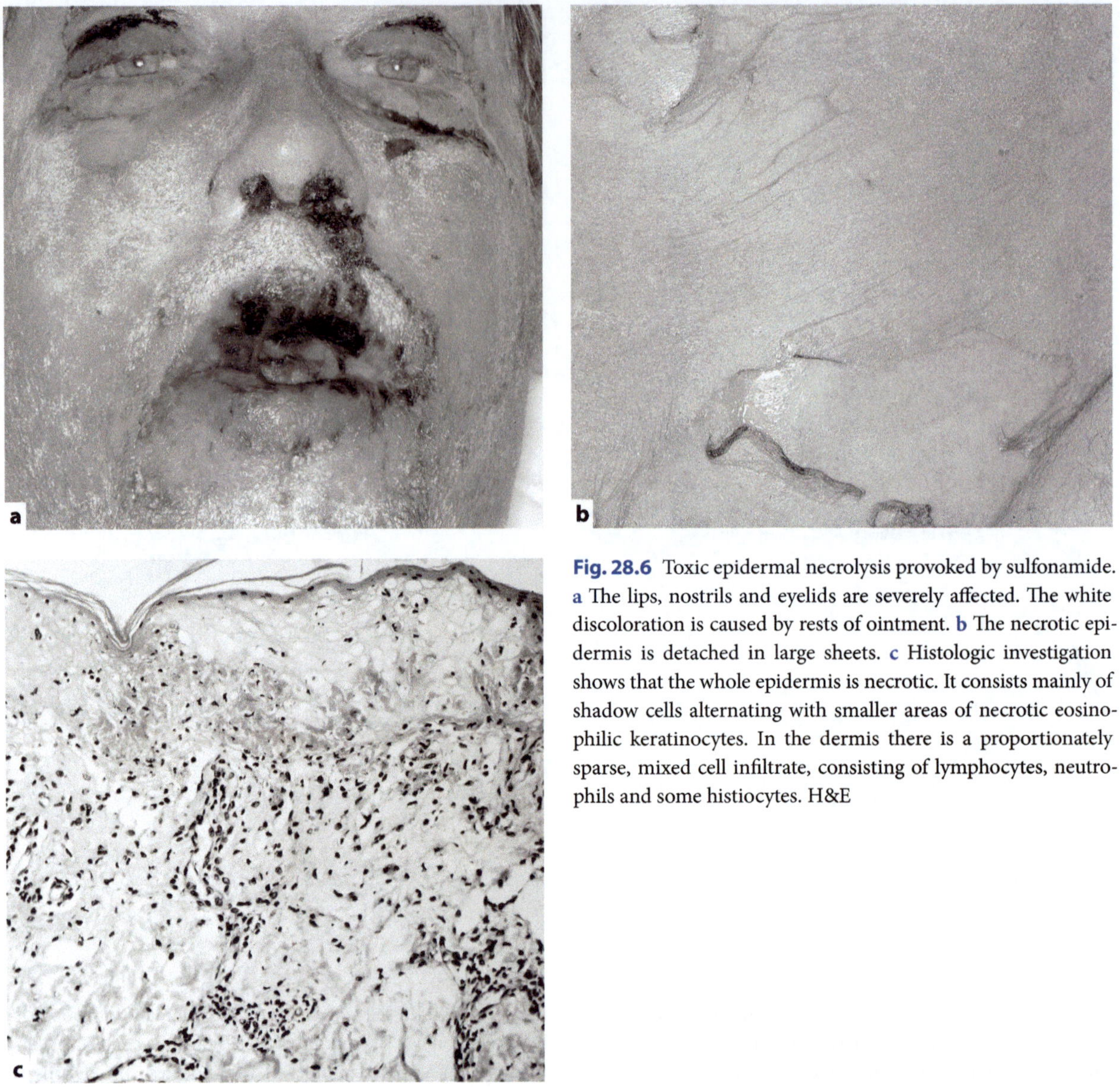

Fig. 28.6 Toxic epidermal necrolysis provoked by sulfonamide. a The lips, nostrils and eyelids are severely affected. The white discoloration is caused by rests of ointment. b The necrotic epidermis is detached in large sheets. c Histologic investigation shows that the whole epidermis is necrotic. It consists mainly of shadow cells alternating with smaller areas of necrotic eosinophilic keratinocytes. In the dermis there is a proportionately sparse, mixed cell infiltrate, consisting of lymphocytes, neutrophils and some histiocytes. H&E

28.5.1 Clinical Appearance

A generalized eruption of hundreds of small, sterile, and non-follicular pustules (less than 5 mm in diameter) suddenly appears on edematous and reddened skin. The lesions are associated with a high fever and massive blood neutrophilia. All symptoms regress spontaneously within 15 days (Roujeau et al. 1991).

28.5.2 Histopathologic Appearance

There are superficial, neutrophilic and spongiotic pustules in the epidermis, and in the dermis infiltrates of lymphocytes; occasionally vasculitis has been observed. In contrast to psoriasis, acanthosis and papillomatosis are usually absent (Roujeau et al. 1991; Sidoroff et al. 2001).

28.5.3 Pathogenesis

AGEP is a cell-mediated immunologic reaction, mostly provoked by drugs, usually penicillins (Roujeau et al. 1991). It has been possible to isolate drug-specific T cells from positive patch tests as well as from the peripheral blood of patients with drug-induced AGEP (Britschgi and Pichler 2002). Also these drug-specific

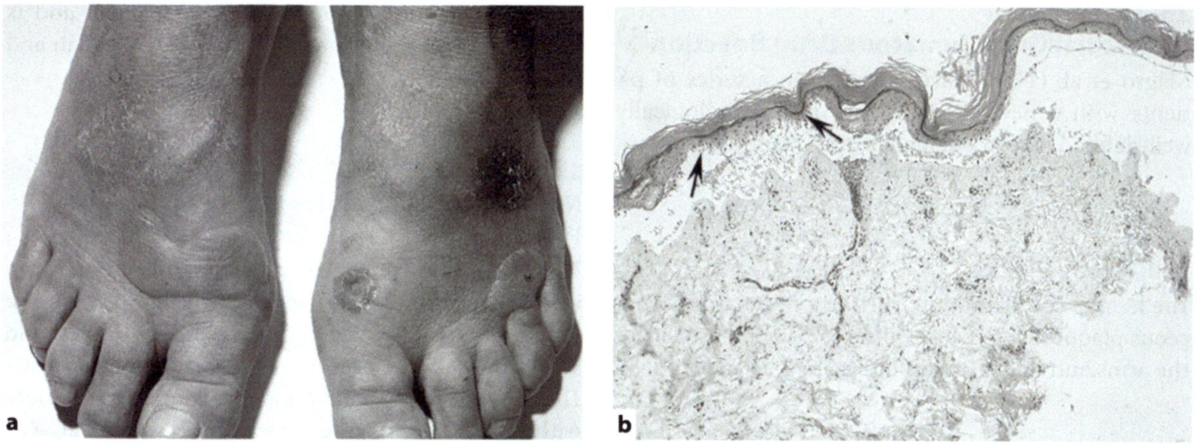

Fig. 28.7 Bullous lesions provoked by nalidixic acid and exposure to sunlight. a Multiple bullae on the dorsal aspect of the feet. b There is a wide subepidermal bulla which in the center cuts through a sweat gland. The roof of the bulla consists mainly of a shrunken and hyperkeratotic epidermis. However, in the area *between the arrows* it is better preserved and displays intracellular edema in the basal cells. The floor is composed of the dermis with well-preserved, distinct papillae. Inflammatory cells are sparse. H&E

T cells have been proven to produce large amounts of IL-8, which is a potent cytokine attracting neutrophils. The authors suggested the possibility that a similar mechanism could explain the presence of neutrophils in psoriasis, which probably is a cell-mediated immunologic disease.

28.5.4 Differential Diagnosis

- *Pustular psoriasis* (Sect. 23.2)
- *Intraepidermal IgA pustulosis* (Sect. 25.2)

28.6 Bullous Skin Lesions due to Photosensitivity Reactions

Only those agents with an absorption spectrum in the range of sunlight are associated with photosensitivity. There are two main forms: *phototoxicity* and *photoallergy*. In phototoxicity, absorption of ultraviolet light produces a reactive drug or metabolite, which by one of two pathways ultimately gives rise to photosensitization (Svensson et al. 2001).

Drug-induced photoallergy is a type IV delayed hypersensitivity reaction. An antigenic drug or its metabolite becomes activated after exposure to ultraviolet light. Examples of orally administered drugs which may cause phototoxic or photoallergic bullous reactions are nalidixic acid, chlorpromazine, tetracycline, thiazides and fluoroquinolone.

28.6.1 Example

Case 9. Drug Reaction Provoked by Nalidixic Acid in Combination with Intensive Exposure to Sunlight

A 55-year-old woman suffered from chronic pyelonephritis and was treated with nalidixic acid. During a sun vacation in Spain, bullae appeared on the dorsal aspects of hands and feet.

A biopsy specimen revealed a wide subepidermal bulla, which contained erythrocytes, but no inflammatory cells. In the central part of the bulla the roof consisted of a shrunken and hyperkeratotic epidermis. At the margin where the epithelium was preserved and in areas close to the bulla, the basal cells showed marked intracellular edema. The floor consisted of dermis with well-preserved papillae and sparse infiltrates of lymphocytes (Fig. 28.7).

28.6.2 Differential Diagnosis

Porphyria cutanea tarda shows a very similar pattern (Fig. 25.12e,f). Investigation excluded porphyria cutanea tarda as the cause in Case 9 and nalidixic acid was considered to be the culprit. The only difference between the lesion seen in the patient in Case 9 and a lesion of porphyria cutanea tarda may be the intracellular edema observed in the basal cells in the patient in Case 9.

28.7 Interstitial Granulomatous Drug Reaction

Magro et al. (1998) have reported on a series of patients with a new clinically and histopathologically well-defined type of cutaneous drug reaction.

28.7.1 Clinical Appearance

The lesions consist of nonpruritic erythematous/violaceous plaques mostly located on the medial aspects of the arms and thighs and in intertriginous areas.

28.7.2 Histopathologic Appearance

In the upper dermis there are diffuse infiltrations of lymphocytes and histiocytes and piece-meal fragmentation of collagen and elastic fibers. Lymphocytes migrate into the overlying epidermis that shows intracellular edema. The presence of atypical (stimulated) lymphocytes has been observed in several cases.

28.7.3 Pathogenesis

Drugs that have been found to be responsible are, among others, calcium channel blockers, angiotensin-converting enzyme inhibitors, beta-blockers and lipid-lowering agents. The pathogenesis is not clear.

28.7.4 Differential Diagnosis

- *Granuloma annulare* is located in the mid-dermis; inflammatory cells do not invade the epidermis.
- *Lymphoma* must be considered if stimulated lymphocytes are observed.

28.8 Skin Lesions Provoked by Penicillamine

Because of several different chemical characteristics, penicillamine has been used in the treatment of very different kinds of diseases, and may give rise to both allergic and nonallergic adverse reactions. For example, penicillamine may combine with metals and is used in Wilson disease (see Glossary) to prevent accumulation of copper in organs and tissues, and in lead poisoning for detoxification. It may dissociate naturally occurring disulfides and macroglobulins such as rheumatoid factor and is used in rheumatoid arthritis, and in cystinuria (see Glossary) to prevent urinary stone formation. It inhibits maturation of collagen and is also used in scleroderma and keloid (Bialy-Golan and Brenner 1996).

28.8.1 Nonallergic Degenerative Lesions Induced by Penicillamine

These lesions are dose-dependent and most often seen in patients with diseases which need high doses for a long time, such as Wilson disease and cystinuria, and sometimes also in patients with rheumatoid arthritis. They are due to the ability of penicillamine to interfere with the maturation of collagen and elastin (Bialy-Golan and Brenner 1996).

28.8.1.1 Clinical Appearance

Besides areas with excessive wrinkling and atrophy, lesions similar to pseudoxanthoma elasticum and elastosis perforans serpiginosa may appear, single, together or in different combinations. Pseudoxanthoma elasticum-like lesions consist of pale-yellow waxy papules and elastosis perforans serpiginosa-like lesions of raised papules, some with a central keratotic plug, arranged in small annular or serpiginous figures. Preferential sites are the back of the neck, axilla and groins (Bolognia and Braverman 1992; Iozumi et al. 1997).

28.8.1.2 Histopathologic Appearance

Investigation of pseudoxanthoma elasticum-like lesions in the dermis reveals large, eosinophilic elastic fibers, which are rough, unevenly thick, and provided with oval spike-like projections. In contrast to normal elastic fibers they are readily visible in routinely stained sections. In general there is no calcification (Burge and Ryan 1988; Iozumi et al. 1997). After protracted treatment with penicillamine, the same kind of changes have also been observed in elastic tissue of internal organs, for example the wall of the aorta and alveolar septa of the lungs (Burge and Ryan 1988). In lesions similar to elastosis perforans serpiginosa, in addition to thickened elastic fibers in the dermis, there are abscesses located in the papillae close to the epidermis. The abscesses consist of necrotic tissue containing degenerated elastic fibers with accentuated basophilic walls and inflammatory cells. Some of them may perforate the epidermis (Meyrick Thomas and Kirby 1985). There may be foreign body granulomas with giant cells. Also in some cases keloid-like formations of collagen without elastic fibers have been observed (Iozumi et al. 1997).

28.8.1.3 Example

Case 10. Elastosis Perforans Serpiginosa Provoked by Penicillamine[1]

A 40-year-old man had been treated for many years with penicillamine for severe cystinuria, known to be present since the age of 17 years. For 5 months he had observed small bluish-red and circinate infiltrates bilaterally at the dorsal axillary border. He had no subjective symptoms.

The biopsy specimen included the whole dermis and some subcutaneous tissue. Abnormal elastic fibers were observed in the whole dermis. In the middle and deep part of the dermis the fibers were rough, uneven, and provided with spike-like projections. In the papillary dermis they seemed degenerated and to be broken up into smaller pieces. Also there were two abscesses. One was located in the papillary dermis, and the other was intrafollicular (Fig. 28.8).

28.8.1.4 Differential Diagnosis

Pseudoxanthoma elasticum. In this hereditary disease the affected elastic fibers are confined to the middle and lower parts of the dermis, are curled up, and do not have spikes. Older lesions contain calcium (Poon et al. 2002).

28.8.2 Allergic Skin Reactions Provoked by Penicillamine

Penicillamine may give rise to urticaria and exanthema or autoimmune bullous dermatoses such as different variants of pemphigus and cicatricial pemphigoid. These kinds of adverse reactions are seen in individuals who already have disturbed immunity such as patients with rheumatoid arthritis (Bialy-Golan and Brenner 1996).

1 Courtesy of Dr. Alf Rausing, Microklin AB, Barsebäck, Sweden

28.9 Bullous Skin Lesions in Acute Drug Intoxication and Coma

Bullous skin lesions in association with drug intoxication are well known and described clinically (Holten 1951-1952; Sorensen 1963; Beveridge and Lawson 1965) as well as histologically (Adebahr 1963; Brehmer-Andersson and Pedersen 1969; Mandy and Ackerman 1970; Arndt et al. 1973; Sanchez Yus et al. 1993). The same types of lesions have also been described in carbon monoxide intoxication (Achten et al. 1971; Torne et al. 1991). Barbiturate is the most common causative drug, but other hypnotic and narcotic drugs have also been reported to be involved, occasionally in combination with alcohol.

28.9.1 Clinical Appearance

In unconscious patients, or in patients who were unconscious shortly before being attended to, well-circumscribed reddened areas or plaques >10 cm in diameter with or without vesicles and/or bullae may be seen. These are usually, but not always, located on areas exposed to pressure and are often symmetrical. Lesions appearing several hours after regaining consciousness have also been observed (Holten 1951-1952). If the patient survives, the skin lesions heal spontaneously.

28.9.2 Histopathologic Appearance

Common to all vesicular/bullous lesions and nonvesicular lesions are more or less complete necrosis of sweat glands and sweat gland ducts below the lesional area. However, in addition to sweat gland necrosis, necrosis in the pilosebaceous units has also been observed (Arndt et al. 1973; Sanchez Yus et al. 1993). Small accumulations of neutrophils, venules with fibrinoid necrosis, and small hemorrhages have been noted around necrotic sweat glands and hair follicles (see also below).

28.9.3 Example

Case 11. Sweat Gland Necrosis in Acute Drug Intoxication

A 25-year-old male student was found alone in a dazed condition in his room. Because of bullous skin lesions he was referred to the dermatology department and

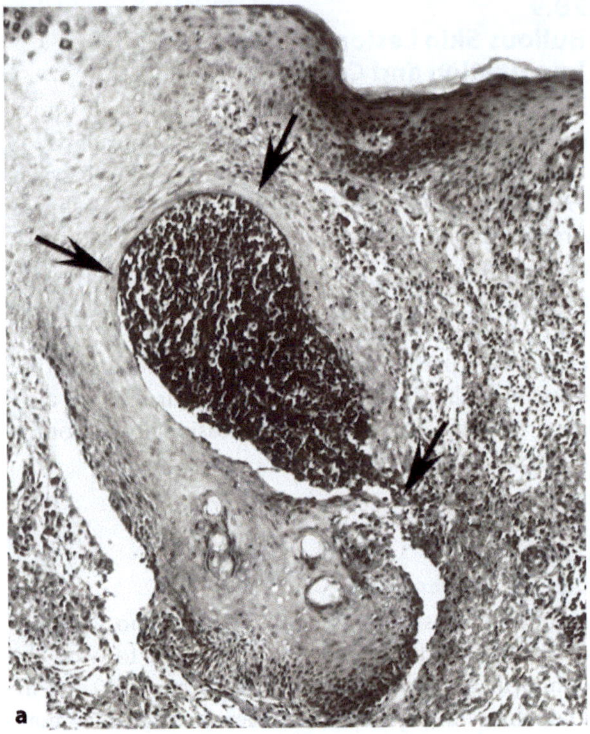

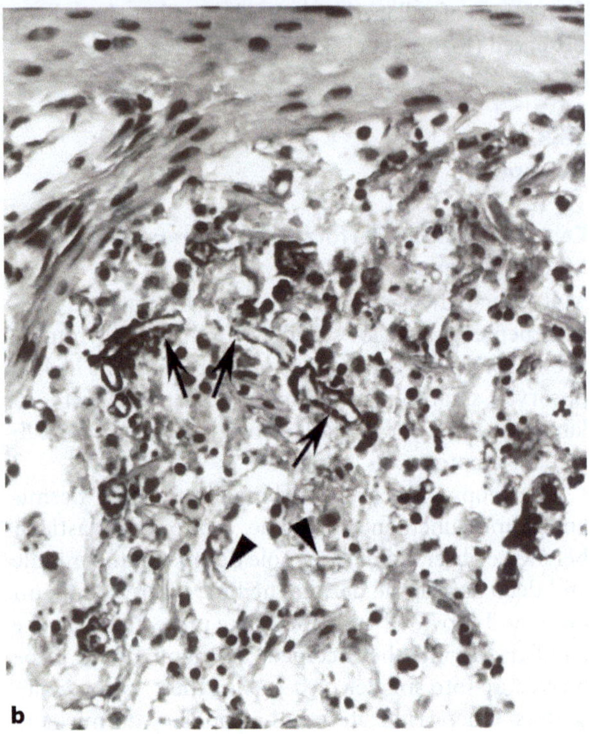

Fig. 28.8 Elastosis perforans serpiginosa-like lesion provoked by penicillamine. **a** An abscess is located in a papilla in close contact with the epidermis (*arrows*). The rete ridge to the left is club-like and contains small hair follicles. There is a narrow passage between the upper dermis and the abscess. The abscess contains abnormal elastic fibers and a dense diffuse infiltrate of inflammatory cells. **b** Close-up shows necrotic tissue with inflammatory cells and abnormal elastic fibers. Some fibers are irregular and thick and have dark accentuated walls (*arrows*); others are thinner, lighter, and have minute, plump projections (*arrowheads*). H&E

hospitalized. Over the right great trochanter was observed a 5×5 cm large well-defined reddish plaque. The surface of the plaque was stuffed with minute vesicles, and also contained a somewhat larger vesicle and a 15×10 mm large bulla (Fig. 28.9a). On the left trochanter there was an 8×8 cm large reddish plaque without vesicles, and on the medial border of each foot a 4×4 cm large bulla. Bullae and vesicles contained clear fluid. A knife biopsy was taken from the lesion on the right trochanter; it included the bulla and normal skin.

Because of a severe drink problem the patient was regularly taking the tranquillizers meprobamate and propiomazine together with disulfiram (a deterrent to alcohol consumption). He reported that for about two weeks he had stopped taking disulfiram and a few days before he was found, had consumed some alcohol. After that he remembered nothing until he was rescued by friends (Brehmer-Andersson and Pedersen 1969).

The biopsy specimen was cut at ten levels (over 100 sections) and stained with H&E and according to vG. The material included a substantial part of subcutaneous tissue and also normal skin. In the affected part there was a large, mainly subepidermal bulla. The floor of the bulla consisted of dermal papillae, which in areas were covered by minimal rests of basal cells. The roof comprised the suprabasal part of the epidermis, which in the central part was disintegrating and shrunken. At the dermal-subcutaneous border below the bulla several scattered groups of sweat glands and ducts were totally or partially necrotic. At different levels in the dermis it was possible to identify parts of necrotic ducts, one of which could be followed to the floor of the bulla. Beside the bulla there were several vertical, club-shaped or pear-like intraepidermal vesicles surrounded by normal epithelium. Some of these contained the remnants of a sweat gland duct at the base. Also a complete acrosyringium with a necrotic duct surrounded by a vesicle was observed. The bulla and vesicles contained eosinophilic exudate and a moderate number of neutrophils. In addition, there was close to the above-described changes in the epidermis a longitudinally cut hair follicle, which could be followed in its entirety, and showed

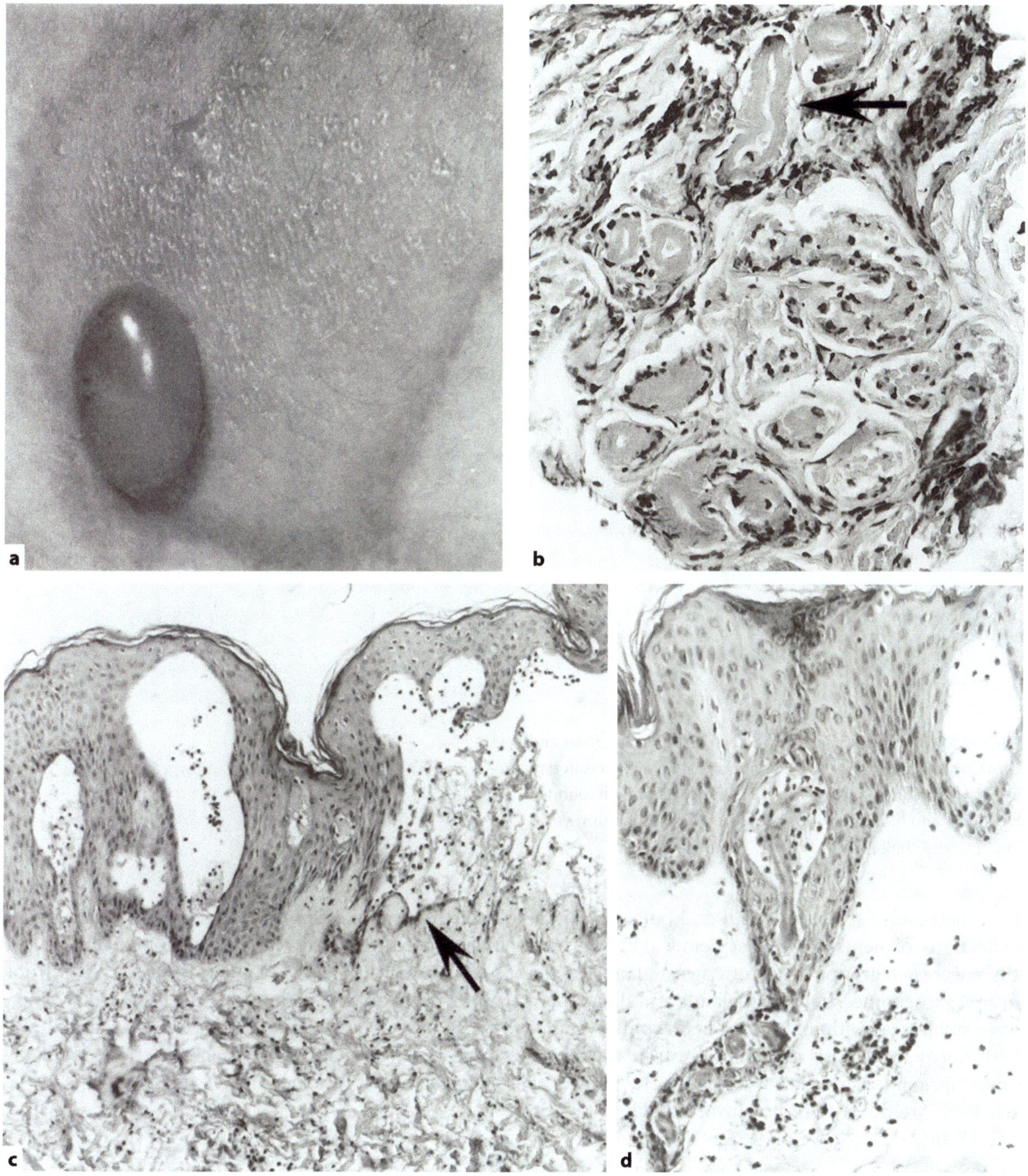

Fig. 28.9 Sweat gland necrosis in acute drug intoxication and coma. **a** A well-demarcated plaque on the right trochanter major shows many minute vesicles and also displays a somewhat larger vesicle and a bulla. **b** There is a group of totally necrotic sweat glands with a necrotic duct at the top (*arrow*). **c** In the left half of the micrograph there are two longitudinally intraepidermal vesicles with the remains of sweat gland ducts at the base. The right half shows a part of the bulla, the floor of which consists of dermal papillae. The *arrow* indicates an area with tiny remains of basal cells. **d** A necrotic sweat gland enters the epidermis. In the lower half of the epidermis the necrotic duct is surrounded by a vesicle and inflammatory cells. To the right there is another longitudinal vesicle, which probably also represents an affected acrosyringium. H&E (**a**, **d** reproduced from Brehmer-Andersson and Pedersen 1969, with permission)

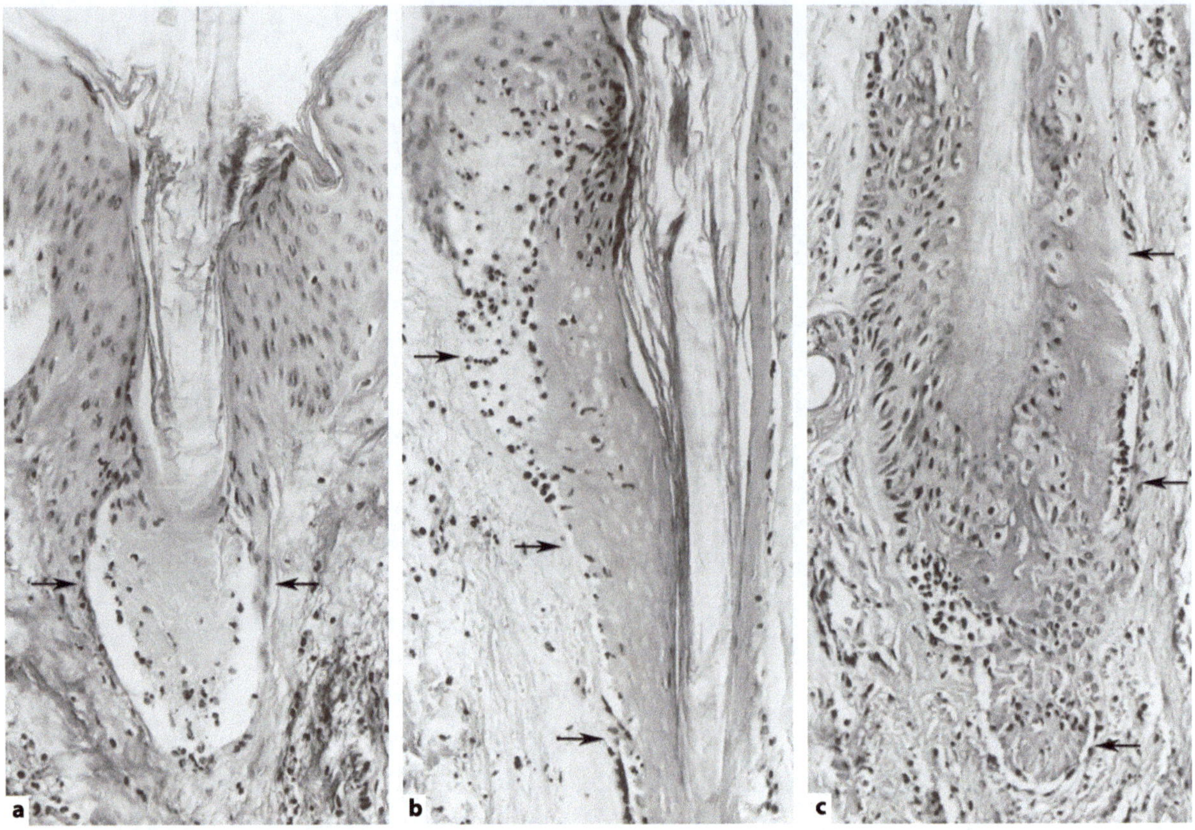

Fig. 28.10 Hair follicle necrosis in acute drug intoxication and coma. The micrographs show necrotic areas (*arrows*) at different levels of the same hair follicle. Necrotic parts are surrounded by edema and infiltrates of neutrophils. **a** Infundibulum; vG. **b** Shaft; H&E. **c** Bulb; H&E

focal necrosis of the root sheath and bulb, and small collections of neutrophils. Just below the hair bulb there were two groups of necrotic sweat glands. In the dermis close to necrotic sweat glands and ducts there were small areas with infiltrate of neutrophils, venules with fibrinoid necrosis and small fresh hemorrhages. These insignificant vascular lesions were judged as reactive. Arterioles were not involved (Fig. 28.9b,c,d and 28.10).

28.9.3.1 Comment

I was confronted with Case 11 early in my career as a dermatopathologist. By chance I did not miss the diagnosis altogether. At the Department for Pathology I had at my disposal a cubicle at one side of a small laboratory. At the other side there was a similar cubicle, into which a young colleague from the Department of Forensic Medicine had just moved. When we met, the first question he asked was: "Do you know that drug-intoxicated and comatose patients can get skin lesions due to sweat gland necrosis?" I did not, and I was skeptical. Could this really be true? When the slides appeared on my desk I was prepared in my mind for sweat gland necrosis, but overlooked the unexpected hair follicle necrosis.

28.9.4 Pathogenesis

The mechanism of the phenomenon is not clear and the interpretation of it differs. The most common view is a decubitus (pressure) ulcer caused by pressure and hypoxia during the unconscious state. This is contradicted by the observations of Holten (1951-1952), who observed lesions appearing even in conscious patients, and in unconscious patients lesions sometimes so widespread that pressure could not possibly explain them all.

The most significant common finding in histologic investigations of both vesicular/bullous and nonvesicular lesions is necrosis of sweat gland units. Furthermore, Adebahr (1963), whose investigation was based on 300 autopsy cases due to barbiturate poisoning, suggested the possibility that the intoxicating drug was excreted via the sweat glands and induced the damage to the surrounding tissue. The clinical photograph in Case 11 shows a well-demarcated plaque which is stuffed with minute vesicles and also contains some larger vesicles and a bulla. In accordance with this, the micrographs demonstrate how necrotic sweat ducts from underlying necrotic sweat glands can be followed through the dermis into the epidermis and become surrounded by a vesicle. These smaller vesicles enlarge, coalesce and form a bulla, which is mainly subepidermal. However, small remains of basal cells on the dermal papillae at the ends of the bulla, also observed by Sanchez Yus et al. (1993), indicate that the bulla from the beginning has been intraepidermal. These findings strongly indicate the important role of the sweat gland units in the development of the vesicular and bullous lesions, and thus highly support the theory of Adebahr.

How then can one explain the fact that even scattered hair follicle units, which anatomically have nothing to do with eccrine sweat duct units, may be affected? It has long been known that drugs may be excreted in the sweat (Brehmer-Andersson and Pedersen 1969). Recently this knowledge has been applied to verify abuse of drugs such as amphetamines, cocaine, and cannabis in sweat samples from drivers (Samyn et al. 2002). Furthermore, an investigation by Lester et al. (2002) has revealed that excretion of cocaine is also possible via sebaceous glands. Probably the concentration of the drug in the excretion is decisive for the development of damage or no damage.

There are two different types of decubitus (pressure) ulcers, one superficial and one deep, neither of which is in accordance with the pattern described above in Case 11. The superficial type is caused by a shear force (friction) on the skin, which gives rise to maceration (necrosis) of superficial skin layers that eventually may lead to ulceration. Deep ulcers arise in deep muscle layers covering a bony prominence and are mainly caused by sustained compression of tissue and vessels (Bouten et al. 2003). Such ulcers develop quickly and the tissue damage, which may include necrosis of both sweat glands and sebaceous glands, is severe (Witkowski and Parish 1982). This is in contrast to the selective damage to some groups of sweat glands and single hair follicles found in intoxicated and comatose patients.

References

1. Achten G, Ledoux-Corbusier M, Thys J-P (1971) Intoxication à l'oxyde de carbone e lésions cutanées. Ann Dermatol Syph 98:421–428
2. Adebahr G (1963) Hautveränderungen bei Schlafmittelvergiftung. Landarzt 30:1302–1307
3. Arndt KA, Mihm MC, Parrish JA (1973) Bullae: a cutaneous sign of a variety of neurologic diseases. J Invest Dermatol 60:312–320
4. Baker H, Ryan TJ (1968) Generalized pustular psoriasis. A clinical and epidemiological study of 104 cases. Br J Dermatol 80:771–793
5. Bastuji-Garin S, Rzany B, Stern RS, Shear NH, Naldi L, Roujeau J-C (1993) Clinical classification of cases of toxic epidermal necrolysis, Stevens-Johnson syndrome, and erythema multiforme. Arch Dermatol 129:92–96
6. Beveridge GW, Lawson AAH (1965) Occurrence of bullous lesions in acute barbiturate intoxication. BMJ 1:835–837
7. Bialy-Golan A, Brenner S (1996) Penicillamine-induced bullous dermatoses. J Am Acad Dermatol 35:732–742
8. Bolognia JL, Braverman I (1992) Pseudoxanthoma-elasticum-like skin changes induced by penicillamine. Dermatology 184:12–18
9. Bouten CV, Oomens CW, Baaijens FP, Bader DL (2003) The etiology of pressure ulcers: skin deep or muscle bound? Arch Phys Med Rehabil 84:616–619
10. Brehmer-Andersson E, Pedersen NB (1969) Sweat gland necrosis and bullous skin changes in acute drug intoxication. Acta Derm Venereol 49:157–162
11. Britschgi M, Pichler WJ (2002) Acute generalized exanthematous pustulosis, a clue to neutrophil-mediated inflammatory processes orchestrated by T cells. Curr Opin Allergy Clin Immunol 2:325–331
12. Burge S, Ryan TJ (1988) Penicillamine-induced pseudo-pseudoxanthoma elasticum in a patient with rheumatoid arthritis. Clin Exp Dermatol 13:255–258
13. Holten C (1951-1952) Cutaneous phenomena in acute barbiturate poisoning. Acta Derm Venereol Suppl (Stockh) 29:162–168
14. Hunziker T, Künzi U-P, Braunschweig S, Zehnder D, Hoigné R (1997) Comprehensive hospital drug monitoring (CHDM): adverse skin reactions, a 20-year survey. Allergy 52:388–393
15. Iozumi K, Nakagawa H, Tamaki K (1997) Penicillamine-induced degenerative dermatoses. Report of a case and brief review of such dermatoses. J Dermatol 24:458–465
16. Lester L, Uemura N, Ademola J, Harkey MR, Nath RP, Kim SJ, Jerschow E, Henderson GL, Mendelson J, Jones RT (2002) Disposition of cocaine in skin, interstitial fluid, sebum, and stratum corneum. J Anal Toxicol 26:547–553
17. Lyell A (1956) Toxic epidermal necrolysis: an eruption resembling scalding of the skin. Br J Dermatol 68:355–361
18. Magro CM, Crowson AN, Schapiro BL (1998) The interstitial granulomatous drug reaction: a distinctive clinical and pathological entity. J Cutan Pathol 25:72–78

19. Mahboob A, Haroon TS (1998) Drugs causing fixed eruptions. A study of 450 cases. Int J Dermatol 37:833–838
20. Mandy S, Ackerman AB (1970) Characteristic traumatic skin lesions in drug-induced coma. JAMA 213:253–256
21. Meyrick Thomas RH, Kirby JD (1985) Elastosis perforans serpiginosa and pseudoxanthoma elasticum-like skin change due to D-penicillamine. Clin Exp Dermatol 10:386–391
22. Miyauchi H, Hosokawa H, Akaeda T, Iba H, Asada Y (1991) T-cell subsets in drug-induced toxic epidermal necrolysis. Possible pathogenic mechanism induced by CD8-positive T cells. Arch Dermatol 127:851–855
23. Naisbitt DJ, Williams DP, Pirmohamed M, Kitteringham NR, Park BK (2001) Reactive metabolites and their role in drug reactions. Curr Opin Allergy Clin Immunol 1:317–325
24. Paquet P, Piérard GE (1997) Erythema multiforme and toxic epidermal necrolysis: a comparative study. Am J Dermatopathol 19:127–132
25. Paquet P, Nikkels A, Arrese JE, Vanderkelen A, Piérard GE (1994) Macrophages and tumor necrosis factor α in toxic epidermal necrolysis. Arch Dermatol 130:605–608
26. Paul C, Wolkenstein P, Adle H, Wechsler J, Garchon, HJ, Revuz J, Roujeau JC (1996) Apoptosis as a mechanism of keratinocyte death in toxic epidermal necrolysis. Br J Dermatol 134:710–714
27. Pichler WJ (2002) Deciphering the immune pathomechanism of cutaneous drug reactions. Allergy 57 [Suppl 72]:34–36
28. Pichler WJ, Yawalkar N, Britschgi M, Depta JP, Strasser I, Schmid S, Kuechler P, Naisbitt D (2002) Cellular and molecular pathophysiology of cutaneous drug reactions. Am J Clin Dermatol 3:229–238
29. Poon E, Mason GH, Oh C (2002) Clinical and histological spectrum of elastotic changes induced by penicillamine. Australas J Dermatol 43:147–150
30. Roujeau JC, Stern RS (1994) Severe adverse cutaneous reactions to drugs. N Engl J Med 331:1272–1285
31. Roujeau J-C, Bioulac-Sage P, Bourseau C, Guillaume J-C, Bernard P, Lok C, Plantin P, Claudy C, Delavierre C, Vaillant L, Wechsler J, Danan G, Bénichou C, Beylot C (1991) Acute generalized exanthematous pustulosis. Analysis of 63 cases. Arch Dermatol 127:1333–1338
32. Samyn N, De Boeck G, Verstraete AG (2002) The use of oral fluid sweat wipes for the detection of drugs of abuse in drivers. J Forensic Sci 47:1380–1387
33. Sanchez Yus E, Requena L, Simon P (1993) Histopathology of cutaneous changes in drug-induced coma. Am J Dermatopathol 15:208–216
34. Shiohara T, Mizukawa Y, Teraki Y (2002) Pathophysiology of fixed drug eruption: the role of skin-resident T cells. Curr Opin Allergy Clin Immunol 2:317–323
35. Sidoroff A, Halevy S, Bavinck JNB, Vaillant L, Roujeau J-C (2001) Acute generalized exanthematous pustulosis (AGEP)—a clinical reaction pattern. J Cutan Pathol 28:113–119
36. Sorensen BF (1963) Skin symptom in acute narcotic intoxication. Dan Med Bull 10:130–131
37. Stubb S, Heikkilä H, Kauppinen K (1994) Cutaneous reactions to drugs: a series of in-patients during a five-year period. Acta Derm Venereol 74:289–291
38. Svensson CK, Cowen EW, Gaspari AA (2001) Cutaneous drug reactions. Pharmacol Rev 53:357–379
39. Torne R, Soyer HP, Leb G, Kerl H (1991) Skin lesions in carbon monoxide intoxication. Dermatologica 183:212–215
40. Witkowski JA, Parish LC (1982) Histopathology of the decubitus ulcer. J Am Acad Dermatol 6:1014–1021
41. Yawalkar N, Pichler J (2001) Immunohistology of drug-induced exanthema: clues to pathogenesis. Curr Opin Allergy Clin Immunol 1:299–303

Chapter 29

Artifacts 29

The term artifact is used here to denote self-inflicted or accidentally induced lesions on the skin and oral mucosa. It is often difficult to prove that self-inflicted lesions (*pathomimia*) made unknowingly or with the intention to mislead are indeed self-inflicted, even though this may be suspected both clinically and histopathologically. In rare cases, the histologic investigation may be decisive, for example if a needle track or injected foreign material is identified in the dermis and/or subcutis. Mostly the pattern is difficult to interpret, but there are some guiding clues indicating friction, scratching, pressure, or burns.

29.1 Friction Blisters and Scratch Marks

Blisters provoked on the palms by unaccustomed manual labor, or on the feet from ill-fitting shoes are probably the most common lesions caused by friction, but are rarely the subject of histologic investigation. Scratch marks mostly indicate severe pruritus. So-called *acquired perforating collagenosis* is a severe form of scratching, which appears in different kinds of diseases. It is most commonly observed in association with chronic kidney failure, but is also described in diabetes mellitus, hypothyroidism, hyperparathyroidism and liver dysfunction (Faver et al.1994).

29.1.1 Clinical Appearance

On hands and feet friction gives rise to vesicles/bullae filled with clear, water-like fluid, and in other areas to superficial ulceration. Scratch marks appear as scattered deep ulcerations all over the body.

29.1.2 Histopathologic Appearance

Friction blisters, located on hands and feet, usually have a characteristic histopathologic pattern. There is a superficial intraepidermal vesicle, the roof of which consists of stratum corneum and one or two rows of granular or necrotic keratinocytes. The remains of the epidermis makes up the floor, the uppermost part consisting of a band of necrotic and vacuolated cells, the lower part of preserved keratinocytes (Fig. 29.1a–c). There is very little inflammatory response. In an early lesion, instead of a vesicle, there is a superficial band of necrotic keratinocytes (Fig. 29.1d). Vesicles located in other areas show a less typical pattern (Fig. 29.2c). Also secondary infection can modify the picture (Fig. 29.2a,b).

Scratch marks are histologically deep ulcerations which include the papillary dermis and sometimes expose damaged collagen bundles. The margins are abrupt and the inflammatory reaction poor (Fig. 29.2d).

29.1.3 Pathogenesis

Sulzberger et al. (1966) studied the development of friction blisters. They were able to evoke blisters on volunteers at all sites of the skin either by linear rubbing (using an instrument constructed for the purpose) or by twist rubbing (using an eraser on an ordinary pencil). However, in most places the vesicle cracked rapidly, and complete fluid-filled blisters did not occur. It was possible to produce the latter only in areas where the skin was taut (i.e., where the lower epidermis is firmly attached to the underlying tissue and at the same time the stratum corneum and the stratum granulosum are thick); those regions are the soles, heels, palms and the dorsal aspect of the fingers. This means that the location of the exposed area modifies the histopathologic pattern. Scratch marks are probably caused by a long pointed nail.

29.1.4 Examples

Case 1. Friction Blisters

A 60-year-old man had suffered from recurrent blisters on the hands for many years. A biopsy specimen including a fresh blister from the palm of the hand revealed a typical friction blister. When asked, the patient admitted that he had himself provoked the lesions by scratching with his nails. On request he scratched up a

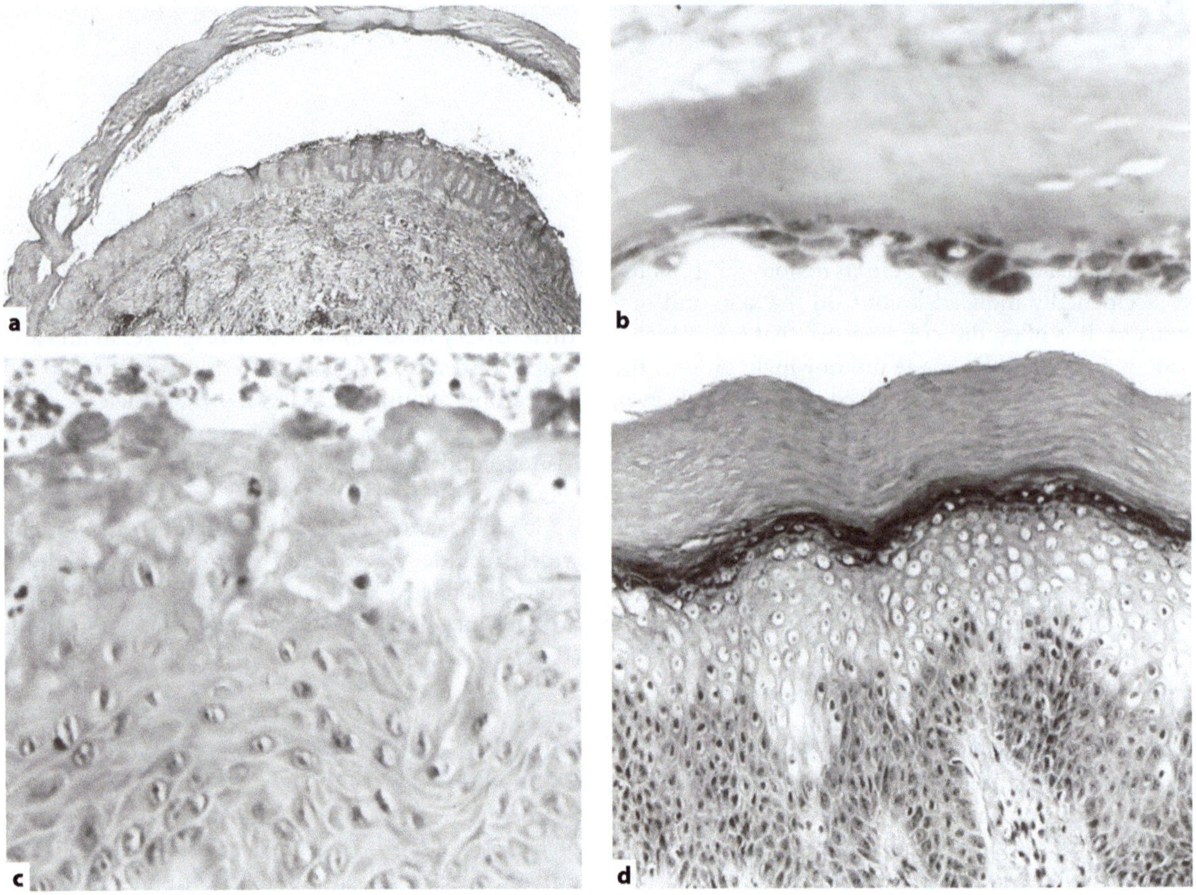

Fig. 29.1 Friction blisters. **a** There is a wide, superficial and intraepidermal vesicle. **b** The roof consists of stratum corneum and one or two rows of granular cells. **c** The remains of the epidermis makes up the floor; the upper part consists of a band of necrotic keratinocytes, the lower part is normal. **d** Friction blister in the making. The cells in the upper two-thirds of the stratum spinosum are faded and vacuolated, while the cells in the lower part are preserved. The stratum granulosum and the horny layer seem to be preserved. H&E

new blister on the palm. This was excised and showed exactly the same histopathologic pattern as the blister first examined (Fig. 29.1a–c) (Brehmer-Andersson and Göransson 1975).

Case 2. Friction Blister in the Making

A 32-year-old general laborer had suffered from spells of small, non-itching blisters on the wrists, dorsal aspect of the hands, lower legs, front of the chest, and face from the age of 18 years. Outbreaks occurred every 1 or 2 months and developed over 1–2 days. The blisters broke after a short while and healed with a scar. No fresh lesions were observed. A month later a few maculopapules with a scratch mark on the top and one with a suspected vesicle were seen on the fingers.

A biopsy specimen was taken from the lesion with the suspected vesicle and cut in series. There was no vesicle, but a broad band of vacuolated and necrotic keratinocytes below the stratum granulosum (Fig. 29.1d).

The pattern was interpreted as a friction blister in the making. When confronted with this possibility the patient did not come back to the next appointment and was lost to follow-up (Brehmer-Andersson and Göransson 1975).

Case 3. Friction Blister with Secondary Infection

A 75-year-old woman now and then suffered from scattered urticaria wheals. A punch biopsy specimen was taken from one such lesion located on the wrist and suspected to have a vesicle on the top.

Histologic investigation showed a thickened epi-

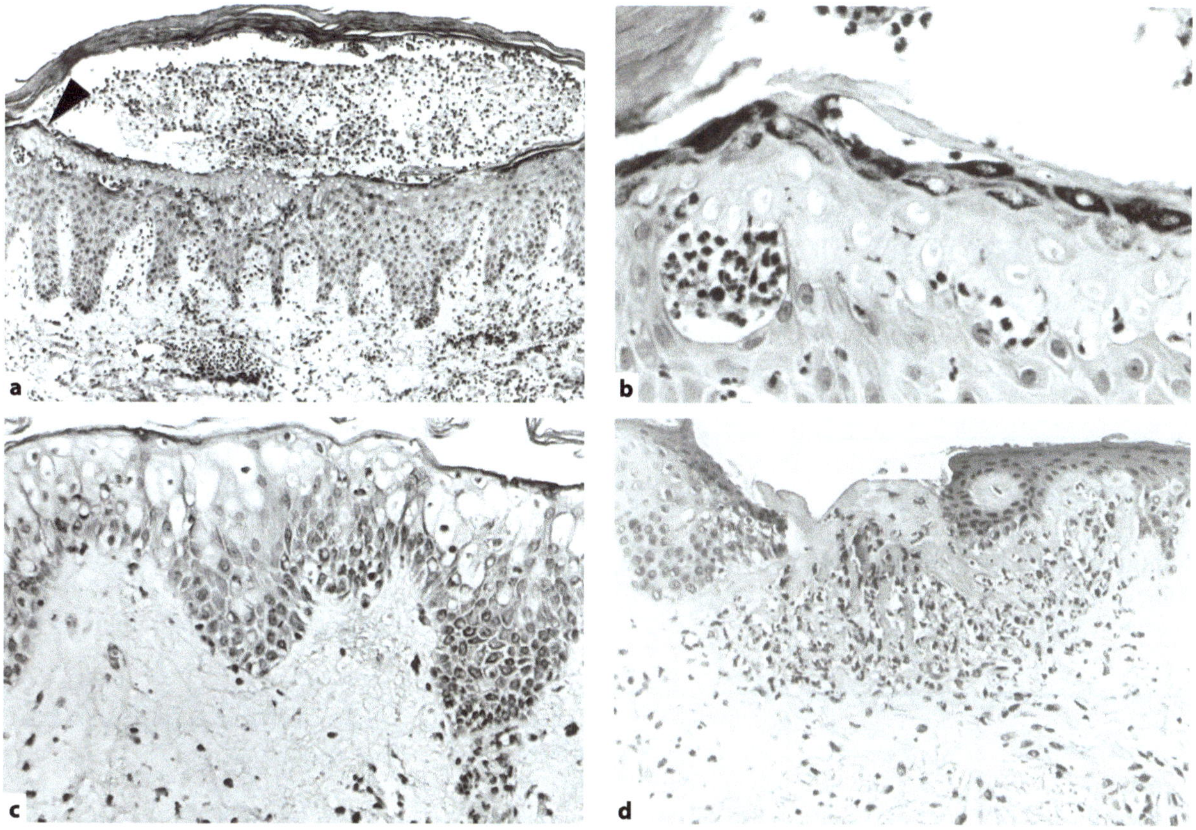

Fig. 29.2 Friction and scratching. **a** Friction blister and secondary infection. There is a wide subcorneal pustule filled with neutrophils. The lower and largest part of the floor has preserved keratinocytes; between this part and the pustule there is an edge composed of stratum granulosum and a band of faded, necrotic keratinocytes. **b** Close-up of the area indicated (*arrowhead*) in **a**. The granular cells seem preserved, but some of them contain a vacuole instead of a nucleus. Between necrotic and normal epithelium there are microabscesses. **c** Urticaria wheal with signs of scratching. The epidermis is slightly acanthotic and, mainly in the upper half, shows vacuolated and faded keratinocytes. In the upper dermis there are conspicuous edema and sparse inflammatory cell infiltrates. **d** Scratch mark. The small but deep ulcer has abrupt margins. The bottom of the ulcer is covered with fibrin and the adjacent part of the dermis is soaked with fibrin and permeated by neutrophils. H&E

dermis with a subcorneal pustule filled with neutrophils and exudate. The floor consisted of the remains of the epidermis. Below the stratum granulosum there was a distinct band of necrotic shadow keratinocytes and scattered small pustules filled with neutrophils. There were perivascular and diffuse infiltrates of lymphocytes with an admixture of eosinophils in the dermis (Fig. 29.2a,b).

The lesion was interpreted as an itching wheal which had been rubbed (indicated by the necrotic band below the stratum granulosum) and was secondarily infected.

Case 4. Urticaria Wheal with Signs of Scratching

This 48-year-old woman for 2 weeks had had itchy papules, which came and vanished, on pressure sites.

Histologic investigation revealed a slightly acanthotic epidermis, the outermost part of which consisted of swollen, faded or vacuolated keratinocytes. There was a conspicuous edema in the dermis with sparse perivascular cell infiltrates composed of lymphocytes with an admixture of eosinophils and neutrophils. Vasculitis was not observed (Fig. 29.2c).

The lesion was interpreted as an urticaria wheal with epidermal injury due to scratching. The epidermal damage was not as distinct as in the previous cases, probably due to the location of the wheal, not specified in the request form.

Case 5. Scratch Mark

A 91-year-old man presented with scratch marks on the legs and shoulders.

The biopsy specimen comprised superficial subcutaneous tissue. In the center of the specimen there was a single small and deep ulceration which included the entire thickness of the epidermis and the underlying papillary dermis. It had abrupt margins and the bottom was covered with fibrin. Also in the area close to the ulceration the dermis was soaked by fibrin and permeated by neutrophils. In the whole specimen there was a slight edema in the upper dermis, dilated venules and a sparse infiltrate of lymphocytes. The rest of the dermis and the included parts of the subcutaneous tissue were normal (Fig. 29.2d).

29.2 Decubitus Ulcers

Deep decubitus ulcers are caused by pressure and are common in disabled and/or debilitated, bedridden patients (Sect. 28.9.4) (Witkowski and Parish 1982; Bouten et al. 2003).

29.3 Hematidrosis

Hematidrosis, hemorrhage in the papillary dermis and terminal sweat gland ducts, also called calcaneal petechiae and black heels, is a kind of pressure trauma that was first described in basket ball players (Crissey and Peachey 1961). Subsequent reports have revealed that this is a rather common kind of injury in teenagers and young adults practicing different kinds of ball games, and has been observed also on the soles, on the knees in nuns, and in the thenar region in golf players (Kirton and Price 1965; Rufli 1980).

29.3.1 Clinical Appearance

On one or both heals there is a black patch which consists of dark dots seemingly located at different levels in the horny layer. The condition is harmless; however, a single lesion may be mistaken for malignant melanoma.

29.3.2 Histopathologic Appearance

Amorphous material, which is not positive for hemosiderin, accumulates in the acrosyringium. Histochemical investigations have proved that the amorphous material is hematoidin, a degradation product of hemoglobin (Kirton and Price 1965; Rufli 1980).

29.3.3 Example

Case 6. Calcaneal Petechiae

A 19-year-old man presented with dark, painful patches on both heels. Clinically the patches seemed to be composed of black dots located at different levels of the stratum corneum. He did not practice any particular sport that could be held responsible for the lesion.

Histologic investigation showed a conspicuously thickened horny layer with many dilated sweat gland ducts. In H&E-stained sections these were filled with orange-colored amorphous material. Scattered dilated ducts containing red blood cells were observed in the upper epidermis. In the dermal papilla below one of these there was a fresh hemorrhage. The rest of the papillae and the upper dermis contained dilated venules and a few lymphocytes. Sweat glands and intradermal sweat ducts were normal (Fig. 29.3). (Dammert et al. 1965)

29.4 Burns

Burns may be caused in different ways, for example by contact with hot objects, hot liquids, steam, fire and electricity. In dermatological practice it is seen in self-inflicted lesions, after therapeutic radiation, at the margins of specimens excised by means of diathermy, and in phytophotodermatitis.

29.4.1 Accidental and Self-Inflicted Burns

The severity of the burn is correlated with the depth of tissue damage. In a first-degree burn only the epidermis is affected. A second-degree burn also includes the superficial dermis, and a third-degree the whole dermis and appendages. First- and second-degree burns are also referred to as partial thickness burns, which means that at least the deeper parts of the dermal appendages, which are able to provide cells for epithelial regeneration, are preserved. A full-thickness burn is equal to a third-degree burn. First-degree burns give rise to erythematous dermatitis, second-degree burns to vesicular and/or bullous dermatitis, and third-degree burns to ulcerations and/or charring.

Histologically a second-degree lesion shows a necrotic epidermis. A typical finding is elongated basal cells, resembling a shoal of fish (Fig. 29.4c,d). In the underlying tissue there is a conspicuous edema. Burns caused by contact with live or grounded electrical con-

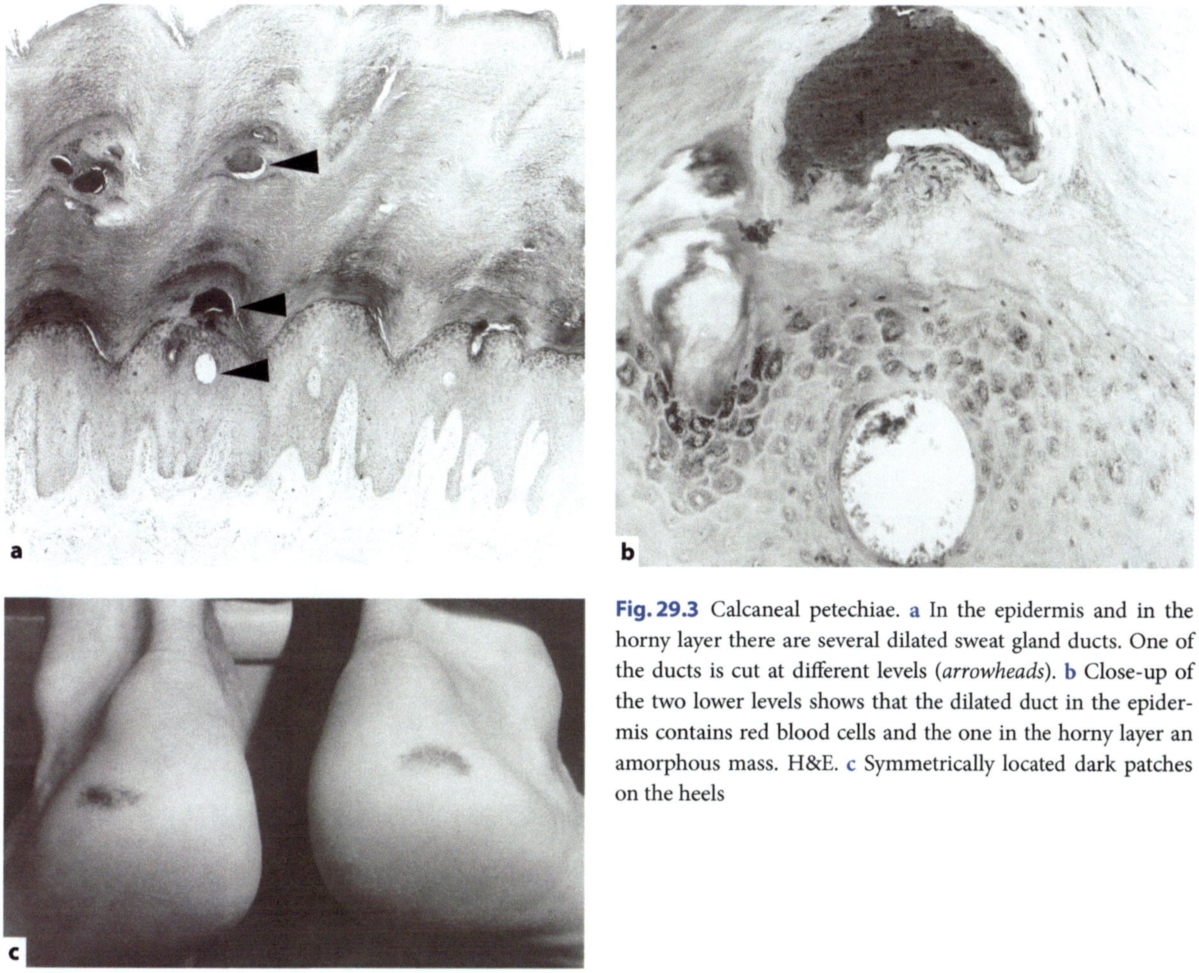

Fig. 29.3 Calcaneal petechiae. a In the epidermis and in the horny layer there are several dilated sweat gland ducts. One of the ducts is cut at different levels (*arrowheads*). b Close-up of the two lower levels shows that the dilated duct in the epidermis contains red blood cells and the one in the horny layer an amorphous mass. H&E. c Symmetrically located dark patches on the heels

ductors carrying high-voltage circuits (i.e., more than 440 V) are ordinarily charred and deep (Fig. 29.4a–c).

29.4.2 Late Therapeutic Radiation Dermatitis

There are two kinds of reactions. Early radiation dermatitis occurs shortly after the treatment and is transient and heals without remnants or with pigmentation or scarring. Late radiation dermatitis, if it occurs, may be evident months or several years later. Now and then the pathologist has to deal with the late variant.

29.4.2.1 Clinical Appearance

Clinically the skin is mainly atrophic, but may show focal hypertrophy. There are irregular areas of hypo- and hyperpigmentation and telangiectases, and sometimes ulceration.

29.4.2.2 Histopathologic Appearance

The typical histopathologic pattern shows an atrophic epidermis together with edema, dilated thin-walled vessels, and areas with hyaline collagen tissue in the upper half the dermis (Fig. 29.5a). Sometimes there are also thick-walled vessels and thrombotic veins in the deep dermis and subcutis (Fig. 29.5b). The changes may be difficult to differentiate from those seen in lichen sclerosus et atrophicus. However, a band-like cell infiltrate below the edematous hyaline area is usually present in lichen sclerosus (Fig. 27.1e).

29.4.3 Phytophotodermatitis

Phytophotodermatitis is caused by contact with crushed plants containing *furocoumarin* followed by exposure to light, and gives rise to bullous skin lesions due to epidermal necrosis (Fig. 29.5c,d).

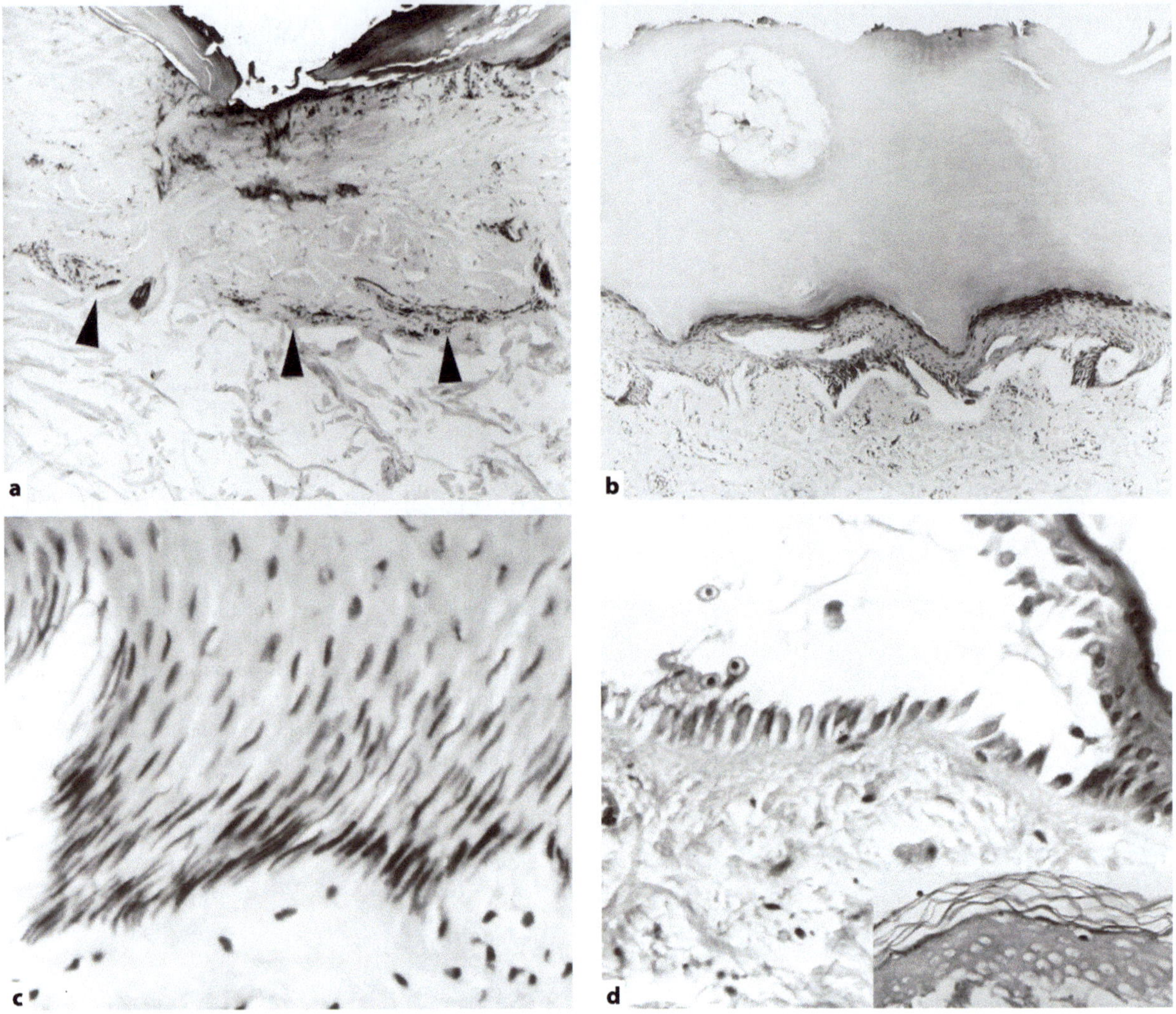

Fig. 29.4 Burns: **a–c** electrical burn; **d** self-inflicted burn. **a** In the center of the injury, the stratum corneum and epidermis are charred, and the adjacent part of the dermis is charred or homogenized due to coagulation. Below this area there is a conspicuous edema. *Arrowheads* indicate the border between coagulated and edematous parts. **b** Close to the center, the horny layer is either coagulated or charred and contains a large vacuole. The remains of the epidermis is severely damaged and with a cleft separated from the dermis. **c** Close-up shows that cells in the basal cell layer and in the rows next to it are elongated and give the impression of a shoal of fish. **d** The micrograph shows the end of a subepidermal vesicle, where a row of longitudinally stretched basal cells is still attached to the dermis; above them there are a few acantholytic cells. The *inset* shows a part of the necrotic epidermis; instead of a nucleus the cells contain a vacuole. H&E

29.4.4 Examples

Case 7. Electrical Burns

A young apprentice had current pass through his body when drilling in an elevator shaft and died close to the accident.

Histologic investigation of the contact surface between the conductor and the skin showed that the epidermis and the subepidermal area were charred, or homogenized due to coagulation necrosis. Below the necrotic area the tissue was markedly edematous. Peripherally to the necrotic area, the epidermis was severely damaged and there was a subepidermal cleft detached from the dermis. Basal cells and adjacent rows of keratinocytes were longitudinally stretched and had a typical shoal of fish appearance (Fig. 29.4a–c).

Case 8. Lesion Probably Caused by a Burning Cigarette

A 39-year-old woman had had a therapy-resistant ulcer on the sole of her foot for 6 months. The ulcer

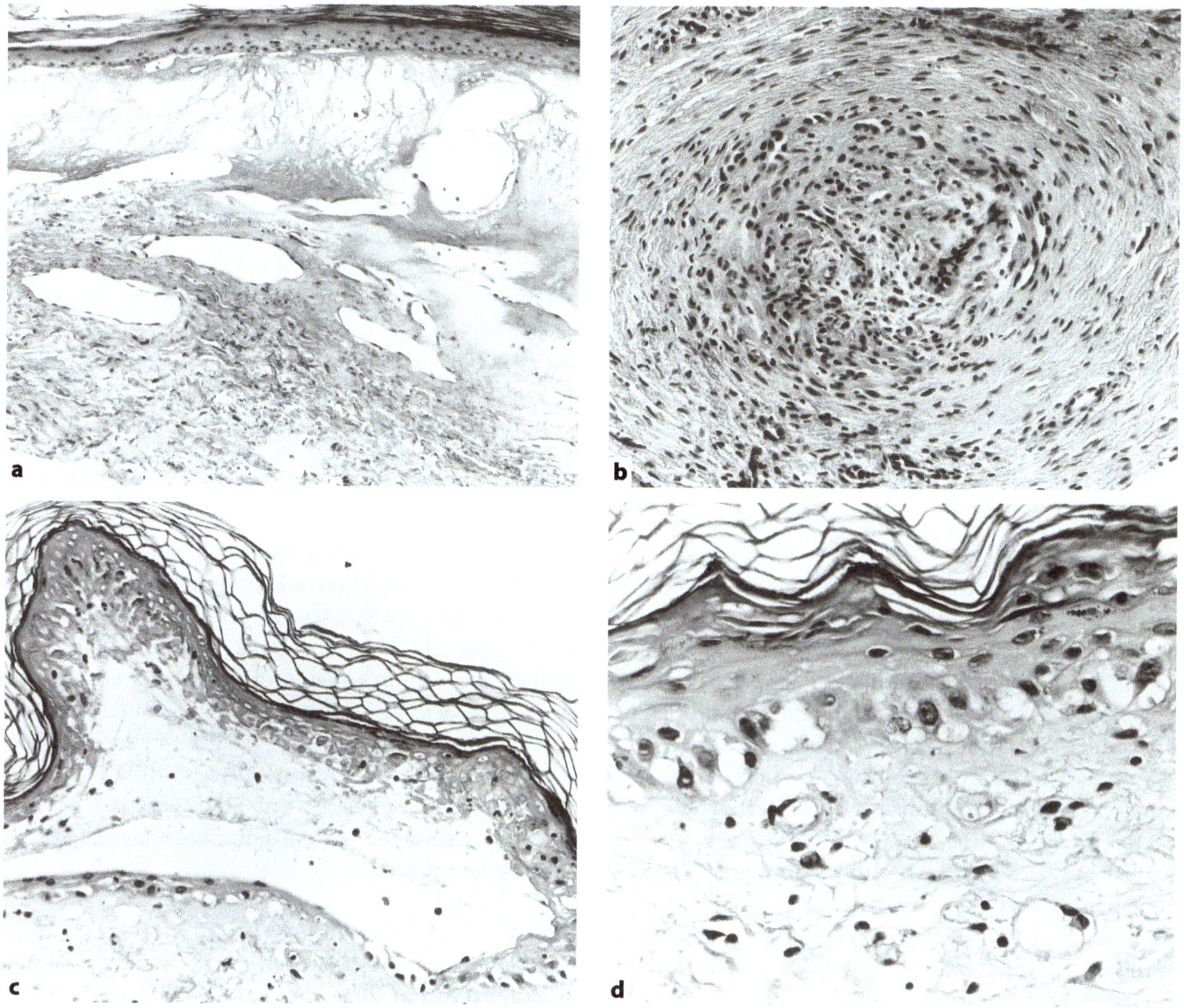

Fig. 29.5 Radiation dermatitis: **a, b** late therapeutic radiation dermatitis; **c, d** phytophotodermatitis. **a** The epidermis is very thin and hyperkeratotic. There is a conspicuous subepidermal edema, below which the dermis is composed of hyaline connective tissue and contains several dilated lymphatics. The two vessels to the left have valves. **b** A large, subcutaneous, thick-walled fibrotic vein is occluded by a thrombus in organization. **c** There is an intraepidermal vesicle. The roof consists of a seemingly normal horny layer with a basket-weave pattern and necrotic epithelial cells, and the floor of one or two rows of cells, some of which are conspicuously vacuolated. **d** Close-up of another area of the same specimen. The epidermis is thin and shows marked vacuolization in the basal cell layer. The subepidermal area is edematous. H&E

healed when a shoe of plaster was applied, but instead two circular blisters appeared above the plaster on the ventral aspect of the lower leg. A biopsy specimen was taken from the margin of one of the vesicles.

Histologic investigation revealed a part of a subepidermal vesicle. The epidermis was necrotic and partially detached from the dermis. At the end of the vesicle there was a row of longitudinally stretched basal cells still attached to the dermis. The upper half of the dermis was edematous and contained a few dilated vessels stuffed with erythrocytes. There were small perivascular infiltrates of neutrophils. The lesion was probably caused by a burning cigarette (Fig. 29.4d).

Case 9. Late Radiation Dermatitis

A 55-year-old woman had received X-ray treatment for ovarian carcinoma 12 years previously. Now the skin on the lower part of the abdomen was atrophic and telangiectatic. The surface showed small crusts and minute red papules, and was in some areas oozing.

The epidermis was very thin and hyperkeratotic. The subepidermal part was conspicuously edematous.

Below the edema, the tissue was hyaline and contained dilated lymphatics. Subcutaneous tissue was not included (Fig. 29.5a).

Case 10. Late Radiation Dermatitis

A 65-year-old man previously treated with whole-body radiation for mycosis fungoides presented with nonspecific dermatitis.

A biopsy revealed a chronic dermatitis with irregular acanthosis, inflammatory cell infiltrates and telangiectases in the dermis. In the subcutis there was a large fibrotic and thrombosed vein (Fig. 29.5b).

Case 11. Phytophotodermatitis

A 76-year-old man had had several bullae on a reddish base for a few days. The lesions were located on the trunk and one arm. A biopsy specimen was taken from the arm.

Histologic investigation revealed several confluent intra- and subepidermal vesicles with a necrotic or conspicuously vacuolated epithelium. In the whole dermis, but most prominently in the upper part, there was a marked edema, dilated lymphatics, and patchy infiltrates of lymphocytes (Fig. 29.5c,d).

Comment. The history given was poor. At first a drug reaction with toxic necrolysis under way was suspected. However, discussion with the referring dermatologist revealed that before the eruption the patient had spent a sunny day lying in the grass stripped to the waist. This indicated the possibility of phytophotodermatitis. No more bullae developed and the lesions healed without sequelae.

29.5 Morsicatio Mucosae Oris

Morsicatio mucosae oris, lesions on the oral mucosa caused by habitual biting or chewing, may be found on the buccal mucosa, the border of the tongue, and on the lips. Case reports with this type of lesion first appeared at the beginning of the 1960s (Kocsard et al. 1962). Later a series of patients with biting lesions was published (Hjørting-Hansen and Holst 1970).

29.5.1 Clinical Appearance

There is flaky desquamation of the mucosa interspersed with erosions and superficial ulceration.

29.5.2 Histopathologic Appearance

The characteristic histopathologic pattern is a superficial band of distorted, irregular, frayed, and bacteria-covered epithelium, superimposed on a normal epithelium (Fig. 29.6c,d).

29.5.3 Examples

Case 12. Morsicatio Buccarum

A 28-year-old woman had been treated for a histopathologically proven condyloma acuminatum in the vagina. A buccal lesion with a laciniated surface was excised for histologic investigation with the question at issue being condyloma.

Histologic investigation showed that the epithelium was divided into a lower and an upper compartment. The lower and main part consisted of an essentially normal epithelium to which an upper part of distorted epithelium with an irregular and bacteria-coated surface was added. The connective tissue contained only a sparse number of lymphocytes. There were no signs of human papilloma virus infection, and PAS staining gave no evidence of candidiasis (Fig. 29.6c).

When asked, the patient admitted that she was a habitual cheek-biter.

Case 13. Morsicatio Linguae

The patient was a 52-year old woman who complained of a smarting and somewhat ragged patch on the right border of the tongue.

The histopathologic pattern was essentially the same as in Case 12. There were no signs of human papilloma virus infection. PAS staining gave no evidence of candidiasis (Fig. 29.6d).

29.5.4 Comment

The epithelium of the buccal mucosa, the ventral surface of the tongue, and the inner surface of the lips do not undergo cornification under normal conditions. The nucleus of the superficial cells becomes pyknotic, but does not disappear, and the flatness of the cells becomes less conspicuous than in the skin. The superficial cells exfoliate. Thus saliva normally contains a large number of rather large, rounded, and regular epithelial cells with a small and centrally located nucleus (Fig. 29.6a,b). The usually light epithelium of these areas is variable. The presence of large, more or less vacuolated and clear cells (balloon cells)

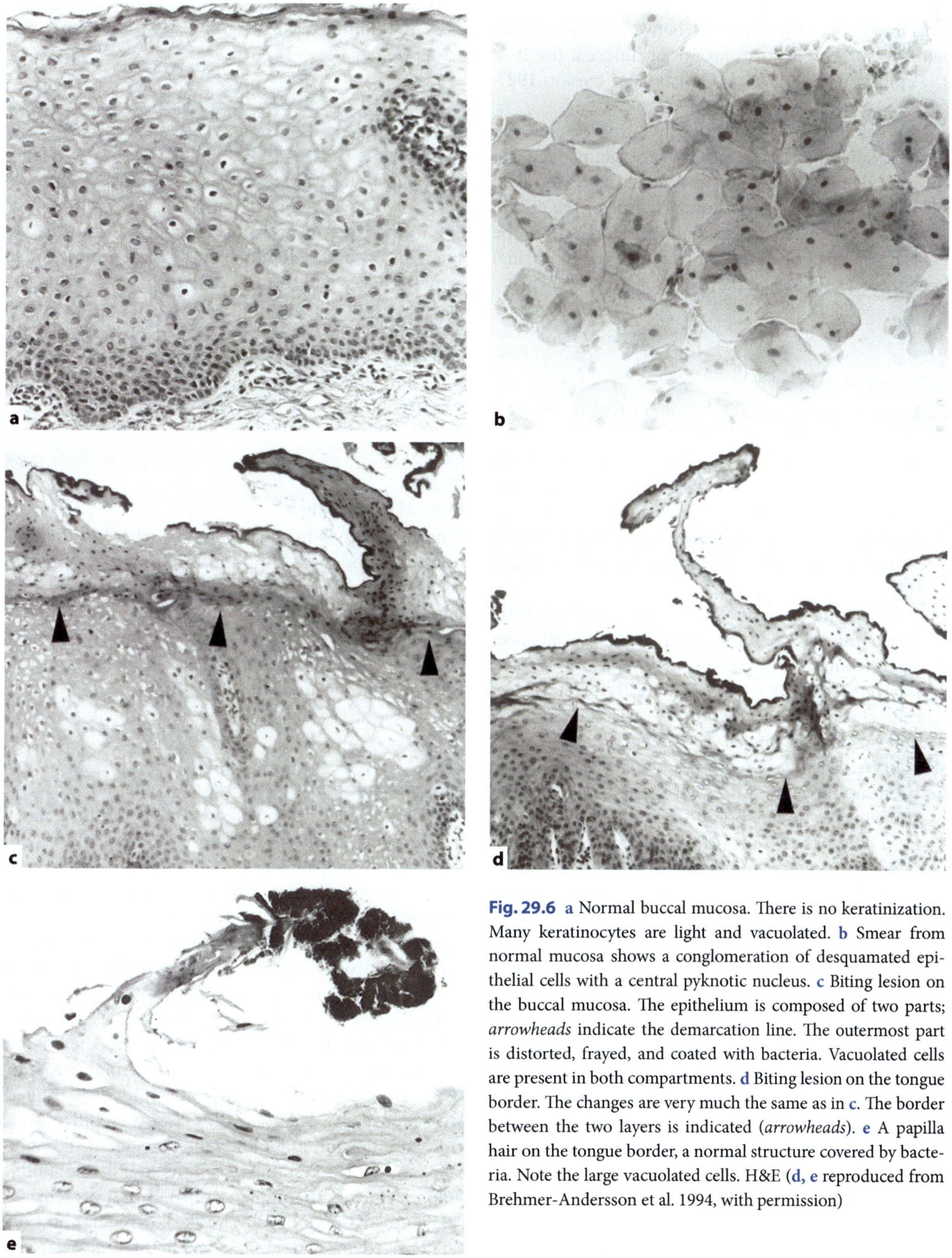

Fig. 29.6 a Normal buccal mucosa. There is no keratinization. Many keratinocytes are light and vacuolated. b Smear from normal mucosa shows a conglomeration of desquamated epithelial cells with a central pyknotic nucleus. c Biting lesion on the buccal mucosa. The epithelium is composed of two parts; *arrowheads* indicate the demarcation line. The outermost part is distorted, frayed, and coated with bacteria. Vacuolated cells are present in both compartments. d Biting lesion on the tongue border. The changes are very much the same as in c. The border between the two layers is indicated (*arrowheads*). e A papilla hair on the tongue border, a normal structure covered by bacteria. Note the large vacuolated cells. H&E (d, e reproduced from Brehmer-Andersson et al. 1994, with permission)

containing a small central nucleus is common. These cells may occupy the main area between the basal cells and the surface, or form groups at different levels of the epidermis (Fig. 29.6c) (Cawson and Eveson 1987; McKee 1989).

The patient is not continuously biting or chewing. This explains the characteristic histologic pattern. Before the damaged part of the epithelium is sloughed off, a brake in the biting allows the rest of the epithelium to be reconstructed from the remains below. The covering layer of bacteria can be seen even in normal oral mucosa and has no pathologic significance.

29.5.5 Differential Diagnosis

- *Normal oral mucosa.* Not infrequently the vacuolated cells normally present in the oral mucosa are mistaken for cells infected with human papilloma virus (HPV). Also small rudimentary filiform papilla hairs, which are normal structures on the tongue border, may be mistaken for a hairy-like projection in lesions caused by biting (Fig. 29.6e).
- *Candida infection* provokes hyper- and parakeratosis. Thus PAS staining is mandatory on all specimens from the oral mucosa.
- *Infections with HPV* (condyloma). In infected areas, cells show atypia (i.e., they have irregular nuclei and vary in form and size) (Ferenczy 1982).
- *Hairy leukoplakia.* Greenspan et al. (1984) described irremovable white, thick, corrugated or "hairy" lesions on the tongue border in patients positive for HIV. Because of the histopathologic pattern (i.e., hyper- and parakeratosis and hair-like projections from the surface) they called the phenomenon hairy leukoplakia (HL). The lesions were most often seen in patients with advanced HIV infection and commonly associated with Epstein-Barr virus (EBV) and *Candida* infections. It was assumed that a clinically typical HL lesion was synonymous with EBV infection. However, clinically typical HL lesions do not always contain EBV-infected epithelium (McMillan et al. 1989; Brehmer-Andersson et al. 1994) and clinically normal-looking epithelium has been proven to contain EBV (Näher et al. 1991; Ammatuna et al. 1998). Consequently, the relation between hyper- and parakeratosis and EBV infection is uncertain. Even early small foci invaded by *Candida* hyphae show conspicuous hyper- and parakeratosis, confined to affected areas. *Candida* infection is probably the main cause of HL. However, HL-like lesions can also be provoked by mechanical injury such as biting and ill-fitting rough dental fillings (McMillan et al. 1989; Brehmer-Andersson et al. 1994)

29.6 Amalgam Tattoo

By amalgam tattoo is meant a patch (macula) of blue–black or blue–gray discoloration on the oral mucosa due to inadvertent insertion of amalgam into the tissue. This occurs in different ways: finely ground amalgam particles may be inserted through a damaged or intact mucosa by high-speed rotary instruments, or fragments of amalgam may be deposited into the sockets during a tooth extraction or into the surgical wound during a retrograde root filling (Weathers and Fine 1974).

29.6.1 Clinical Appearance

Amalgam tattoos may be found anywhere in the oral cavity, but the most common locations are the gingival, alveolar, and buccal mucosa. Usually there is only one lesion up to 2 cm in diameter (Buchner and Hansen 1980). It is mostly a clinical diagnosis. The most common reason to take a biopsy or make an excision is to rule out melanocytic lesions.

29.6.2 Histopathologic Appearance

Histologic investigation shows finely ground amalgam as fine, black or dark-brown granules diffusely scattered in the papillary and reticular lamina propria and in the submucosa. Characteristically, densely aggregated granules are also seen along and between collagen bundles (Fig. 29.7a). In the submucosa, granules are found around striated muscles, nerves and small vessels, and also in the wall of vessels (Fig. 29.7c), and in the lumen of minor salivary glands. The epithelium is normal and does not contain granules. There is no or very little inflammatory response. Amalgam granules are not doubly refractive and cannot be identified with any special stains. In this way they differ from iron and melanin granules, which are about the same size, and in H&E-stained sections are also a similar color. Hemosiderin pigment is usually not present.

Fragments of amalgam are dark, irregular and different-sized foreign bodies, which may give rise to dense infiltrates of inflammatory cells with many giant cells of both types (amalgam granulomas) (Weathers and Fine 1974; Buchner and Hansen 1980).

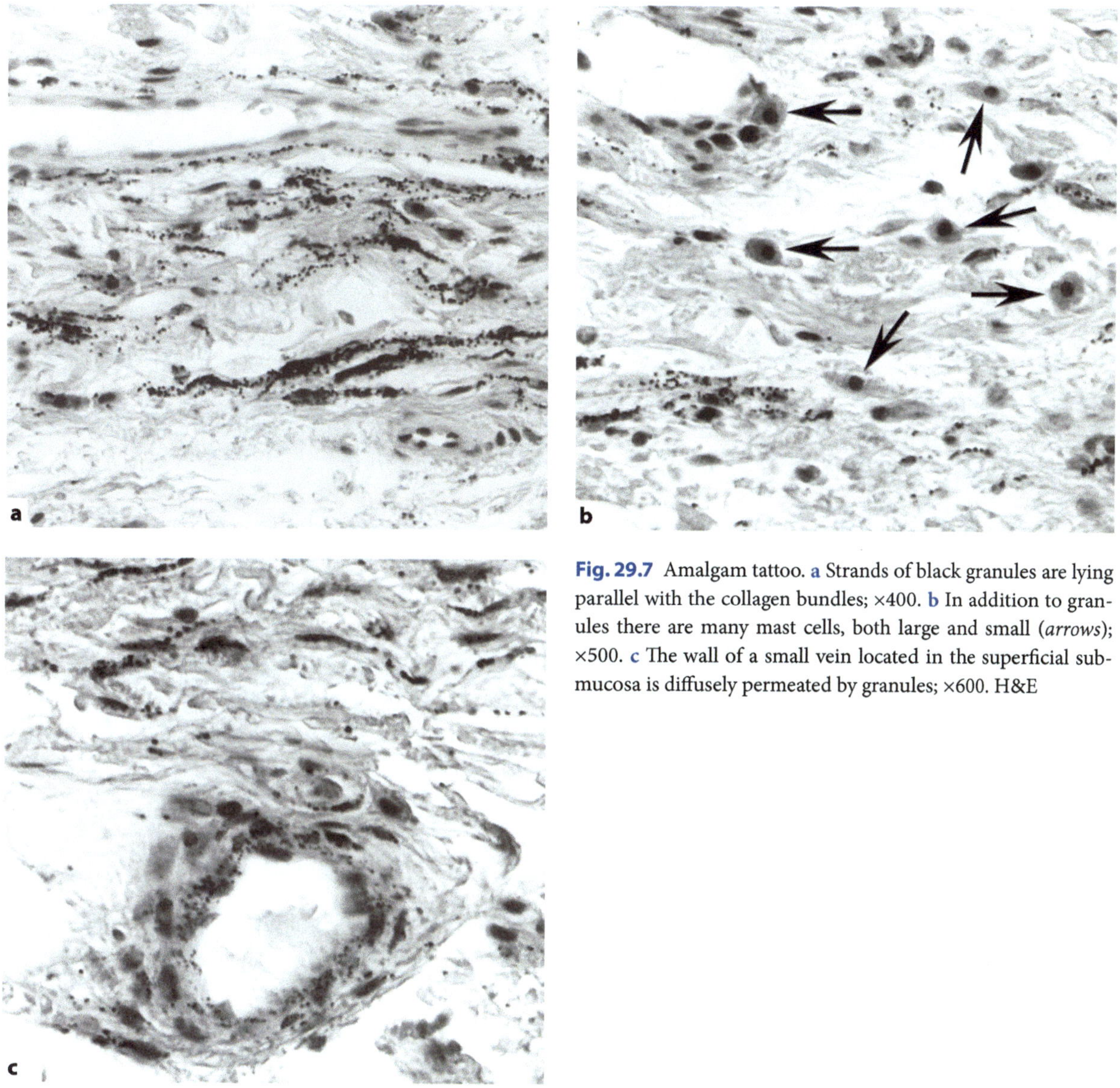

Fig. 29.7 Amalgam tattoo. **a** Strands of black granules are lying parallel with the collagen bundles; ×400. **b** In addition to granules there are many mast cells, both large and small (*arrows*); ×500. **c** The wall of a small vein located in the superficial submucosa is diffusely permeated by granules; ×600. H&E

29.6.3 Example

Case 14. Amalgam Tattoo

A 67-year-old woman presented with a bluish patch in the oral mucosa, suspected to be due to amalgam implantation. It was excised.

Histologic investigation revealed diffusely scattered black fine granules in a characteristic pattern in the lamina propria. In the submucosa, granules were observed around nerves and vessels, and also in the vessel walls. There were only sparse infiltrates of inflammatory cells, many of which were mast cells. In comparison with normal oral mucosa and biting lesions as well, the number of mast cells was notably large. Staining for melanin and iron pigments was negative (Fig. 29.7).

29.7 Chemical Burns in the Oral Mucosa

Chemical burns in the oral mucosa may be caused by accidentally drinking a solution of a corrosive substance such as caustic soda, or by misuse of drugs such as betel nut chewing. Fresh lesions show necrosis of the epithelium. Continuous use of drugs gives rise to fibrosis/sclerosis of the underlying tissue, which may be conspicuous in betel nut chewing.

Because of its stimulating effect betel chewing is an ancient habit regularly practiced in areas where the

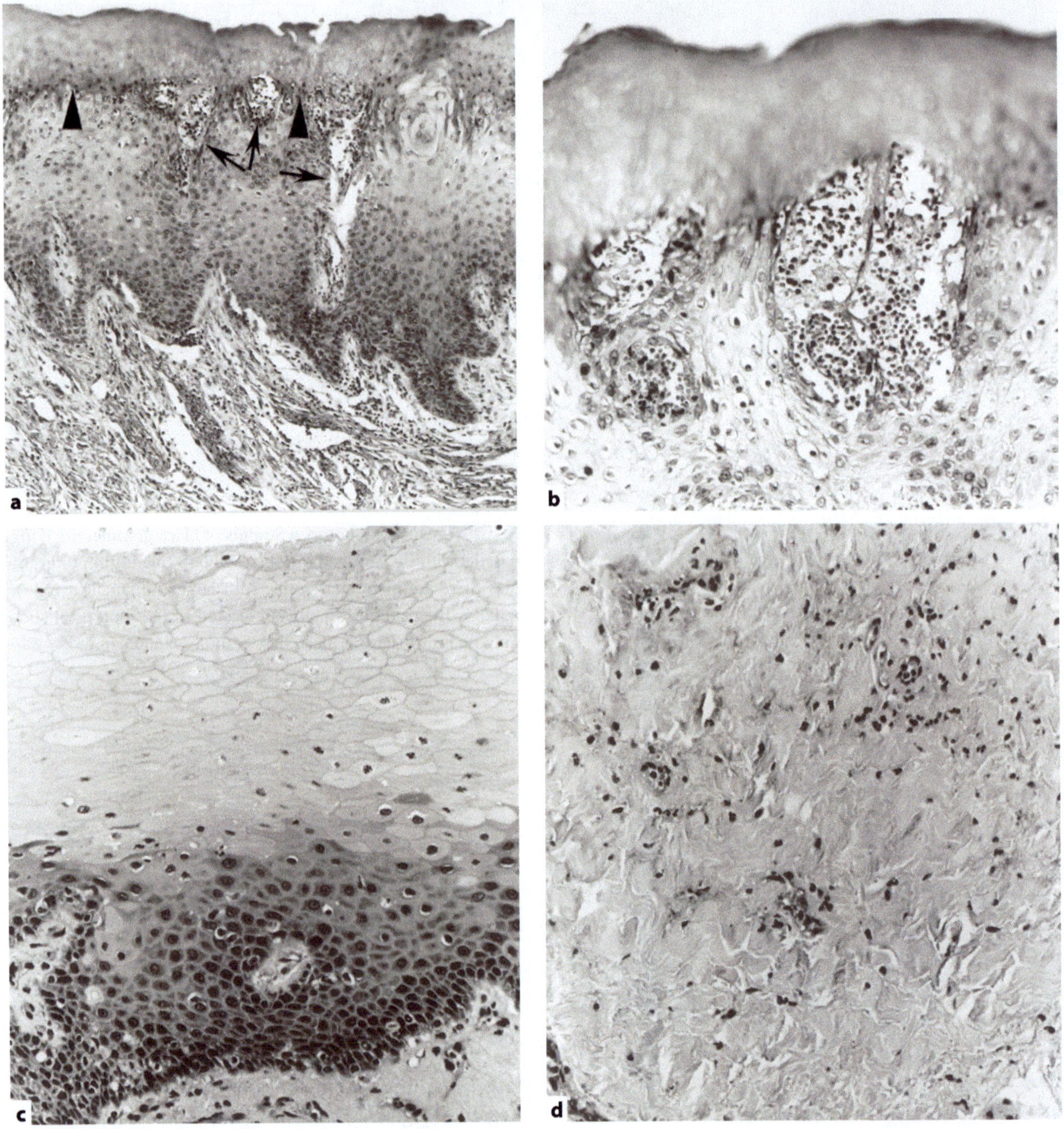

Fig. 29.8 Chemical burns: a, b lidocaine-adrenaline application; c, d betel nut chewing. a The thickened gingival epithelium has a superficial necrotic band. *Arrowheads* indicate the demarcation line and *arrows* show papillae filled with red blood cells. b Close-up of another area of the same specimen shows the necrotic epithelium above the blood-filled papillae, which are hugged by edematous rete ridges. c Thickened oral epithelium, the outermost two-thirds of which is necrotic and consists of shadow cells. In the transition zone some cells contain a pyknotic nucleus. d The lamina propria and submucosa are made up of sclerotic connective tissue that contains scattered capillaries and a sparse number of lymphocytes. H&E

betel palm, *Areca catechu*, is cultivated (i.e., a belt running from East Africa over India, South East Asia, Indonesia and the Philippines to New Guinea). In spite of undesired side effects there is an increasing use in the West. The betel quid is composed of the sliced or crushed core of the areca palm fruit mixed with a soft paste containing slaked lime (calcium hydroxide) and wrapped in a leaf from the vine betel pepper. Sometimes an aromatic spice or tobacco is added. Calcium hydroxide converts the active component of the betel seed, arecoline, into arecaidine which together with the active component of the betel pepper leave is absorbed into the circulation via the oral mucosa. Important adverse reactions are erosion and ulceration of the oral mucosa due to the caustic effect of the lime, and subsequent fibrosis of the submucosa and muscles, which in advanced cases may impair opening of the mouth. Also the incidence of oral squamous cell carcinoma is increased in betel-chewing individuals (Norton 1998; Pettersson et al. 1998).

29.7.1 Examples

Case 15. Lesion Caused by Lidocaine-Adrenaline Solution

A 54-year-old surgeon himself extracted a severely aching tooth. Two weeks later he consulted a dentist as the pain continued. The dentist found that the tooth socket was nearly filled up with granulation tissue and looked fine, but recognized that the mucous membrane around the socket was eroded, and thus took a biopsy.

Histologic investigation showed that the upper third of the epithelium formed a sharply demarcated band of eosinophilic or conspicuously faded and vacuolated cells. In the lamina propria hemorrhages, dilated vessels and patchy infiltrates of neutrophils were seen (Fig. 29.8a,b).

A self-inflicted lesion was suspected. Asked what he had done, the patient related that for long periods of time he had pressed pads of cotton wool soaked with a solution of lidocaine-adrenaline against the area to mitigate the pain. The astringent effect of the adrenaline on the vasculature may have explained the injury.

Case 16. Betel Nut Chewing[1]

A 29-year-old woman, a native of India, consulted for a chewing problem and reduced ability to open her mouth. She also complained of daily headache and pain in the right jaw joint. Clinical examination showed that she was able to open her mouth no more than 20 mm. There were white streaks on the buccal mucosa and the soft palate. Also the mucosa felt hard and fibrous. For 3 years the patient had chewed betel together with a considerable quantity of chilli pepper. A biopsy specimen from the oral mucosa was taken from the area close to the right ramus mandibulae.

Histologic investigation disclosed that either a superficial band of the epithelium or the entire epithelium was necrotic and composed of shadow cells, which lacked nuclei or contained a pyknotic one. The epithelium was mostly thickened, but sometimes thin and in small areas ulcerated. The lamina propria and submucosa were thickened and composed of densely packed collagen bundles with only few fibroblasts and sparse perivascular infiltrates of lymphocytes and neutrophils. The fibrosis also involved the underlying musculature (Fig. 29.8c,d).

References

1. Ammatuna P, Capone F, Giambelluca D, Pizzo I, D'Alia G, Margiotta V (1998) Detection of Epstein-Barr virus (EBV) DNA and antigens in oral mucosa of renal transplant patients without clinical evidence of oral hairy leukoplakia (OHL). J Oral Pathol Med 27:420–427
2. Bouten CV, Oomens CW, Baaijens FP, Bader DL (2003) The etiology of pressure ulcers: skin deep or muscle bound? Arch Phys Med Rehabil 84:616–619
3. Brehmer-Andersson E, Göransson K (1975) Friction blisters as a manifestation of pathomimia. Acta Derm Venereol 55:65–71
4. Brehmer-Andersson E, Lucht E, Lindskog S, Ekman M, Biberfeld P (1994) Oral hairy leukoplakia: pathogenetic aspects and significance of the lesion. Acta Derm Venereol 74:81–89
5. Buchner A, Hansen LS (1980) Amalgam pigmentation (amalgam tattoo) of the oral mucosa. A clinicopathologic study of 268 cases. Oral Surg Oral Med Oral Pathol 49:139–147
6. Cawson RA, Eveson JW (1987) Oral pathology and diagnosis. Gower Medical Publishing, London
7. Crissey JT, Peachey JC (1961) Calcaneal petechiae. Arch Dermatol 83:501

1 Courtesy of Dr. Barbro Lund Rozell, Huddinge University Hospital, Stockholm. Sweden

8. Dammert K, Brehmer-Andersson E, Ahlquist J, Niemi KM (1965) Calcaneal petechiae. A histopathologic study. Proc Fenno-Scand Ass Derm 81–85
9. Faver IR, Daoud MS, Su WPS (1994) Acquired reactive perforating collagenosis. J Am Acad Dermatol 30:575–580
10. Ferenczy A (1982) Benign lesions of the cervix. In: Blaustein A (ed) Pathology of the female genital tract. Springer-Verlag, New York, pp 136–155
11. Greenspan D, Greenspan JS, Conant M, Petersen V, Silverman S Jr, De Souza Y (1984) Oral "hairy" leukoplakia in male homosexuals: evidence of association with both papilloma virus and a herpes-group virus. Lancet ii:831–834
12. Hjørting-Hansen E, Holst E (1970) Morsicatio mucosae oris and suctio mucosae oris. An analysis of oral mucosal changes due to biting and sucking habits. Scand J Dent Res 78:492–499
13. Kirton V, Price MW (1965) "Black heel". Trans St. John's Hospital Dermatol Soc 51:80–84
14. Kocsard E, Schwarz L, Stephen BS, D'Abrera VSE (1962) Morsicatio buccarum. Br J Dermatol 74:454–457
15. McKee PH (1989) Pathology of the skin with clinical correlations. Gower Medical Publishing, London
16. McMillan MD, Boyd NM, MacFadyen EE, Ferguson MM (1989) Oral hairy leukoplakia-like lesions in an HIV-negative male: a case report. N Z Dent J 85:121–124
17. Näher H, Gissmann L, von Knebel Doeberitz C, von Knebel Doeberitz M, Greenspan JS, Greenspan D, Petzoldt D, Edler L, Freese UK (1991) Detection of Epstein-Barr virus-DNA in tongue epithelium of human immunodeficiency virus-infected patients. J Invest Dermatol 97:421–424
18. Norton SA (1998) Betel: consumption and consequences. J Am Acad Dermatol 38:81–88
19. Pettersson B, Svanberg I, Tunón H (1998) Nötter Etnobiologisk läsebok. (in Swedish) Studenlitteratur, Lund
20. Rufli T (1980) Hyperkeratosis haemorrhagica. Hautarzt 31:606–609
21. Sulzberger MB, Cortese TA, Fishman L, Wiley HS (1966) Studies on blisters produced by friction. I. Results of linear rubbing and twisting technics. J Invest Dermatol 47:456–465
22. Weathers DR, Fine RM (1974) Amalgam tattoo of oral mucosa. Arch Dermatol 110:727–728
23. Witkowski JA, Parish LC (1982) Histopathology of the decubitus ulcer. J Am Acad Dermatol 6:1014–1021

Chapter 30

Glossary

abscess A localized and circumscribed collection of pus in tissues (Fig. 14.1b).
acantholysis Loss of coherence between keratinocytes that may be primary (i.e., caused by direct damage to the desmosomes as in vesicular/bullous dermatoses of the pemphigus group) (Figs. 25.1 and 25.6), or secondary (i.e., the consequence of damage to the keratinocytes as in herpes virus and bacterial infections) (Fig. 20.1).
acanthosis Thickening of the epidermis with elongation of the rete ridges (Fig. 23.1).
acrosyringium The epidermal part of the sweat gland duct. It is also called the intraepidermal sweat duct unit (Fig. 25.8b).
anaphylatoxins The common name for the complement factors C3a, C4a and C5a (Sect. 4.2.1).
angiogenesis The formation of new blood vessels (neovascularization) from already existing vessels both in the embryo and in the adult
apoptosis A kind of cell death (Chapter 6; Figs. 6.1, 24.2b and 28.4). The term is Greek meaning the dropping off or falling off of petals from flowers and leaves from trees.
bacterial index See *slit-skin smears*.
Birbeck granules Membrane-bound rod- or tennis racquet-like organelles observed by means of electron microscopy in the cytoplasm of Langerhans cells.
Caldwell-Luc operation An intraoral surgical opening into the maxillary sinus to remove abnormal tissue. Named after the American physician George W. Caldwell (1834–1918) and the French laryngologist Henri Luc (1855–1925).
carrier molecule The large molecule in an antigen complex, consisting of one large and one small molecule (hapten). The non-antigenic hapten becomes antigenic in combination with the carrier molecule (Sect. 4.1 and 4.5).
cell adhesion molecules (CAMs) Multifunctional integral membrane protein and glycoprotein molecules that allow cell to cell and cell to matrix interactions and signal transduction (Fig. 4.2).
cell line A cell line is composed of oncogenically transformed cells which in culture are able to grow indefinitely, if adequately provided for. One such cell line is the HeLa cell line which was obtained in 1952 from a human cervical adenocarcinoma and since has been used in scientific investigations (Lodish et al. 2000).
chemokines Cytokines (see Sect. 4.1.5).
classification of fungal and bacterial organisms See Table 30.1.
clone of cells A group of genetically identical cells; for example, T cells reacting to a specific antigen.
Crohn disease An inflammatory bowel disease which mostly involves the colon and the distal part of the ileum, but may involve any part of the alimentary tract including the oral and anal mucosa. In the bowel all layers of the wall may be affected and in the fully developed lesions there are dense infiltrates of inflammatory cells, ulcerations, abscesses and fistulas. In addition, in involved and in otherwise non-involved areas,

Table 30.1 The principle of classification of fungal and bacterial organisms

Organism	Order	Family	Genus	Species	Strain
Trichophyton mentagrophytes	Moniliales	Moniliaceae	*Trichophyton*	*mentagrophytes* (subgroups: anthropophilic, zoophilic)	*T. mentagrophytes* cultured from a given person
Borrelia afzelii	Spirochaetales	Spirochaetaceae	*Borrelia*	*afzelii*	*B. afzelii* cultured from a given person

there are small epithelioid cell granulomas in 50% of cases. Epithelioid cell granulomas in the oral mucosa may for a long time be the only sign of the disease.

cystinuria Hereditary disease. Disturbance of reabsorption of cystine and three other amino acids in the kidneys leading to continual formation of kidney stones.

cytokines See Sect. 4.1.5.

cytoskeleton The cytoskeleton is composed of a complex network of filaments that provides structural integrity to the cell, but allows cells to move and change shape, and also provides anchoring sites for proteins.

denaturation of protein In contrast to normal protein, the protein molecules are uncoiled. Injury to cells such as heat or ischemia may cause denaturation. That is what has occurred in the white of a boiled egg.

dendritic cells Cells which have numerous thread-like cytoplasmic processes. They do not phagocytose. *Interdigitating dendritic cells* are present in lymphoid and non-lymphoid tissue and are similar, if not identical, to Langerhans cells in the skin. They present antigen to $CD4^+$ T cells. *Follicular dendritic cells* are present in the germinal centers of lymphoid follicles in lymph nodes, spleen, and in lymphocytomas, e.g. borrelial lymphocytomas in the skin. Follicular dendritic cells have Fc receptors for immunoglobulin G (IgG) and are capable of trapping antigen bound to antibodies (see also Sect. 4.1.2).

desmosomes and **hemidesmosomes** Desmosomes are intercellular bridges which connect keratinocytes with other keratinocytes (Figs. 5.7 and 22.1a). Hemidesmosomes connect keratinocytes with the lamina densa in the epidermal–dermal junction area (Fig. 25.1).

direct microscopy Method used by dermatologists to identify fungal hyphae at the consultation. Scrapes from the suspected lesion are put on a glass slide and a solution of potassium hydroxide is added. The mixture is gently heated. A coverslip is applied over the softened material. Under the microscope translucent septate hyphae and arthrospores may be identified. Today this kind of diagnostic investigation is made in the laboratory using the optical brightener Blancophor (Rüchel and Schaffrinsi 1999).

endarteritis obliterans Thickening and fibrosis of the intima of small arteries followed by narrowing of its lumen. This is due to migration of smooth muscle cells into the intima from the media and is seen, for example, in areas with chronic inflammation.

estrus The restricted period of sexual receptivity in female mammals (other than human females).

exocytosis Migration of lymphocytes from the dermis into the epidermis.

fibrinoid necrosis Fibrin-soaked necrotic tissue that stained with H&E becomes shiny eosinophilic, with vG yellow, and with PAS red, seen for example in leukocytoclastic vasculitis (venular neutrophilic vasculitis), rheumatic nodules and sometimes in granulomas caused by mycobacteria (Figs. 7.11 and 15.1c).

genome the complete set of genes in the chromosomes of an individual.

germinal centers The active center of a lymphoid follicle (Fig. 18.2).

glabrous skin The term has a double meaning. It is used synonymously for areas with vellus hair and areas where all kinds of hair are missing. The latter areas include the palms and soles, the lower and lateral surfaces of the fingers and toes, the upper surface of the third phalanx of the fingers, the lips, the glans penis, the prepuce, and the internal surface of the labia majora. The use of the term glabrous skin is therefore avoided in this book.

gram stain Bacteria may be divided into two major groups with respect to their reaction on staining with crystal violet. After staining with a solution containing crystal violet and then decolorizing with ethanol, one group of bacteria retains the violet color and is said to be gram-positive, and the other loses the color and is said to be gram-negative. Named after the Danish physician Hans C.J. Gram (1853–1938).

granzyme B granules See *perforin granules.*

hapten See *carrier molecule.*

hemidesmosomes see *desmosomes and hemidesmosomes.*

high endothelial venules High venular endothelium indicates that the endothelial cells are activated and able to transiently bind to leukocytes (Fig. 18.1a). The phenomenon is seen in lymph nodes and in inflammatory tissue. In lymph nodes it is required for recirculation of lymphocytes, and in inflammatory tissue it takes part in the recruitment of leukocytes to inflamed areas.

histiocyte See *monocyte/histiocyte/macrophage.*

hydropic degeneration Intracellular accumulation of fluid; gives rise to degeneration and cell death.

immunoblotting A variant of immunoelectrophoresis.

immunoprecipitation A technique for isolation of a specific kind of molecule from a solution by binding the molecules to an antibody and then rendering the antigen–antibody complex insoluble (Abbas and Lichtman 2004).

incontinentia pigmenti A hereditary disease that has three stages. The first stage appears in the neonatal period of life. Linear erythematous vesicular/bullous lesions occur mainly on the extremities. The histopathologic pattern is that of an acute dermatitis with marked eosinophilia. The eruption subsides and leaves verrucous lesions (the second stage), which later flatten out leaving pigmentation (the third stage).

interdigitate The term means interlock and interrelate as the fingers of a clasped hand.

interleukins A common term for a group of multifunctional cytokines produced by a variety of lymphoid and nonlymphoid cells (see Sect. 4.1.5).

Kaposi sarcoma The disease was described in 1872 by the Austrian dermatologist Moritz Kaposi Kohn (1837–1902). It is a type of multifocal sarcoma appearing in the skin and probably derived from lymphatic endothelial cells in the dermal microvasculature. In the Western world in the past Kaposi sarcoma was a rare and slowly developing disease. Today it is well known as an aggressive disease with widespread lesions in untreated patients infected with HIV.

Kimura disease In 1948, the Japanese pathologist Tetsuji Kimura reported an unusual disease, thought to be a chronic inflammatory disease of unknown cause (Chun and Ji 1992). The clinical findings are subcutaneous nodules, preferentially in the head and neck area, combined with lymphadenopathy and blood eosinophilia. Histologically there are dense subcutaneous infiltrates of lymphocytes with follicular reactions and eosinophilia. The disease is very rare in the Western world.

Köbner (Koebner) phenomenon Refers to the appearance of typical efflorescences in skin diseases such as lichen planus and psoriasis on previously uninvolved skin and is caused by slight traumata (i.e., scratching and pressure). Named after the German dermatologist Heinrich Köbner (1838–1904).

Langerhans cells Dendritic cells. Named after the German pathologist Paul Langerhans (1847–1888) (see Sect. 4.4.2).

lepromin test A test used in leprosy. A suspension of heat-killed *Mycobacterium leprae* is injected into the dermis. A positive reaction is either a nodule that appears after 48–72 hours, or an ulcerated nodule that appears after 3–4 weeks. It is not a diagnostic test, but a method to reveal the immune status of the patient with respect to *M. leprae*. In a patient with known leprosy a positive test indicates the tuberculoid end of the spectrum; a negative the lepromatous end.

liquefaction degeneration Conversion of tissue into a fluid (liquid form). Synonym: hydropic degeneration.

livedo reticularis Persistent cyanotic discoloration of the skin with a typical network pattern (Fig. 7.9). It is a symptom not a diagnosis. It is caused by obstruction of arterioles and small arteries and is observed in both neutrophilic and lymphocytic/monocytic arterial vasculitis, and in arteriolosclerosis.

macrophage See *monocyte/histiocyte/macrophage*.

MHC antigen The HLA antigen complex includes the most important antigens involved in the rejection of tissue grafts; in humans they were first detected on lymphocytes and therefore called the *human leukocyte antigen* (HLA) complex. The most important HLA antigens are coded by genes located in a small region on chromosome 6 and designated the *major histocompatibility complex* (MHC). The MHC gene products are classified into three categories. Class I and II genes encode cell surface proteins, and class III genes encode components of the complement system. Class I antigens are expressed on all nucleated cells and platelets, and are encoded by three closely linked loci: HLA-A, HLA-B, and HLA-C. Class II antigens are coded for in a region called HLA-D, which has three subregions: HLA-DP, HLA-DQ, and HLA-DR. Class II MHC molecules are mainly expressed on antigen-presenting cells such as macrophages, dendritic cells, and B cells. However, expression of MHC class II molecules can be induced by INF-γ on other cell types such as endothelial cells, fibroblasts, and keratinocytes. $CD4^+$ helper T cells can recognize antigen only in the context of self-class II molecules, and are therefore referred to as class II restricted T cells.

monocyte/histiocyte/macrophage Monocytes are bone marrow-derived cells, which enter the circulation, from where they migrate into tissues. In tissues they mature and become histiocytes with the capacity to phagocytose (Sect. 5.1.7; Fig. 5.2).

Munro microabscesses Minute aggregates of neutrophils in the horny layer, often seen in active lesions of psoriasis. Named after the English dermatologist William J. Munro (1863–1908).

naive lymphocytes B and T cells which are committed or specifically responsive to a particular antigen, but not yet introduced to it.

natural killer cells (NK cells) A type of lymphocyte which lack both T and B cell receptors. They are somewhat larger than ordinary lymphocytes and make up 10–15% of the lymphocytes in the peripheral blood. They are able to lyse (disintegrate) some types of tumor cells and virus-infected cells without previous sensitization, probably because these cells have a disturbed or reduced expression of class I MHC molecules. All normal nucleated cells express class I MHC molecules, which have an inhibitory effect on NK cells. However, NK cells are also able to lyse target cells coated with IgG because they have a surface receptor which binds to the Fc receptor of the IgG molecule.

nuclear fragments (dust) Nuclear fragmentation most often befalls neutrophils, as in neutrophilic venular vasculitis (leukocytoclastic vasculitis), but may also happen to eosinophils, as in eosinophilic cellulitis, and to monocytes as in monocytic vasculitis (Figs. 7.3a, 26.2b and 7.11b).

oxidative stress By oxidative stress is meant damage to cells caused by reactive oxygen species (ROS), which include free radicals (i.e., atoms or molecules which have in their outer orbit an unpaired electron) and peroxides. The free radicals superoxide anion radical ($\cdot O_2^-$), hydroxyl ions ($\cdot OH$) and hydrogen peroxide (H_2O_2) are produced in small amounts during normal cell metabolism. Because of their ability to kill bacteria, they are also created over short periods in larger amounts (respiratory bursts) in neutrophils and macrophages during phagocytosis. Free radicals are unstable, highly reactive, and highly toxic. Under normal conditions they are rapidly removed from the cell through different pathways. If not cleared, they may cause cell damage. Free radicals may also be produced from toxic agents provided from the environment and metabolized in the liver. For example, inhaled vapor from the chemical carbon tetrachloride (CCl_4) is transported to the liver, where it is metabolized and gives rise to the free radical metabolite ($\cdot CCl_3$), highly toxic to liver cells.

papillomatosis Finger-like or verrucous epithelial projections above the surrounding surface due to irregular thickening of the epidermis and papillary dermis (Fig. 25.7a).

parakeratosis The presence of nuclear remains in the horny layer in combination with the absence or underdevelopment of the stratum granulosum (Fig. 23.1c).

Pautrier microabscesses Darier-Pautrier abscesses were originally described by Darier (1892) as small intraepidermal accumulations (nests) of lymphocytes which had migrated into the epidermis from the dermal infiltrates in patients with mycosis fungoides. At least in the Anglo-American literature, the phenomenon is generally called only Pautrier abscesses, which surprised Pautrier himself (Steffen 2003). It was a great surprise to me as well when in the 1960s I studied the literature on mycosis fungoides and found that Pautrier did not write anything about this type of abscess. However, by chance I later came across an obituary on Pautrier, written in English and signed F.R.B., in a journal now unknown to me. This obituary revealed that Lucien Marie Pautrier (1876–1959) studied medicine in Paris and specialized in dermatology. From 1903 to 1914 (when he entered the army and served as a medical officer until the end of the war) he was engaged at the Dermatology Clinic at the Hôpital St. Louis in Paris. He made important contributions to the development of systematic teaching of dermatology and his case presentations with histological demonstrations earned the particular praise of Jean Ferdinand Darier (1856–1938). Thus Darier was senior to, and also the teacher of, Pautrier. In 1919, Pautrier was appointed Professor of Dermatology at the Faculty of Medicine in Strasbourg, and the obituary reads: "over the succeeding twenty years it was the brilliance, the personality and the inspiration of this remarkable man that made Strasbourg famous and admired throughout the dermatological world. Young dermatologists came from all over the world to study under Pautrier and received there their lifelong inspiration.... From his students and assistants he demanded careful, accurate work: in return he gave brilliant guidance, encouragement and a very genuine affection. The whole atmosphere in his clinic was a delightful combination of enthusiasm, scientific endeavor and warm-hearted friendliness". I think that it was his young, "post-war" pupils who created the concept *Pautrier abscesses* and, as his apostles, spread it all over the world.

perforin granules Granules present in cytotoxic T cells and natural killer (NK) cells. Like factor 9 of the complement cascade, perforin granules form channels into the cytoplasm of the target cells, through which *granzyme granules*, present in the toxic T and NK cells, are transported into the target cells. Granzyme granules contain enzymes, the activity of which finally leads to apoptotic death of the target cells (Figs. 24.1 and 28.4).

polymerase chain reaction (PCR) A technique to amplify and thereby make possible the identification of small amounts of specific molecules present in the tissue. An example is virus antigen incorporated in the genome of DNA virus-infected human cells. First the target DNA in the infected material is split up into fragments by means of a restriction enzyme and heat-denatured at 95°C. The latter causes the double-stranded DNA spiral to break up into two single strands. An excess of synthetic short pieces (primers, oligonucleotides) of a given virus DNA and a heat-resistant DNA polymerase are added to the material and the temperature is reduced to 60°C. If the synthetic primers match with the virus that had infected the material they hybridize with their complementary sequences in the genomic DNA. With heat-resistant DNA polymerase added, the hybridized primers serve as primers for the synthesis of new double-stranded virus DNA. By heating again to 95°C the newly formed double-stranded virus DNA breaks up into single strands, which hybridize with synthetic oligonucleotides, present in excess, and on cooling synthesize new virus. The process may be repeated many times; with every round the amount of virus DNA is doubled (Lodish et al. 2000).

professional antigen-presenting cells To this group belong macrophages, dendritic cells (i.e., Langerhans cells in the skin, interdigitating dendritic and follicular dendritic cells in lymph nodes and other lymphoid tissue), and B cells. The latter ingest protein antigens and display them to helper T cells. This interaction stimulates the secretion of antibodies (Abbas and Lichtman 2004).

promontory sign This phenomenon was first focused on by Gottlieb and Ackerman (1982) in patients suffering from early Kaposi sarcoma and HIV infection; however, it was later shown to be present in richly vascularized lesions of other causes (Brehmer-Andersson et al. 1986; Brehmer-Andersson et al. 1998) (Fig. 7.18e,f).

pseudopodium Pseudopodia are temporary protrusions of the cytoplasm enabling the cell to move over a surface or embrace and phagocytose foreign material.

reticular degeneration Network or strings composed of cell membranes from otherwise dissolved epithelial cells, seen in vesicular dermatitis, pustular dermatitis, and herpes vesicles (Fig. 20.2a).

Ridley index See *Slit-skin smears.*

salt-split-skin technique A biopsy from perilesional skin is taken and placed in 1 *M* NaCl solution for 24 hours. This preparation splits the skin between the epidermis (layer 1) and the lamina lucida (layer 2), and can be used for both direct and indirect immunofluorescence.

sensitized lymphocytes Immunocompetent (specifically primed) B and T lymphocytes, which have been confronted with their specific antigen.

Sjögren syndrome A disease of unknown cause which is characterized by keratoconjunctivitis sicca and xerostomia in combination with an autoimmune disease, such as rheumatoid arthritis and systemic lupus erythematosus. Named after the Swedish ophthalmologist Henrik S.C. Sjögren.

slit-skin smears (bacterial index, Thangaraj and Yawalkar 1987) Technique used in leprosy to count bacilli in tissue. Material is taken from the most active-looking lesion and from normal-looking skin (usually the ear lobe). The skin is gripped between the thumb and forefinger to press out the blood. The pressure should be maintained to render the area bloodless until the smear is taken. With a sterile small-bladed scalpel a 5-mm long incision is made. The blade is then turned at right angles to the incision and the wound is scraped firmly two or three times in the same direction so that a drop of dermal tissue fluid collects on the tip. This material is gently smeared over a circular area about 7 mm in diameter on a clean, new, unscratched glass slide, and can then be stained. The bacterial index is a measure of the density of leprosy bacteria present in smears taken from several lesions located at different sites. In Ridley's logarithmic calculation the scale ranges from 0 to 6+. It is based on the number of bacilli seen in an average microscopic field of the smear using the ×100 objective. Thus: 0 = no bacilli in any of 100 fields; 1+ = 1–10, on average, in 100 fields; 2+ = 1–10, on average, in 10 fields; 3+ = 1–10, on average, in each field; 4+ = 10–100, on average, in each field; 5+ = 100–1000, on average, in each field; and 6+ = more than 1000, on average, in each field. The bacterial index is the sum of the plus numbers divided by the number of investigated sites.

spongiosis Intercellular edema in the epidermis. The desmosomes are stretched and become visible under the light microscope (Fig. 22.1a).

TCR (T cell receptor) The TCR is a membrane receptor. It has two chains of polypeptides, which in most T cells are composed of one α chain and one β chain. They both have a constant region and a variable region and are both active in the recognition of peptide antigens presented to them by antigen-presenting cells also expressing MHC antigen. Due to the process of recombination of genes during the maturation of T cells, the variable region of α and β chains requires the ability to respond to a very high number of different specific antigens. The TCR is connected to the CD3 molecular complex that is involved in signal transduction. A small fraction of TCRs have one γ and one δ chain. They recognize a variety of antigens not displayed together with MHC molecules. They are abundant in epithelia. Their specificity and function are not known (Abbas and Lichtman 2004).

telangiectasia Permanent dilatation of arterioles, capillaries, and venules, which clinically gives rise to focal or widespread red or bluish-red lesions (Fig. 11.1).

Tzanck test A vesicle is opened with care, and its contents, including the sediment at the floor, secured with a small, blunt curette. The material obtained is smeared on a glass slide, air-dried and then stained by the Giemsa method. For Mayer staining the material should be fixed immediately in 95% alcohol (for a minimum of half an hour and a maximum of 24 hours).

vasculogenesis (see also *angiogenesis*).

vector An animal that carries and transfers an infectious agent from one host to another (Chapters 18 and 19).

virion The virus particle (virion) is composed of the *nucleoid*, the genetic material, and the *capsid*, a protecting protein shell. A virion can survive outside the cell in crystalline form and is capable of infecting living cells. Some viruses, such as HSV and VZV, also have an *envelope*. This is a lipoprotein bilayer that surrounds the capsid. When new virions have been produced inside the cell they bud through the membrane of the host cell and become coated with the envelope. The lipids are derived from the host cell and the virus encodes the protein.

von Willebrand factor (vWF) vWF is secreted from endothelial cells and is the carrier of factor VIII, a complex crucial for coagulation and promotion of the adhesion of platelets to subendothelial collagen in the event of injury. Impairment of the complex gives rise to hemophilia. Named after the Finnish physician Erik A. von Willebrand (1870–1949).

Wegener granulomatosis A systemic necrotizing arteritis which affects small and medium-sized vessels in the upper and lower respiratory tracts, eyes and kidneys, and gives rise to a granulomatous inflammatory cell infiltrate. Named after the German pathologist Friedrich R. Wegener (1907–1990).

Wilson disease A hereditary disease due to a defect in the metabolism of copper. It gives rise to progressive accumulation of copper in, among other organs, the liver, brain and kidneys and is followed by degenerative changes of these organs. Named after the English neurologist Alexander K. Wilson (1877–1937).

References

1. Abbas AK, Lichtman AH (2004) Basic immunology. Functions and disorders of the immune system. Saunders, Philadelphia
2. Brehmer-Andersson E, Torssander J, Tengvar M (1986) Extensive hemangiomatosis of the extremities with the same histopathological pattern as the early lesion of Kaposi's sarcoma. Acta Derm Venereol (Stockh) 66:449–451
3. Brehmer-Andersson E, Hovmark A, Åsbrink E (1998) Acrodermatitis chronica atrophicans. Histopathologic findings and clinical correlations in 111 cases. Acta Derm Venereol 78:207–213
4. Chun SI, Ji HG (1992) Kimura's disease and angiolymphoid hyperplasia with eosinophilia. Clinical and histopathologic differences. J Am Acad Dermatol 27:954–958
5. Darier M (1892) (in discussion on Philippson ML) Histologie du mycosis fongoïde typique. Bull Soc Fr Dermatol Syph 3:528–539
6. Gottlieb GJ, Ackerman AB (1982) Kaposi's sarcoma. An extensively disseminated form in young homosexual men. Hum Pathol 13:882–892
7. Lodish H, Berk A, Zipursky SL, Matsudaira P, Baltimore D, Darnell J (2000) Molecular cell biology. W.H. Freeman, New York
8. Rüchel R, Schaffrinski M (1999) Versatile fluorescent staining of fungi in clinical specimens by using the optical brightener Blankophor. J Clin Microbiol 37:2694–2696
9. Steffen C (2003) The man behind the eponym. Lucien Marie Pautrier–Pautrier's microabscess. Am J Dermatopathol 25:155–158
10. Thangaraj RH, Yawalkar SJ (1987) Leprosy for medical practitioners and paramedical workers. Ciba-Geigy, Basle

Subject Index

E

F

G

H

I

J

K

L

M

N

O

P

R

S

T

U

V

W

Z

MIX
Papier aus verantwortungsvollen Quellen
Paper from responsible sources
FSC® C105338

If you have any concerns about our products,
you can contact us on
ProductSafety@springernature.com

In case Publisher is established outside the EU,
the EU authorized representative is:
Springer Nature Customer Service Center GmbH
Europaplatz 3, 69115 Heidelberg, Germany

Printed by Libri Plureos GmbH
in Hamburg, Germany